Living, Dying, Grieving

Dixie L. Dennis, PhD, CHES
Interim Dean
College of Professional Programs & Social Sciences
Austin Peay State University
Clarksville, TN

JONES AND BARTLETT PUBLISHERS
Sudbury, Massachusetts
BOSTON TORONTO LONDON SINGAPORE

World Headquarters
Jones and Bartlett Publishers
40 Tall Pine Drive
Sudbury, MA 01776
978-443-5000
info@jbpub.com
www.jbpub.com

Jones and Bartlett Publishers Canada
6339 Ormindale Way
Mississauga, Ontario L5V 1J2
Canada

Jones and Bartlett Publishers International
Barb House, Barb Mews
London W6 7PA
United Kingdom

Jones and Bartlett's books and products are available through most bookstores and online booksellers. To contact Jones and Bartlett Publishers directly, call 800-832-0034, fax 978-443-8000, or visit our website www.jbpub.com.

Substantial discounts on bulk quantities of Jones and Bartlett's publications are available to corporations, professional associations, and other qualified organizations. For details and specific discount information, contact the special sales department at Jones and Bartlett via the above contact information or send an email to specialsales@jbpub.com.

Production Credits
Acquisitions Editor: Shoshanna Goldberg
Production Director: Amy Rose
Associate Editor: Amy Flagg
Editorial Assistant: Kyle Hoover
Production Editor: Tracey Chapman
Marketing Manager: Jessica Faucher
V.P., Manufacturing and Inventory Control: Therese Connell
Composition: Paw Print Media
Cover Design: Brian Moore
Photo Research Manager and Photographer: Kimberly Potvin
Senior Photo Researcher and Photographer: Christine McKeen
Cover Image: © Christina Tisi-Kramer/ShutterStock, Inc.
Printing and Binding: Malloy, Inc.
Cover Printing: Malloy, Inc.

Library of Congress Cataloging-in-Publication Data
Dennis, Dixie.
Living, dying, grieving / Dixie Dennis.
p. cm.
Includes bibliographical references and index.
ISBN-13: 978-0-7637-4326-0 (pbk.)
ISBN-10: 0-7637-4326-7 (pbk.)
1. Death. 2. Grief. 3. Terminal care. I. Title.
HQ1073.D465 2009
306.9—dc22

2008009648

6048
Printed in the United States of America
12 11 10 09 08 10 9 8 7 6 5 4 3 2 1

Brief Contents

Contents

Preface

Most people can expect to live to about 75 or 80 years of age. And although most of you are probably too busy living to worry about dying, you might have questions about the topic. Maybe you have wondered, "What's it like to die?" or "What am I supposed to do or say when someone I love dies?" or "How can I cope if someone I love dies?" These are good questions to ask because, in the act of asking, you have begun the search for answers that are true and helpful; some of these answers will be found in this textbook.

More than 200 years ago, one of America's founding fathers, Benjamin Franklin, said that nothing in life is certain except death and taxes. Although many books have been written to teach Americans about taxes, few have been designed and written to help Americans find answers to questions about death. Most likely, you were about 9 years old before you came to understand that death is final and that it happens to every person. Your childhood cartoon and video game heroes frequently fell down "dead" and jumped up again. Now that you have a mature understanding of death, you know that death is real and that no one who is really dead jumps back up again. Yet, just like in childhood, a mature understanding of death is not always easy—even for adults. In Chapters 2 and 7, definitions of death and dying are presented as well as information about the different types of death and the stages of dying. Reading about historical and cultural perspectives of death (Chapter 3) likely will be very interesting for you. In Chapter 13, you will read about how children and adolescents view death, and in Chapter 14, you will learn about how adults' views of death have changed over the years.

You might have questions regarding how to truly live the one and only life that you have been given. Did you ever wonder why many adults, who must "know" that they are going to die one day, do not try to enjoy every minute of their lives? Wouldn't a mature understanding of death mean that people make sure that they *really* live? Similarly to not living life to the fullest, not all people make plans about dying. In Chapters 8 (End-of-Life Issues) and 11 (Death-Related Tasks and Decisions), you will find examples of ways in which people can prepare for what is inevitable.

You do not have to wait to begin taking care of the business of dying. Ideally, you can begin today and reevaluate your plans throughout your life. Among other tasks covered in this book, some basic ones that allow you to plan for your eventual death include making a will, expressing medical wishes in an "advance directive," deciding whether to become an organ donor (Chapter 11), and planning your funeral and burial or cremation (Chapter 12).

Much of this textbook is devoted to issues associated with aging (particularly Chapter 6). Targeting elders is important, because older people are more likely to die than younger people. Eighty percent of Americans live past age 65. You should be in that percentage, especially if you do not smoke (the number one preventable cause of death for Americans), maintain a healthy weight, exercise, reduce stress, and drink alcohol in moderation—if at all. In Chapter 15, you will find important facts about suicide and death by violence, both of which are high in incidence among youth. In Chapter 4, you will learn about the American healthcare system, information that is helpful regardless of your age.

Do you have questions about the death of others around you (Chapter 9)? The news media routinely sensationalizes death, making it possible for you to view it as something that impersonally happens to others. But if those others are your family members or your friends, your loss can be devastating. If someone you love has died, you know that your feelings and reactions were different depending on many factors. Was the person your best friend? Did the person love you unconditionally? Did you love the person unconditionally? Did you spend much time with the person?

Even if you have never experienced the death of someone you love, you have probably had "little deaths" throughout your life. Examples of these little deaths, or life losses, include the loss of a job, ending a relationship, losing the "big game," or possibly enduring the divorce of your parents—or your own divorce. Whether you experience "little deaths" or death of a loved one, all loss involves grief. Grieving is covered extensively throughout this textbook, particularly in Chapter 10.

You might have heard about physician-assisted suicide (PAS). This topic is covered extensively in Chapter 5. Also in this chapter is information about euthanasia. A topic in which students report being interested is the possibility of life after death. Do you believe that is possible? After reading Chapter 16, you will know how others view this prospect.

As you read this textbook, you might realize that education about death, or "death education," is really "life education" (see Chapter 1). Possibly, you can lessen any fears you might have about death by learning that dying is merely a natural change that is similar to the change from fall to winter. After reading the last chapter, Chapter 17, you likely will resolve many issues about death; at this point you might realize that this course is one of the most important courses you have taken or ever will take.

Finally, the use of the activities at the end of the chapters—critical thinking, class activities, books to read, and movies to see—serve to make this text come alive. Read, watch, wonder, question, feel, speak, forgive, love, plan, but most of all, live!

Acknowledgments

In dedication to my husband, Dr. Brent G. Dennis, who, because of his belief in me, helped me do and be what God intended.

In honor of my children (Trace [wife Lisa], Suzanne [husband David], J. Michael, and Jon) and my grandchildren (Griffin, Bailey, and Lauren), all of whom are more beautiful/handsome, gifted, and loving than I could have thought possible.

In memory of my parents and Mama Mae, who *lived* and *died*, and in whose absence I still *grieve*.

Thank you to Robert Runck of Editorial Associates, Inc. for the developmental edit on this edition.

Thank you also to the reviewers of this edition. Your voices, criticism, and support have truly made this a better text:

- Patricia J. Fanning, PhD, Bridgewater State College
- Susan R. Adams, ACADC, LCSW, University of Central Arkansas and University of Arkansas at Little Rock
- Dr. Chris Newcomb, Bethune-Cookman University
- Beth Canfield-Simbro, PhD, MPH, CHES, Mount Union College
- Lesa Rae Vartanian, PhD, Purdue University, Fort Wayne
- Angela L. Wadsworth, PhD, University of North Carolina Wilmington
- Linda L. White, PhD, San Houston State University
- Jeffrey K. Clark, HSD, Ball State University
- Laura Kathryn Jones, PhD, Southern Oregon University
- Jonathan C. Davis, PhD, LMFT, Samford University

Why Study Death and Dying?

Remember friend as you pass by,
as you are now, so once was I.
As I am now, so you shall be,
so prepare for death and follow me.
—Tombstone Inscription in Bowling Green, Kentucky

Objectives

After reading this chapter, you will be able to answer the following questions:

- What is thanatology?
- Why is it important for people to have knowledge of death and dying?
- What publications are available for learning about death and dying?
- What is the status of death education in training health professionals?
- What disciplines are concerned with death and dying, and how is research on death and dying conducted?

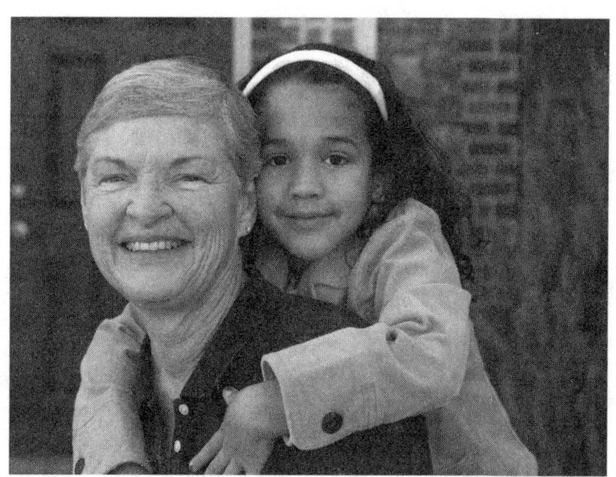

Death is part of life. Death comes to the young, the old, the happy, the sad, the poor, the wealthy, the ready, the not-so-ready, the saint, the sinner, the wise, and the unwise. Each year, 2.3 million people die in the United States and 55 million die throughout the world. Every person born before 1880 has died, and nearly everyone alive today will die before the end of the twenty-first century (Gillick, 2000).

Because death, dying, and bereavement are fundamental aspects of the human experience, education about these topics should be an essential part of the academic course curriculum at all levels (International Work Group, 1994). The study of behavior related to death, dying, and bereavement is called **thanatology**, which is formed from the Greek word for *death*, "thanatos," and the phrase for *the study of*, "ology."

Understanding what death is and how it affects you is a process whereby fear of the unknown may be lessened. This knowledge can help develop a more positive perspective of other life issues, such as job loss, being dumped by a lover, illness, and separation from loved ones, such as through divorce, military service, children growing up and moving out, or friends and relatives who have moved and are living elsewhere.

On a personal level, knowledge of death and dying can help relieve feelings of guilt—for example, from having feelings about not having done what one could have done after the death of a loved one. Moreover, this knowledge can help us in cultivating our relationships with others.

Expressing Grief

Knowledge about death and dying also can help you express grief. In the nineteenth century, the accepted way to grieve was a step-by-step process to eliminate feelings of grief. More recently, during the past 30 years or so, new and more positive models of grief have come forward, suggesting that grief:

- can be a growth experience (Schneider, 1994).
- need not be emotional in content (Martin & Doka, 2000).
- as "anticipatory mourning" is a response by patients, families, and even professional caregivers to losses encountered during a life-threatening illness, such as Alzheimer's disease (Rando, 2000).
- can involve continuing bonds by which the bereaved maintain a connection to the dead and develop a new relationship with that person (Klass, Silverman, & Nickman, 1996).
- is a process of developing and confiding an account or narrative of the relationship with a lost loved one (Harvey, 1998).

These newer concepts for expressing grief are often helpful to caregivers and counselors as well as to survivors and can help professionals who deal with death in their work, such as nurses and emergency room (ER) personnel.

Other Social Issues

On a broader level of understanding, with better knowledge of the issues of death and dying you can review, and perhaps revise, your attitudes toward such social issues as care of the aged and dying, euthanasia, the conduct and cost of funerals, and cremation. Furthermore, knowing how death and dying are viewed and experienced in other cultures can deepen our understanding of those cultures.

Publications Dealing with Death and Dying

Several notable books and journals that are focused on death and death-related issues have appeared since the 1950s. Gorer (1965) and Feifel (1959) made early attempts at calling attention to these once-taboo topics (Vovelle, 1980). Best-selling treatments of death-related issues (Albom,

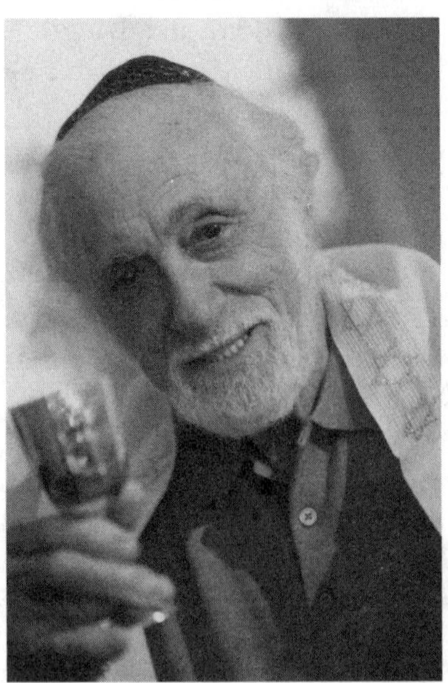

1997; Mitford, 1963) have been popular among general audiences.

One publication, Kübler-Ross's *On Death and Dying* (1969), remains a focus of major attention, both laudatory and critical. Kübler-Ross suggested that people who are dying typically progress through stages of denial, anger, bargaining, depression, and acceptance before they die. Her ideas have helped medical personnel, caretakers, friends, and family respond to a dying person in a more helpful way.

Currently, thanatology is the sole focus of three major professional journals: *Death Studies; Omega: The Journal of Death and Dying;* and *Mortality*. Related topics, such as hospice care and suicide, also are discussed in other healthcare journals.

Death Education

Until the 1970s, educators avoided teaching about death and dying. The topic was not examined by students in medical schools or schools of theology. These students eventually worked with the dying and the dead. Soon thereafter, though, classes in thanatology began to appear in large numbers. Results of a survey by Cummins (1978) involving some 1200 colleges revealed that 75% offered courses on death and dying, mainly in departments of sociology and social work, but also in psychology, religious studies, and health education. Although secondary education has lagged behind, school shootings, among other events, have encouraged an increase in the number of high-school classes in death education and suicide prevention.

Ratner and Song (2002), among other commentators, said that courses on death and dying should not be elective, but, because death and dying affect everyone, required or integrated into the coursework for all majors. Elective courses do not reach very many students. Requiring all students to take a general death and dying course, or integrating the material into the various disciplines, reinforces the fact that death and dying are part of everyone's future.

Goals and Context of Death Education

What should the goals of death education be? The following are a few possible goals:

- Reducing anxiety about death
- Enhancing the ability to cope with the death of the self and of others
- Improving the ability to engage with death professionals: medical, funerary, and governmental
- Enhancing health professionals' ability to deal more effectively with terminal patients

How might death education best be taught? In a course organized as a small seminar, students could:

- explore attitudes and appropriate language through introductory readings and discussion.
- discover community activities and resources by interviewing professionals in the field.
- present reports on such topics as children's views of death and dying, euthanasia, and suicide.

Such a course could become a full program of death education for students interested in practical applications of philosophy, as well as for professionals such as nurses and educators (Amend, 1976).

Approaches for Study

Thanatology is an interdisciplinary field. Various academic disciplines contribute to the study of death and dying, including anthropology, biology, health education, history, law, philosophy, psychology, social work, sociology, and theology. Of these, sociology (along with its cousin, social-psychology) might offer the broadest perspective on death.

The sociological perspective of death assumes that concerns about, and experiences of, death, dying, and bereavement are influenced by social environments. Death influences religions, philosophies, political ideologies, the arts, and medical technologies. Death sells newspapers and insurance policies and enters into the plots of television programs.

Death is one way that societies are measured. For example, comparison of cross-cultural death and life-expectancy rates is used to gauge social progress. Also, national homicide rates often are used to judge the stability of social structures, and death rates of different social groups typically are compared to establish social inequalities.

You can rightly assume that an increased understanding of death and dying helps you to be more accepting of life and its consequences. However, that is not the case for all knowledge related to death and dying. Paradoxically, research results suggest that enhanced death-of-self awareness has a different effect on individuals. When this death-related awareness is increased, it appears that in-group solidarity is intensified, out-groups become more despised, and prejudice and religious extremism escalate (Rosenblatt, Greenberg, Solomon, Pyszczynski, & Lyon, 1989).

Research Related to Death

It is difficult to establish controls when conducting research on death and dying. Only controlled experimentation can produce cause-and-effect results. Most research about death and dying is conducted in situations in which control conditions are impossible and/or unethical. Most research on death and dying is conducted in places where normal activities are underway, such as hospitals, nursing homes, classrooms, playgrounds, and in the streets. Also, this type of research usually is conducted by observation, interviews, and surveys. The types of studies include both *longitudinal studies*, in which a group is followed over time, and *cross-sectional studies*, in which people are compared at the same time.

Studies also can be *prospective*, in which the researcher returns to the same group later to chart changes, and *retrospective*, which involves comparing past history with present circumstances. For example, in a prospective study, a group of young people are evaluated for characteristics hypothesized to be predictive and subsequently tracked to determine when and why they died. In a retrospective study, one group of elders dying of a particular disease is compared with a similar but healthy age group to see what background factors may have contributed to the different outcomes.

SUMMARY

- The study of behavior related to death, dying, and bereavement is called *thanatology*.
- Understanding death and dying and how they affect you can be used to substitute for fear of the unknown; to relieve feelings of guilt; to help express grief; to enlighten your attitudes on care of the old and dying, euthanasia, funerals, and cremation; and to deepen our understanding of other cultures.
- Thanatology is an interdisciplinary field. Contributing disciplines include anthropology, biology, health education, history, law, philosophy, psychology, social work, sociology, and theology.
- Research on death and dying is usually conducted through observation, interviews, and surveys.

AWARENESS OF DEATH AND MORAL VIEWS

In an experiment to determine the effect of awareness of one's own death on one's moral views, 11 municipal judges were asked to write about their own deaths, including what they thought would happen physically and what emotions were evoked in thinking about their deaths (Rosenblatt et al., 1989). A control group of 11 other judges were not asked to engage in this exercise. Both groups of judges were then asked, on the basis of a case brief, to set bond for a prostitute. Those judges who had thought and written about their deaths set an average bond of $455. The judges in the control group set bonds averaging $50.

Looking Ahead

As you work through this book, consider the following questions, particularly with the understanding that the number of people over age 65 is growing rapidly, with those over 85 growing the fastest of all. Consider the specific questions below regarding how you believe people will experience and view death and dying differently fifty years from now.

1. Fifty years from now, what do you think will be different about death and dying?
2. How will changes affect businesses that deal with dying and death (e.g., funeral homes, health care, care of the aged)? Explain.
3. How will death rituals (e.g., funerals) change? Explain.
4. What changes might occur in last resting places? Explain.
5. What sorts of support groups and services do you envision?
6. What medical developments do you foresee?

References

Albom, M. (1997). *Tuesdays with Morrie*. New York: Doubleday.

Amend, E. W. (1976, May 1). *The academic study of death and dying*. Paper presented at the Southwestern Psychological Association, Albuquerque, NM.

Cummins, V. A. (1978, September). *Death education in four-year colleges and universities in the U.S.* Paper presented at the Forum for Death Education and Counseling.

Feifel, H. (1959). *The meaning of death*. New York: McGraw-Hill.

Gillick, M. (2000). *Lifelines: Living longer, growing frail, taking heart*. New York: Norton.

Gorer, G. (1965). *Death, grief, and mourning*. New York: Doubleday.

Harvey, J. (1998). *Perspectives on loss: A sourcebook.* Philadelphia: Taylor & Francis.

International Work Group. (1994). *Statement of assumptions and principles concerning education about death, dying, and bereavement.* London, Ontario, Canada: International Work Group on Death, Dying, and Bereavement.

Klass, D., Silverman, P. R., & Nickman, S. L. (Eds.). (1996). *Continuing bonds: A new understanding of grief.* Washington, DC: Taylor & Francis.

Kübler-Ross, E. (1969). *On death and dying*. New York: Touchstone.

Martin, T. L., & Doka, K. J. (2000). *Men don't cry, women do: Transcending gender stereotypes of grief.* Philadelphia: Brunner/Mazel.

Mitford, N. (1963). *The American way of death.* New York: Simon and Schuster.

Rando, T. A. (2000). *Clinical dimensions of anticipatory mourning*. Champaign, IL: Research Press.

Ratner, E. R., & Song, J. Y. (2002, June 7). Education for the end of life. *Chronicle of Higher Education, 48*, B12.

Rosenblatt, A., Greenberg, J., Solomon, S., Pyszczynski, T., & Lyon, D. (1989). Evidence for Terror Management Theory I: The effects of mortality salience on reactions to those who violate or uphold cultural values. *Journal of Personality and Social Psychology, 57,* 681–690.

Schneider, J. M. (1994). *Finding my way*. Burnsville, NC: Compassion Books.

Vovelle, M. V. (1980, January). Rediscovery of death since 1960. *Annals of the American Academy of Political and Social Science*, *447*, 89–99.

What Does It Mean to Die?

The boundaries which divide Life and Death are at best shadowy and vague.
Who shall say where the one ends, and where the other begins?
—Edgar Allan Poe

Objectives

After reading this chapter, you will be able to answer the following questions:

- Before the twentieth century, where did most people die? Why did this change?
- What is the technological imperative, and how does it affect the dying process?
- What are the various types of death, and how are they defined?
- What happens to the body after death?
- Why do some people argue for new definitions of death?

Living involves experiencing loss. Think about how many losses you already have experienced in your life. Did you ever lose an important game or match? Some people lose their jobs. Has one of your best friends ever moved away? You, along with some of your friends, have probably experienced the loss of a love relationship. As sad as these losses can be, there is another painful loss—the ultimate loss—the death of someone you know or to whom you are close.

Death as Commonplace

Today, Americans cope with death much differently than they did at the turn of the nineteenth century. Death used to be a familiar part of every family's life. Most people lived on farms, and death, particularly of animals, was commonplace.

Almost without exception, people died at home. Because there were no **funeral homes** (places where the dead body is prepared for viewing and burial) or **funeral directors** (persons who prepare the dead body for viewing and burial), family members and close friends prepared the dead body for viewing and burial on home property.

When a member of the family died, the family notified everyone in the community by word of mouth. In some communities, a church or town bell rang to indicate that someone had died. A typical way to inform family members who lived far away that a loved one had died was horse-drawn mail service. The death-announcement envelope usually was trimmed in black to alert the receiver that a death notice was inside. Also, death notices were placed in local newspapers, but they were very different from today's versions. See the following examples of nineteenth-century death notices:

> **February 11, 1878:** Mrs. Richard Crafton, her brother, and her five children, were headed in a buggy to Deerlick, North Carolina, to visit her mother in Logan Co.; while crossing the Forked River at Lewisburg, the horse backed the buggy into the river. The children all drowned, but the two adults were saved.

> **August 16, 1880:** Jonathan Marcus Ladd was found dead about one-half mile north of his house in Hopkinsville, Illinois. It is the verdict of a jury that he died by a pistol and murdered by an unknown party. Although erratic, Ladd had been a successful farmer.

> **July 3, 1852:** Barney M. Senick died in Morgantown from a self-inflicted gunshot. Probable cause given by one family member was his stormy marriage.

Following the Civil War, many death practices changed (Laderman, 1996). For example, **embalming**—the process of replacing the blood in a dead person's vessels with a preservative—was introduced to the funeral process so that the bodies of soldiers who died far from home during the Civil War could be preserved well enough to transport them to their hometowns for **funeral services**—services to commemorate the dead person—and burial by their families. The rise of the funeral industry soon followed. Not only had the aftermath of the war changed attitudes about embalming and the funeral industry, but progress in medicine had removed the death of loved ones and dead bodies from the direct experience of most people.

In addition to the fact that today dead bodies and burial services are handled almost exclusively by funeral directors, more people are now dying at older ages than in the past, when infant mortality was rampant. People are living longer because of advances in medicine, and death is less often a sudden event, and in many cases, the dying process is prolonged.

Today, death typically takes place behind closed doors, most often in nursing homes and hospitals. A dying person usually spends his or her last days in a hospital, and after death, the body is discreetly removed out of sight to a funeral home and made presentable for viewing. Death, as a reality, has receded from everyday life and, therefore, has become almost a mystery.

Making death a mystery only stimulates curiosity about it, especially on the part of children. Adults typically believe that children should be protected from firsthand observation of death in order to protect their supposed innocence. Many adults fear that knowledge about death will harm children emotionally, but experience has shown that children do not react well to being kept in the dark. Children almost always know more than adults think they do; yet, without age-appropriate knowledge about death, children tend to construct terrifying fantasies about what is happening.

In Other Words

As if to lessen the harshness and reality of death, many people, instead of saying *die* or *dead* or *died*, use euphemisms or slang. The following are some common euphemisms for *death*:

- Bit the dust
- Bought the farm
- Deceased
- Departed
- Expired
- Kicked the bucket
- Passed on
- Six feet under

Some euphemisms are specific to a particular religion. For example, understanding that death is a transition or a natural returning to the beginning, a religious person might say, "She's gone home," or "He's asleep in Christ," or "He returned to dust."

Technological Imperative

A major factor affecting attitudes toward death is the **technological imperative**. This idea is used to imply that what a person can do, he or she therefore must do, especially with regard to advances in medical treatment. How has this notion affected people's expectations regarding life and death? Often, loved ones want everything done to keep someone close to them alive—no matter how intrusive and painful it might be for the dying person.

Not uncommon is the phenomenon of resisting the acceptance of death, because in many instances it can be postponed. But what sorts of terrible end-of-life experiences might such delays bring to the dying person? How more peaceful might death be if it is seen as inevitable and acceptable?

Before the medical advances of the twentieth century, defining and deciding when death occurred was not an issue. Many medical advances have created major ethical dilemmas and highly publicized legal, even legislative, fights over decisions to "pull the plug." The technological imperative leads people to consider how death should be defined.

Death Defined

Although death is final, the actual moment of death is not always easy to determine. In years past, a person was pronounced dead when his or her heart stopped beating. Current technology, however, has changed that. Today, the heart can continue beating even though the person cannot think, eat, or breathe on his or her own. Thus, more precise definitions of death are needed.

As will be discussed in more detail in Chapter 11, methods for conclusively defining when a person is irrevocably dead have become important in deciding when to remove organs from an organ donor. Many people are troubled by **autopsies**, after-death examinations to determine the cause of death, and removing organs for donation. Families, therefore, often overrule a donor's life decision to donate organs. In general, the ambivalence of society's attitudes about organ donation often creates controversies over when and how death is determined.

The process of dying takes place in stages. These stages include clinical death, brain death, and cellular/biological death.

Clinical Death

In **clinical death**, the heartbeat stops. Oxygen carried by the blood no longer circulates throughout the body. The good news is that revival is possible. Immediate **cardiopulmonary resuscitation (CPR)**, which involves mouth-to-mouth breathing and chest compressions, can bring a person back to life. To avoid irreversible brain damage, however, CPR must begin within about 4 minutes of when the heartbeat first stopped. To prevent brain death, CPR must begin within approximately 15 minutes. Time is critical.

Cortical Death

Akin to brain death (described next in this section), **cortical death**, also called **persistent vegetative state (PVS)**, is a permanent brain-dead condition, accompanied by severe brain damage, in which a person has progressed to a state of wakefulness without detectable awareness. The Karen Quinlan and Teri Schiavo cases (discussed in Chapter 5), with their attendant media coverage and the extended grief they brought upon their families, have caused many people worldwide to decide to communicate clearly their wishes about how they want their lives to end. In short, these cases caused many people to rethink their own definitions of exactly what death is.

Brain Death

Brain death is determined by testing a patient's response to stimulation of motor responses by purposefully administering pain in all extremities (Sullivan, Seem, & Chabalewski, 1999). If the brain is dead, a patient does not feel a pain response. Before this testing procedure, the patient is checked to determine that no muscle relaxants, opiates, or barbiturates have been administered or ingested in the past 24 hours. The patient's body temperature also is checked to make sure it is not too far from normal. These conditions can reduce reflexes.

The patient is considered brain dead if all of the following conditions exist:

- No response to verbal or visual commands.
- Flaccid body, with no movement, restraint, or hesitation when arms and legs are raised and allowed to fall.
- Pupils of the eyes are fixed when a bright light is shined into them.
- The patient has no **oculocephalic ("doll's eye") reflex**. The eyes remain fixed when the head is turned from side to side (see Figure 2.1).
- A cotton swab dragged across the cornea produces no eye blink.
- No response motion of the extremities exists when the eyebrow ridge is compressed with the thumb.
- The patient has no **oculovestibular reflex** (violent eye twitching) when ice water is injected into both ear canals.
- No gag reflex is produced by movement of a breathing tube in and out, as will happen in a comatose patient.
- **Apnea** (inability to breathe spontaneously) is present. The following procedure is used to test for apnea:
  - Disconnect the ventilator.
  - Administer oxygen.
  - Look for spontaneous respiration.
  - Measure blood chemistry after 6 minutes and reconnect the ventilator.

Most medical authorities call for 6 hours to elapse between the first and second clinical determination of brain death in adults (Sullivan et al., 1999). For children up to 1 year, 24 to 48 hours is recommended (University of Missouri, 2008).

Many physicians ask for additional tests before pronouncing brain death. The two most common procedures are the **electroencephalogram (EEG)** and the **cerebral blood flow (CBF)**. The EEG measures brain voltage. Even a patient in a deep coma will show some electrical activity in the brain; however, a dead brain will not. In a CBF test, a radioactive isotope is injected into the bloodstream. Blood flow into the brain is measured with a radioactivity counter. No blood flow means the brain is dead. In a third test, an injection of 1 mg of atropine IV is used to increase the heart rate. Heart rate will rise dramatically in a patient with an intact brain, but nothing will happen if the patient is brain dead.

Figure 2.1 TEST FOR DOLL'S EYE REFLEX.

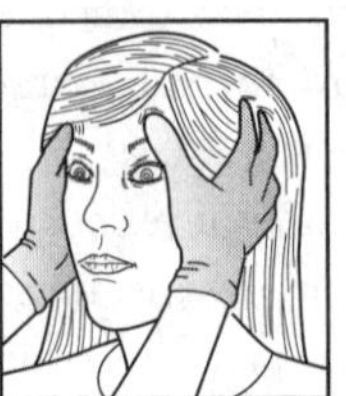
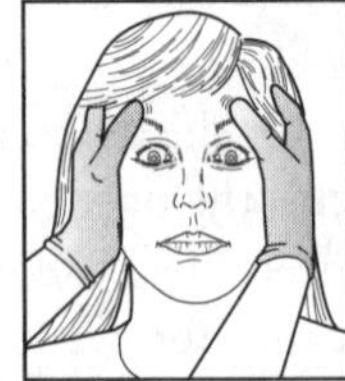
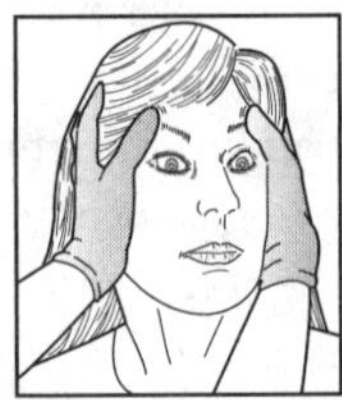

Source: Modified from Springhouse *Nursing: Interpreting Signs & Symptoms*. Lippincott Williams & Wilkins, 2007.

The Federal Uniform Determination of Death Act (UDDA)

With advances in medical technology, it is now possible to keep some parts of the dying body alive. This ability of modern medicine to modify the natural process of dying forces many people to think again about how to define death and develop new ways to decide when death has taken place.

Prior to 1981, each state was free to adopt its own basis for determining death, but life-extending medical advances created a need for a common definition. The Federal Uniform Determination of Death Act (UDDA) was passed in 1980 and approved by the American Medical Association in 1980 and by the American Bar Association in 1981. In the Act, it is specified that an individual is dead if he or she has sustained either irreversible cessation of circulatory and respiratory functions or irreversible cessation of all functions of the entire brain, including the brain stem. An electroencephalogram (EEG) is used to measure brain activity (see Figure 2.2). A determination of death must be made in accordance with accepted medical standards.

The purpose of the UDDA was to make state laws uniform in their definitions of what constitutes death. Although through this act a general legal standard for determining death was created, it did not offer any medical criteria for doing so. Also, determining the time of death depends on the individual case and, if in doubt, is usually resolved by experts testifying in court.

Advice to Health Professionals

The descriptive terminology used by most nurses and doctors to describe someone who is brain dead but on a ventilator can be confusing to the person's family. Saying that the person is on "life support" implies that the person is still alive. Family members also might think that their loved one will get better if he or she is treated or sent to rehab.

Even using the term *brain dead* can be misleading, because it suggests that only the brain is dead, and everything else is alive. This misconception can be made worse when the issue of organ donation is considered. Saying that a loved one is being "kept alive" to permit organ harvest and then "allowed to die" suggests to many family members that their loved one is alive and not really dead. Using such terms as *mechanical ventilation* or *artificial respiration* might be better descriptions of the patient's state, because these terms do not imply that life is present in any form.

Figure 2.2 AN ELECTROENCEPHALOGRAM (EEG).

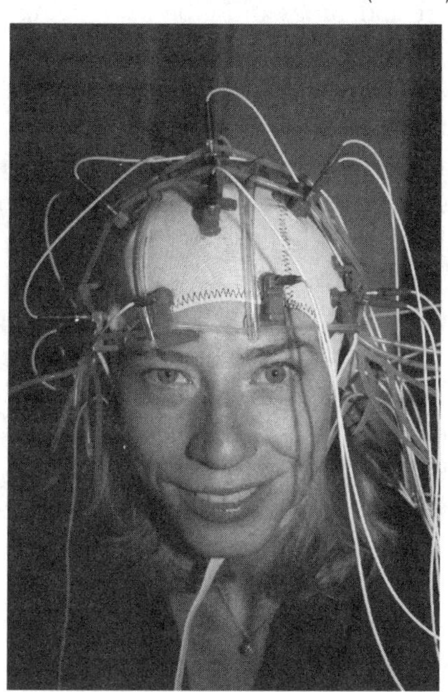

Brain Death and Organ Donation

Understanding what brain death means can be an important influence on the decision to donate tissues and organs for transplant. If a dead person is judged suitable to serve as an organ donor, mechanical ventilation is continued to maintain viability of the soon-to-be-harvested organs. Every family should be offered the chance to donate, but not until the loved one is pronounced dead and the family has had time to accept the death. If the family does not give consent, ventilation should be stopped and the dead person given the postmortem care dictated by the hospital protocol.

One reason some people are reluctant to donate organs is the common belief that all the body's parts should be subjected to the appropriate funerary rites. Consistent with that belief is that a missing part would mar the reassembly expected in some later existence.

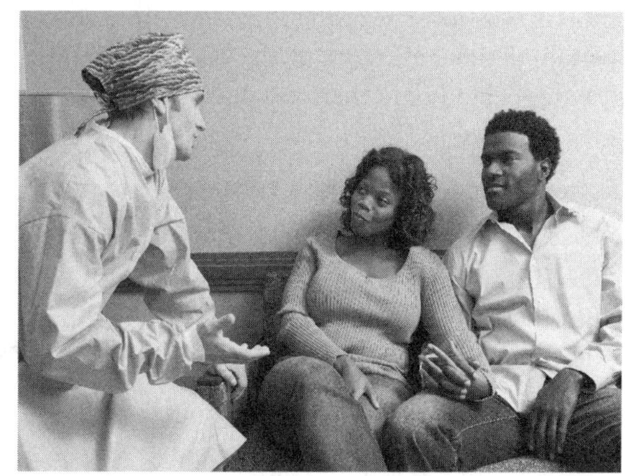

Attitudes Toward Organ Donation in Non-Western Cultures

Organ donation is not universally accepted across cultures. The boundary between life and death has been a puzzle to many cultures for a long time. Moreover, in many non-Western cultures, death is viewed as a natural social event, not a medical one. From a traditional Japanese perspective, for instance, a human being is both alive and dead, an integrated body, mind, and spirit. Removing an organ from a brain-dead person is viewed as a disturbance of this natural integrated unit. Many Japanese believe that a dead person goes to the next world as a soul with its own body, senses, and feelings and, as such, the dead body must remain whole. If parts are missing, the soul will be unhappy in the next world. Many other non-Western and aboriginal cultures also are uncomfortable with organ donation (Bowman & Richard, 2004).

Questions & Answers

Question: Is brain death the same thing as a coma?

Answer: Brain death is different from a coma. A person can "come out of" a coma, but brain death is an irreversible, permanent loss of all functions of the brain.

What Happens After Death?

At death, the eyes lose reflexes. The person's body temperature falls, a phenomenon called **algor mortis**. Because blood no longer circulates throughout the body (**livor mortis**), the face takes on a bluish tint and other parts appear purple-red.

Within a few hours after death, the body takes on a bloated appearance due to the accumulation of gases the body can no longer eliminate. **Rigor mortis**, or muscle stiffening, sets in. Over a period of time, all parts of the body decompose, leaving behind only the teeth and skeleton.

Questions & Answers

Question: Once the final stage of death (cell death) occurs, can any more growth occur in a dead body?

Answer: Cell death marks the point at which a person's death can be no longer reversed, and at this point growth is no longer possible.

Redefining Death

In the United States and other developed countries, brain death is accepted as the definition of death, even if the heart is still beating and the lungs have been kept going by a ventilator. A beating heart and functioning lungs allow for organs to be harvested for transplant. These medical advances cause heartache for many people, even for professionals. Lock (2001) described the distress that is frequently experienced by doctors and nurses working in Intensive Care Units (ICU) because death is now legally defined as lack of brain activity. A body might be brain dead, but the heart and lungs must be kept going for its organs to be harvested. So, in essence, that body dies twice, first when the brain stops, then when the heart stops.

Lock (2001) supports organ transplantation. She also argues for extending the definition of brain death to include people in a long-term persistent vegetative state (PVS). Lock maintains that to increase organ donation numbers, people should move away from talking about "gift of life," because it is typically too emotionally charged for the families involved.

Lock (2001) argues that there are larger implications to this new definition of death. She believes that the definition of brain death should be reconsidered, taking into account broader cultural, legal, medical, and political considerations. Lock warns of the possible consequences of allowing advances in biotechnology to proceed without limit.

Lock (2001) has researched attitudes toward organ donation in the United States and Japan. With the introduction of immunosuppressant drugs to prevent tissue rejection, organ transplantation has become standard medical practice in Western countries. In Japan, however, brain death is not widely accepted, organ donation is unpopular, and organ transplantation is rare. Culturally, organ donation in Japan collides with Japanese people's understanding of gifts as based on family bonds and social ties rather than on individual need.

Summary

- Before the turn of the nineteenth century, death was a familiar part of life. People died at home. Family members prepared the body at home for viewing and burial. Following the Civil War, death practices changed when the bodies of soldiers were embalmed so that they could be sent home for burial. The rise of the funeral industry changed attitudes about embalming, and medical advances largely removed the death of loved ones and dead bodies from the direct experience of most people.
- Today, death is often considered a taboo subject. Many people use euphemisms or slang instead of saying *die, dead,* or *died.* Euphemisms such as "departed," "passed on," and "kicked the bucket" are used. In a religious connotation, "asleep in Christ" and "returned to dust" are common sayings.
- The process of dying takes place in stages, namely clinical death, brain death, and cellular/biological death. In clinical death, the heartbeat stops. If administered soon enough, CPR can revive a person in that state. Brain death is now the generally accepted definition of death, even if the heart is still beating and the lungs have been kept working by a ventilator, which allows for organs to be harvested for transplant. Brain death is determined medically by testing if a patient has a typical response to stimulation of motor responses from purposefully administered pain in all extremities. When the brain is dead, a patient feels nothing. In cellular/biological death, the cells begin to die soon after the brain dies, but different parts of the body die at different rates.
- In the Federal Uniform Determination of Death Act (UDDA), it is specified that a person is dead if he or she has sustained either irreversible cessation of circulatory and respiratory functions or irreversible cessation of all functions of the entire brain, including the brain stem. A determination of death must be made in accordance with accepted medical standards.
- Margaret Lock argues that the definition of brain death should be reconsidered, taking into account cultural, legal, medical, and political considerations. In Japan, for example, brain death is not widely accepted, organ donation is unpopular, and organ transplantation is rare.

Additional Resources

Books

Lock, M. (2001). *Twice dead: Organ transplants and the reinvention of death.* Berkeley: University of California Press. This book documents the moral and political responses of the public and of professional medical people to brain death and to organ transplantation.

Spignesi, S. J. (1994). *The odd index.* New York: Plume Publishers. Not for children, this book covers lists of unusual things, such as trivia about religion and death, steps in a medical–legal autopsy, euphemisms for sexual intercourse, a list of body parts that people pierce (including fingernails), methods of execution and torture throughout the ages, 20 alleged cases of backwards phrases in recordings, reasons to believe that Paul McCartney is dead, movie anachronisms, longest movies ever made, unusual foods from around the world, and a list of foods that contain the most cholesterol.

Movie

The Notebook. (2005). This movie is about love, aging, and the boundaries between life and death.

Critical Thinking

1. List three superstitions, rituals, or attitudes that reflect your family's views of death and dying.

2. Write an essay setting forth your views of organ donation and the values you believe are responsible for these beliefs.

CLASS ACTIVITY

You have just found out that you are dying. Write a "goodbye" letter to a loved one. Then have your instructor pair you with a class member (not your best friend) who will read your goodbye letter and write a response. Read the response and write a reaction paper about what you felt and learned.

REFERENCES

Bowman, K. W., & Richard, S. A. (2004). Cultural considerations for Canadians in the diagnosis of brain death. *Canadian Journal of Anesthesia, 51*, 273–275.

Laderman, G. (1996). *The sacred remains: American attitudes toward death, 1799–1883.* New Haven, CT: Yale University Press.

Lock, M. (2002). *Twice dead: Organ transplants and the reinvention of death.* Berkeley: University of California Press.

Sullivan, J., Seem, D. L., & Chabalewski, F. (1999). Determining brain death. *Critical Care Nurse, 19*(2), 37–46.

University of Missouri. (2008). Health Care Web page. Retrieved January, 2008, from www.muhealth.org

Chapter 3

Cultural and Historical Perspectives on Death

Can I see another's woe,
and not be in sorrow too?
Can I see another's grief,
and not seek for kind relief?
—William Blake

Objectives

After reading this chapter, you will be able to answer the following questions:

- Does culture affect the expression of grief?
- How do different cultures give meaning to death?
- How do death rituals vary across cultures?
- How do views toward the afterlife vary across cultures?
- How do views of death vary across various American subcultures?
- What are some non-Western views of death?
- What festivals are held to celebrate the dead from different cultures?

The ways in which people respond to death varies by culture and by historical period. What is universal to all cultures, though, is the effort to make sense of death, to give it meaning.

People from many cultures regard death as a part of everyday life, and even celebrate it, usually on the assumption that those dead are off to a better life after this one. At the other extreme are cultures, such as twenty-first-century Western ones, where death has become a mysterious and dreaded matter, hidden away in hospitals and funeral homes.

Affiliation and Grief by Culture

Mourning in small, closely knit societies differs from mourning in large, more loosely knit societies in which primary membership is the nuclear family. In small social networks (e.g., those in a rural village), members identify with people outside the nuclear family. Death disrupts the social structure, so mourning focuses on rearranging social roles. For example, many adults already care for a child in a small social network, so when a parent dies other adults easily move into the parental role. In more complex, loosely knit social networks (e.g., those in an industrialized city), individual deaths do not usually significantly affect the larger social system, so grief is an individual and family matter (McLennan, Akande, & Bates, 1976).

The way people grieve is shaped by culture; nevertheless, a universal pattern exists. Disrupted close relationships seem to produce similar patterns of grief. When less important relationships are ended by death, grieving behavior is influenced to a greater extent by the culture. Also, socialization prepares individuals to respond to death in a certain way. When death occurs, socialization guides the actual grief response. The individual has a prior perception of grieving behavior that is not changed by the actual experience of a death (Catlin, 1993). In the funerary practices of Australian aboriginal societies, for instance, mourning is less an individual emotion than a duty imposed by the wider social group. Mourners weep not because they are sad, but because they feel obliged to weep out of respect for ritual custom and because they are swept along by crowd behavior (Durkheim, 1915/1976).

As another example of cultural differences, death attitudes between Americans and Spaniards differ around affiliation. In the American culture the individual is emphasized. Although interrelatedness and social welfare are not entirely absent, they are always measured against a national cult of self-reliance. Americans, being more autonomous than Spaniards, are not personally affected to the same extent, but react to the pain of a loved one's death by moving away from others.

In contrast, the social fabric of Spain is more tightly woven than it is in the United States. Spain is a nation sharply divided by region and class, but family and community ties are central to individual identity. Being more closely affiliated with one another, Spaniards experience the death of a loved one as a blow to personal well-being or self-esteem, and they tend to move toward others in times of loss.

Death Acceptance and Denial

People from all human societies are aware of and reflect on death, but differences exist regarding how they explain and give meaning to it (McLennan, et al., 1976). Differences even exist between family members of the same culture. For example, many American families differ in how to give meaning, and memorial, to their loved one's death, depending on whether family members live in a city or more rural setting.

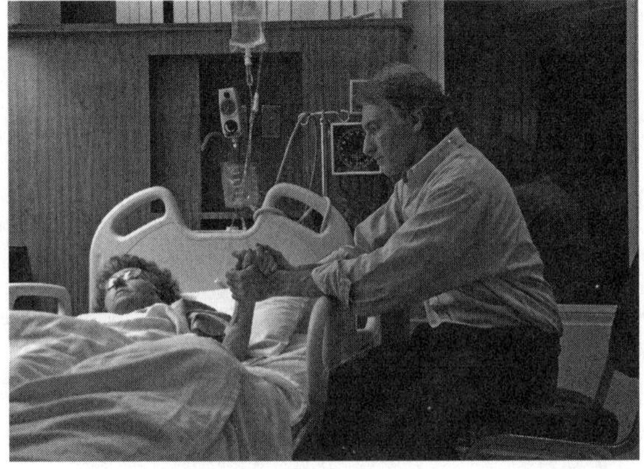

In Western societies, fragmented family ties and scattered communities typically have diluted the emotional and social supports that generally cushion the impact of death. People now die in hospitals and other institutional settings, and commercial funeral arrangements remove ritual from grief and mourning. Death is a mystery for most Westerners, representing an unknown to be feared. Individuals in Asian societies tend to have lower levels of anxiety about death than in the West and, as such, seem to view death as one of life's realities to be accepted.

Member of some cultural societies are comfortable displaying feelings surrounding the death of their loved ones. For example, in the traditional Turkish culture, mourners run through the streets screaming their pain and anger at the dead person for leaving them. In Bali, women are strongly discouraged from crying, whereas in Egypt, women are considered abnormal if they do not incapacitate themselves in demonstrative weeping (Wikan, 1988). In traditional China, women wail, but men sit silently (Watson & Rawski, 1988).

Religious beliefs can lessen anxiety over death, but in many developing nations other factors also are important. These other factors include supportive extended family and community networks and more frequent encounters with death as a result of poorer living and health standards and shorter life expectancies.

In Nigerian and other West African societies, for example, death of a family member is viewed as a family crisis of major proportions, yet death is accepted as universal and inevitable, and families maintain a ritual mourning period as a means of coping with their stress, grief, and loss. The extended family receives friends and other mourners over a period of many days; they discuss the death and talk about the dead person; they recall episodes from the past; and they tell each other how much they will miss their loved one, all the while crying freely (Folte & Deck, 1988; Gijana, Louw, & Mangani, 1989; Peil, 1991).

Rituals of Death

The history of death and dying rituals is older than civilization itself. Archeological evidence of ritual burial ceremonies dates as far back as the Neanderthal, 150,000 years ago. Archeologists have found decorated shells, primitive tools, animal antlers, and flower fragments next to Neanderthal corpses, indicating some type of ritual (Harder, 2001).

A proper send-off of the dead is important in some societies. Some societies believe that the correct funeral rites ensure that the spirit of the dead person has a successful journey. If the funeral rites are performed incorrectly, an angry spirit might bring grief to the living, for instance, by causing death by violence or in childbirth.

Many cultures consider death as simply a change in circumstance, a transition from this world to some other world. In such cultures, funeral rituals are intended to help the dead in their journey. In Hungarian peasant communities, for example, the substance of the dead person generally crosses a bridge over a river or a sea to reach the other world. Before crossing, the soul must pay a toll (Bloch & Parry, 1982; Gennep, 1960; Hertz, 1960). This scenario echoes the Greek and Roman myth of Charon, the boatman who ferries those dead across the River Styx on their way to the underworld.

On the night of the Hungarian death vigil, the dead person is dressed with clothes that are later given to the needy as charity. The dead person's favorite belongings are placed in the tomb next to the body, because the dead person is believed to need them in the afterlife. The dead soul might be fed with the steam of food placed on the windowsill of the death house. The soul must be fed in this symbolic way to make the ritual authentic, because the dead cannot actually eat.

Superstitions to ward off fear appear to be universal. Kübler-Ross (1969) believed that rituals surrounding death began as a means to keep bad spirits away from dead loved ones. For example, the tradition of placing a **tombstone**, or grave marker, on a grave might have originated in the wish to keep bad spirits deep in the ground.

The following are some superstitions regarding the signs of approaching death:

- If you sweep under the bed of a sick person, he or she will die.
- Breaking a mirror brings death to a family.
- When a bird flies in the house, it signals death.
- If you attend a funeral while you are pregnant, your baby will be born dead.
- Death will come if you dream of a wedding.
- If you sneeze at the table with your mouth full of food, you will die.

Death's Aftermath

Melanesian societies believe that no one returns to this life, even if he or she enters another sphere: "However strong their desire, men dare not hope for themselves 'a death like that of the moon or the sun, which plunge into the darkness of Hades, to rise again in the morning, endowed with new strength.' Those who die will return to life, but in another world or as other species" (Hertz, 1960, p. 74).

The notion of enduring bonds between the living and the dead is exemplified in Balinese society, wherein the community unites in a joint venture. In this society, continuing contact is believed essential to ensure the well-being of the living (Warren, 1993). Family loyalties extend beyond death, as ancestors are called upon to intercede with the gods to preserve the well-being of the living. When determining causes of death, traditional Balinese cultures look to nature (the moon), social interactions (anger or envy), or retribution from ancestors (not conducting proper funeral rites). Balance in nature and community is very important, given the power and mystery of the natural world.

Names of the Dead

In some cultures, people avoid using the name of a dead person. This practice is intended to prevent the dead from being disturbed and can extend to denying living persons with the same name continued use of the name. In other words, the living person must take on another name. The Penan Geng of Borneo follow this practice (Brosnius, 1995–1996). Death names are given to the kin of a dead person. A person might take on a series of names during his or her lifetime, signifying several types of relationships to dead kin.

At the other extreme of discontinuing the use of a name is the practice wherein the dead person's name might be honored by giving it to a newly born child. This practice allows the name to live again. Sometimes, the name of a dead child is given to one born later. Among Hawaiians, children might be named by ancestors or by the gods, the names being communicated via dreams by the mother-to-be (Handy & Pukui, 1972).

Western History

In the West, the end of the Middle Ages and the advent of the Renaissance led to consideration of individual death. Up to that point, all (or at least all good) Christians were assured by the Catholic Church that resurrection and entry to Heaven followed death. Later, people began to worry that if they misbehaved on Judgment Day they might go to Hell instead.

The famous lines by John Donne refer to the bell rung in a particular way in Christian churches from medieval times until the seventeenth century, and in primitive tribes and Oriental cultures, to take note of a passing. Ringers in the seventeenth century used the number of strokes to announce the age, gender, and social status of the dead person.

The seventeenth-century Puritans were intensely afraid of death, because they were never sure if they would go to Heaven as part of God's elect or to Hell, proclaimed by their preachers as a place of eternal torment. Puritans believed that election by God of Heaven-bound persons was predetermined, thus they had no opportunity to affect the outcome. They could only study their own lives for signs that they had been selected. Later in the century, in the face of social changes that diluted their theocratic grip, Puritans developed elaborate funeral ceremonies to emphasize their religious views. These included sending gloves as funeral invitations, ringing of church bells, a procession to the graveyard, elaborately carved gravestones with verses extolling the dead person's moral and religious character, and costly funeral rings given to guests who returned to the home for a meal following the funeral (Stannard, 1977).

The Romantic period of the 1800s led to a general emphasis on memorials and on elaborate funerals and mourning customs. Queen Victoria of England epitomized this custom by her lifelong

THE BELL TOLLS FOR THEE

No man is an island, entire of itself; every man is a piece of the continent, a part of the main. If a clod be washed away by the sea, Europe is the less, as well as if promontory were, as well as if a manor of thy friend's or of thine own were. Any man's death diminishes me, because I am involved in mankind; and therefore never send to know for whom the bell tolls; it tolls for thee.

—John Donne, from Meditation XVII, *Devotions Upon Emergent Occasions*

Danse Macabre

The Bubonic plague of the 1200s to 1300s, which killed one-fourth of Europe's population, gave rise to various artistic expressions of the emergent fear of sudden death, collectively labeled *danses macabre* (Dances of Death). Modern examples of these dances include E. A. Poe's *The Masque of the Red Death* (which can be taken today as a metaphor of death by AIDS as well) and Ingmar Bergman's classic film *The Seventh Seal.* The skeletons of Halloween are another modern remnant of the *danse macabre.*

devotion to her late husband. She wore a black bonnet and communed with him at his grave until her death in 1901 (LaMont, 1994).

The dawn of the twentieth century brought World War I. The mechanization of war and medicine that resulted took death and dying away from the home and community and put it into the hospital. Death became a private family matter (Aries, 1974).

Death in American Cultures

Death customs in America vary by culture. Presented in this section is information related to Native Americans, Hispanic Americans, Irish Catholics, African Americans, and Asian Americans.

Native Americans

Native Americans have been represented by as many as 500 different tribes over the history of the United States, and with them came many and varied customs and practices with regard to death. Some of these customs and beliefs, however, are common and have persisted to the present day.

One persistent custom among Native Americans is reverence for the dead. Most Native Americans believe that the dead guard the living and guide them to the spirit world. Native American burial places are, therefore, sacred. This tradition has caused recent problems with respect to the bones of prehistoric people found by archeologists on the west coast of the United States, which have been taken to museums for study. Tribes claiming these prehistoric people as descendants have demanded their return and reburial.

Early Native Americans believed in evil spirits. To drive these spirits away, they shot arrows into the sky. Today, the military practices a similar ritual in firing guns into the air during a military funeral.

Contemporary views of death and the afterlife vary among Native Americans. One tribe might avoid the dead altogether; another might hold elaborate ceremonies to encourage the spirit of the dead person to move on and not linger (Mandelbaum, 1959). For instance, among some tribes the ghost of the dead person is believed to linger after death, so an elaborate funeral ceremony is required to usher the ghost onward (Margolin, 1978). Even so, ghosts may linger. For some tribes, such ghosts act as guides and protectors; for others, such as the Navajo and Apache, ghosts are malign, causing sickness and death (Cox & Fundis, 1992).

Depending on the tribe, what happens after death is viewed in different ways. Some see life as circular, following the repeating pattern of natural

> To us the ashes of our ancestors are sacred and their resting place is hallowed ground . . . the dead are not powerless. . . . There is no death, only a change of worlds.
>
> —Seattle, nineteenth-century Northwest Native American tribal leader (Deloria, 1973/1994, pp. 176–177)

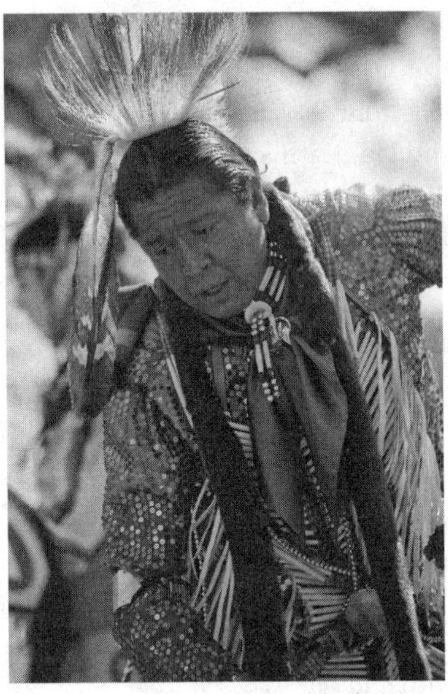

seasons, rather than a linear path (Hultkrantz, 1979; Oswalt, 1986). With this view, what happens after death is not of great consequence, and many Native Americans are always ready for death, sometimes even welcoming it, as did some tribal warriors engaged in war (Steiger, 1974).

Other tribes believe that a person has four souls and that these souls die in stages. The last stage comes about a year after death, so graves are tended for that long, but then ignored, because nothing of the dead person is left behind (Witthoft, 1983).

The Native American view of death as a natural and inevitable occurrence extends to the view of medical (or shamanistic) intervention. Rather than viewing death as a defeat, as do many medical professionals, the use of medicine is believed by many Native Americans to be a treatment for the spirit as well as the body.

Hispanic Americans

Hispanic Americans are the largest subculture in the United States. They originate from Puerto Rico, Mexico, Cuba, and countries in Central and South America. When it comes to attitudes and practices associated with death and dying, family and religion are very important. Families are usually tight-knit and a center of emotional support (Kalish & Reynolds, 1981). Planning and care of the dying remain in family hands (Thomas, 2001).

The great majority of people in the Hispanic American subculture are Roman Catholic (Clements et al., 2003). Thus, the teachings and rituals of Catholicism are strong influences on how many Hispanic Americans approach dying and death. Many Mexican Americans hold to earlier Native American beliefs about the cyclical interrelationship of life and death. Death is *not* seen as something fearful and avoidable. For Puerto Ricans, a fatalistic view of dying and death seems to lessen the intensity of grief (Grabowski & Frantz, 1993; Munet-Vilaro, 1998).

Rituals for the dead might include open caskets, a requiem mass, and a procession to the gravesite. A Catholic **novena**, a nine-day period of saying a rosary, by the family usually follows in the home.

Irish Catholics

A traditional **wake** is typical of Roman Catholic Irish communities. With a typical wake, the body of the dead person is dressed (usually by funeral directors) and returned to the family home for public display prior to burial so that mourners can pay their respects and say farewell. The Irish wake is an expressive and celebratory marking of death, in which the life of the dead person is recollected in cheerful ways, such as singing, dancing, and storytelling (Brennan, 2005).

African Americans

In the United States, African Americans are more likely to die at home than their white counterparts. In part, this situation is because many families resist putting ill or elderly loved ones into nursing homes, because they lack confidence in medical care (Thomas, 2001; Waters, 2001). In line with this distrust is a lack of interest in after-death matters such as advance directives and organ donation (both explained in Chapter 11) and the use of hospice (explained in Chapter 4) (Griener, Perera, & Ahluwalia, 2003; Tschann, Kaufmann, & Micco, 2003).

What happens at an African American funeral is viewed as an affirmation of the individual. The dying person is interested in knowing a terminal prognosis and takes a personal interest in funeral planning and mourning behavior (Hayslip & Peveto, 2004). In African American culture, it is significant how many people attend the funeral, how fancy the casket is, and so on (Holloway, 2003). Reflecting the importance of narrative in most cultures, storytelling is an important part of grieving for African Americans (Rodgers, 2004). African American survivors typically depend on family, friends, and church associates for support in dealing with death and grief (Clements et al., 2003).

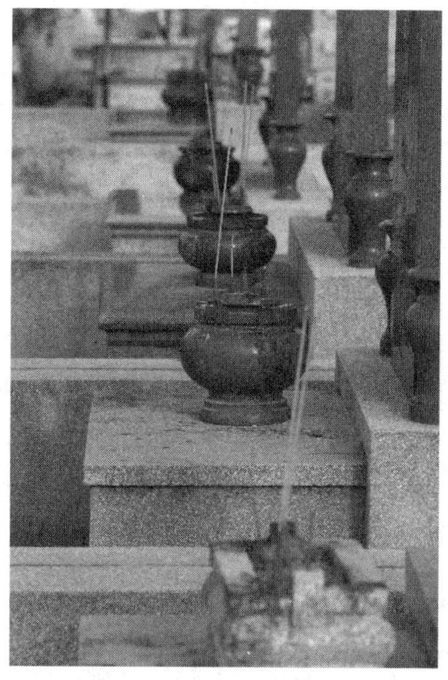

Asian Americans

Asian Americans trace their ancestry to China, Japan, Korea, Hawaii, Samoa, Thailand, Vietnam, and Cambodia. In most Asian cultures, discussions of death are discouraged due to the belief that talking about bad events, such as death, will actually cause them to happen (Thomas, 2001). This reluctance extends to not telling a terminally ill family member that he or she is dying. In fact, death is an outright taboo subject among some Chinese Americans (Tanner, 1995).

Across all Asian American groups, decision making often is in the hands of the senior family members (Crowder, 2000). Attitudes toward physician-assisted suicide (PAS; see Chapter 5), however, differ from one group to another. For example, Chinese and Japanese Americans approve of PAS in large numbers, but depending on religion and degree of assimilation, other groups are less enthusiastic or even disapproving (Braun, Tanji, & Heck, 2001).

Funeral rituals also tend to vary among Asian Americans, again depending on the degree of assimilation, but they are always important. For Chinese Americans, the dead remain part of the family, defining the values by which the family lives and creating the shared identity of living

A Chinese Funeral in America

The family of the dead person visits the mortuary (the place a dead body is prepared for viewing and burial) on the first day. The family forms a receiving line to receive visitors. Family members line up in order of importance, with the oldest son first, and so on. The casket is surrounded by food and items such as a paper house, paper servants, and paper money.

The next day, a service is held at the mortuary, perhaps presided over by a Protestant cleric. A Western-style band then begins to play as the procession leaves the mortuary and proceeds through Chinatown. "Spirit money" (plain paper) is thrown from the hearse to ward off evil spirits. At the gravesite, flowers are thrown into the grave and on top of the casket. The food and paper items that surrounded the casket at the mortuary are burned at the gravesite so that they will accompany the dead person into the afterlife. Finally, the funeral party attends a longevity banquet, which is an opportune place for offering support to the survivors (Crowder, 2000).

members of the family. Thus ancestor worship among Chinese Americans is strong, and funerals are a major ritual of passage from this life to another (Crowder, 2000). Continuing attention to graves also is important, with the well-being of survivors depending, in part, on properly maintaining an ongoing family relationship with the dead person (Hirayama, 1990).

Death in Non-Western Societies

Regarding death and dying issues, differences and similarities exist among members of other cultures living outside the United States. Presented in this section is information specific to Africa, China and Japan, and India and Nepal.

Africa

In black Africa, the traditional belief is that the dead are not really dead; they continue an afterlife of spirit activity, in which they have special powers allowing them to change appearance, as well as inhabit the bodies of people and animals. These spirits are significant only to kin, to whom they are as likely to be benevolent as malicious. For this reason, the spirits of the dead are feared. When the spirits are forgotten or neglected, they manifest their anger by sending calamities on their descendants. Their anger is usually appeased through prayer and ritual offerings. In many black African societies, ancestral veneration is a central tradition, and even though there is no uniform system of ancestor worship, there are many common elements (Nyamiti, 2007).

Some black Africans believe that naming a descendant for an ancestor allows the ancestor to continue to live in his or her descendant. But the ancestor will continue to survive as an ancestor only if he is not forgotten; that is, if the descendants communicate with the spirit regularly through prayer and ritual offering. No one can be an ancestor of an individual who is not kin. Although there are cases where ancestral relationship is not founded on family ties but on membership in a religious or secret society, the relationship rarely, if ever, goes beyond the tribe.

In some black African communities, a person without offspring cannot become an ancestor. Thus, these Africans desire to have many children who will remember them and with whom they can ritually communicate. For living kin, an ancestor is believed to procure benefits, such as health, long life, and the begetting of children.

Ancestors are said to desire frequent or regular contact with their earthly relatives and are even believed to visit them through mediums (e.g., snakes, hyenas, or caterpillars) or by direct possession. In fact, the living and their ancestors form a solidarity lived and expressed through prayers and rituals. Visits to the graves of ancestors, the leaving of food and gifts, and the asking of protection serve as important parts of these traditional rituals.

No one can attain ancestral status without having led a morally good life, according to traditional African moral standards. An ancestor is regarded as a model of conduct in the community and a source of tribal tradition and stability. In some tribes, proper burial with appropriate funeral rites is a necessary condition for ancestral existence, although this tradition is not universal. Some societies do not bury the dead, but simply throw them into the bush.

China and Japan

In Asia, like other non-Western societies, the ancestors live on, having a central place in the family and continuing to have relationships with the living (Rösch-Rhomberg, 1994). Life embraces both the living and the dead, even to the garments worn at Chinese funerals, which show the degree of kinship of the mourners to the dead.

The Japanese consider the spirits of the dead a continuing part of family and community life. A dead person's spirit only gradually fades away as time goes on, but the dead, especially in rural areas, are a continuing solace to the living (Kristof, 1996).

Japanese family members and priests perform funeral rites wherein the dead person is transformed into a revered ancestor, a source of beneficence and guidance to the survivors. The living and the dead depend on each other. For example, the living perform the necessary funeral rites, and the dead bless the living. Thus, one must have heirs; otherwise, no one will be there to perform the necessary rites of ancestry. The Japanese typically continue to honor the dead with rites at a shrine in the home as well as careful tending of the gravesite.

Feng-shui is a Chinese custom not only for decorating a living room, but for such things as housing the dead. Chinese cemeteries usually are on a slope, preferably with mountains to the rear and a sea in front and a view of fertile fields left by the dead person to his descendants. Chinese who travel overseas are required to make arrangements to ensure that, if they die outside China, their remains will be sent back to be buried in family plots. This practice was a special concern of the Chinese track-laying laborers who built the U.S. transcontinental railway in the nineteenth century.

India and Nepal

In India and in other southeastern Asian cultures, the soul of the dead person is a major participant in what happens after death. Complex funeral ceremonies are performed to propitiate deities so that the soul has unhindered passage to heaven. Sometimes, especially in a Buddhist funeral ceremony, the soul itself needs to be convinced that it no longer belongs to the mortal world and it needs to get ready to travel to the other world (Lama, 2007).

Hindus believe that to ensure quick salvation, one must die lying on the bank of a sacred river. Any river will do, because all rivers are sacred to Hindus, although some are more sacred than others. Many Hindu holy shrines are built along famous riverbanks. Banaras, situated along the river Ganges, is the holiest of them all. Even today, pious Hindus in India move to Baneras in old age for the sole purpose of waiting to die on the bank of the Ganges.

Hindu custom requires the body to be cremated (see Chapter 12) as soon as all family members have had a chance to view it, so that the soul is not tempted to linger. The ashes are placed in an urn for scattering in a special year-end ceremony. (Note that Buddhists prefer to disperse the ashes immediately over the river.) Ideally, the ashes should be scattered in or around holy rivers. Those who can afford it travel to Baneras and scatter the ashes in the Ganges. Those who cannot afford to travel dispose of the ashes in a nearby local river.

The typical Hindu mourning period is 11 days, but in some parts of India, Hindus mourn for 13 days. Part of each meal, intended to nourish the dead person's soul, is served on a banana leaf and laid out in the open. If crows eat it, it has been accepted.

For Buddhists, the final ceremony can occur any time within a year. According to Buddhist tradition, the last day of the ceremony is the day when the soul, until now still living in the house, departs on its journey to eternity.

Reincarnation

Many Asians subscribe to the expectation of reincarnation. Reincarnation is a Hindu–Buddhist philosophy of an eternal birth–death–birth cycle during which a soul moves from body to body (Reincarnation, 2007). A good life results in rebirth to a higher-quality life form, and a bad life to a lower-quality life form. This forward and backward progression is based on the Law of Karma, in which good deeds are rewarded and bad deeds are punished. The ultimate goal in the Karmic cycle is for the soul to progress to the highest level of existence and become as one with the universe.

Reincarnation has entered Western thought through New Age teachings. Many Christians even believe in reincarnation; remarkably, nearly 60% of U.S. adults believe in reincarnation (Moore, 2005). Reincarnation appeals to Western New Age thinking because the idea offers additional chances to get life right. With reincarnation, persons can go through this life however they want and, if need be, get it right in the next.

Festivals Celebrating the "Departed"

The *Bon* Festival, which is held during three days in August, is a Japanese Buddhist holiday to honor the "departed" spirits of one's ancestors.

This holiday has been celebrated in Japan for more than 500 years, and it has evolved into a family reunion holiday during which people from big cities return to their hometowns and visit and clean their ancestors' graves.

The *Qingming* is a traditional Chinese festival usually occurring around April 5. Along with Double Ninth Festival, which coincides with the ninth day of the ninth month in the Chinese calendar, it is a time to tend to the graves of loved ones who have died. In addition, in the Chinese tradition the seventh month in the Chinese calendar is called the Ghost Month, in which ghosts and spirits come out from the underworld to visit earth.

During the Nepali holiday of *Gai Jatra*, every family who has experienced the death of a family member during the previous year makes a *gai,* which is a construction of bamboo branches, cloth, paper decorations, and portraits of the dead person. It is called the *Gai Jatra* (Cow Pilgrimage) because in Nepali tradition a cow leads the spirits of the dead into the next land. Depending on local custom, either a live cow or a construct representing a cow is used. The festival also is a time to dress up in costume, including costumes involving political commentary and satire.

The Day of the Dead (*el Día de los Muertos*) has been celebrated in Mexico and other Latin countries since pre–Columbian Aztec and Mayan times. This celebration usually takes place on November 1 (All Saints Day) or November 2 (Souls Day; Salvador, 2003). Celebrants typically approach the Day of the Dead joyfully, with an emphasis on honoring the lives of those who have died and celebrating death as the beginning of a new stage in life. A common symbol of the holiday is the skull (the *calavera*), which celebrants represent in masks called **calacas**. Skulls made of sugar are a gift for both the living and the dead. Other foods related to the holiday include *pan de muerto* (bread of the dead), a sweet egg bread made in various shapes.

Families usually clean and decorate the graves of loved ones with *ofrendas* (offerings) such as orange marigolds called *Flor de Muerto* (Flower of the Dead) to attract the souls of the dead, toys for dead children (*los angelitos,* little angels), and bottles of *tequila, mezcal, pulque,* or *atole* for adults. *Ofrendas* also are placed in homes as a welcoming gesture for the dead person. Some families build altars or small shrines in their homes, spending time around the altar praying and telling anecdotes about the dead person. In some locations, celebrants wear shells on their clothing so that when they dance, the dead will wake up because of the noise.

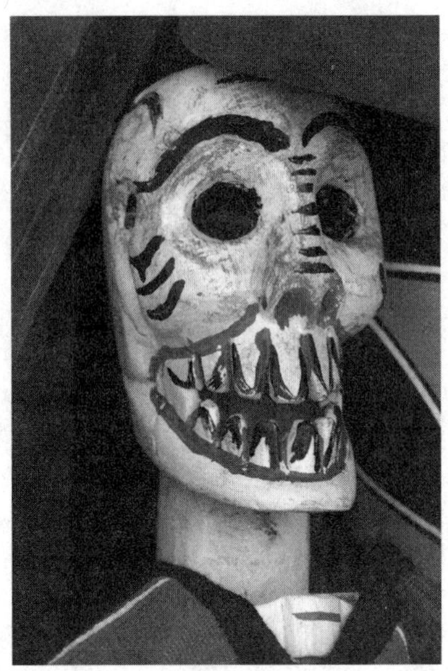

Summary

- The ways in which people respond to death varies by culture and within cultures.
- In all cultures, religious beliefs can lessen death anxiety.
- The history of death and dying rituals are older than civilization itself. Archeological evidence of ritual burial ceremonies date as far back as the Neanderthal, 150,000 years ago.
- In Western societies, fragmented family ties and scattered communities have diluted the emotional and social supports that cushion the impact of death. The Romantic period of the 1800s led to an

emphasis on memorials and on elaborate funerals and mourning customs. The mechanization accompanying World War I, along with new medical practices, took death and dying away from the home and community and put it into the hospital.

- Early Native Americans believed in evil spirits. Views of the afterlife vary among Native Americans. Some see life as circular, following the repeating pattern of natural seasons, rather than linear. In this belief, what happens after death is not of great consequence.
- Hispanic Americans believe family and religion are very important in dealing with death. Catholicism is a strong influence on how Hispanic Americans approach dying and death. A Catholic novena is held by the family for the dead person.
- African Americans generally die at home, in part because their families resist putting them into nursing homes when ill or elderly and because they lack confidence in medical care. An African American funeral usually consists of an affirmation of the individual and usually is judged to be "successful" based on how many people attend, how fancy the casket is, and so on. Storytelling is an important part of grieving.
- In black Africa, ancestor-worship is widespread. Ancestors are believed to procure benefits, such as health, long life, and the begetting of children, for their kin. No one can attain ancestral status without having led a morally good life. An ancestor is regarded as a model of conduct in the community and a source of tribal tradition and stability.
- Asian Americans are reticent to discuss death, believing that talking about bad events will cause them to happen. Death is an outright taboo subject among some Chinese Americans. This reluctance extends to not telling a terminally ill family member that he or she is dying.
- Chinese cemeteries, following the customs of *feng-shui*, usually are on a slope, preferably with mountains to the rear and a sea in front and a view of fertile fields left by the dead to his descendants.
- The Japanese continue to honor the dead with rites at a shrine in the home as well as careful tending of the gravesite.
- In India and in other southeastern Asian cultures, the soul of the dead is a major participant in what happens after death. Complex funeral ceremonies are performed to propitiate deities so that the soul may be given unhindered passage to heaven. Hindus believe that to ensure quick salvation, one must die lying on the bank of a sacred river and be cremated and spread into the river. Hindu customs require the body to be cremated as soon as all family members have had a chance to view it, so that the soul is not tempted to linger. For Buddhists, the final ceremony of the spreading of ashes can occur any time within a year.
- Reincarnation is a Hindu–Buddhist philosophy of an eternal birth–death–birth cycle, during which a soul moves from body to body. A good life results in rebirth to a higher-quality life form, and a bad life to a lower-quality life form. This forward and backward progression is based on the Law of Karma, in which good deeds are rewarded and bad deeds are punished. The ultimate goal in the Karmic cycle is for the soul to progress to the highest level of existence and become as one with the universe. Remarkably, nearly 60% of Americans believe reincarnation is possible.
- Since pre–Columbian Aztec and Mayan times, the Day of the Dead (*el Día de los Muertos*) has been celebrated in Mexico and other Latin countries. Celebrants typically approach the Day of the Dead joyfully, with celebration of the death as the beginning of a new stage in life.

Additional Resources

Books

Barley, N. (1997). *Grave matters: A lively history of death around the world.* New York: Henry Holt and Company. Examined in this book are the many ways in which cultures around the world deal with death and give it meaning. In this book, myths about death, ways to mourn, joking at funerals, postmortem videos, cannibalism, headhunting, and royal mortuary rituals are covered.

Geary, P. J. (1994). *Living with the dead in the Middle Ages.* Ithaca, NY: Cornell University Press. In this book, 12 essays are presented. Among others, topics include saints, cults, and the role of the dead in negotiating the claims of contending interest groups.

Smith, R. J. (1974). *Ancestor worship in contemporary Japan.* Stanford, CA: Stanford University Press. The author traces the changes that have taken place in the ways the Japanese people revere their ancestors, who is chosen to be so honored, and the reasons for the changes.

Watson, J. L., & Rawski, E. S. (1988). *Death ritual in late imperial and modern China*. Berkeley: University of California Press. This book presents a discussion of how uniformity in funeral rituals in China from 1500 to 1911 contributed to uniformity in the overall Chinese culture, despite substantial ethnic, linguistic, and regional differences.

Movie

Elizabethtown. (2005). The plot of this movie is built around an elaborate memorial for a Kentucky patriarch.

Critical Thinking

1. Do you believe that you are able to communicate with a loved family member after his or her death? If yes, how do you believe you should go about it?
2. Do you think that a dead person, with whom you were once close, can continue to have an influence on your life? If so, in what ways?
3. After the death of a relative, how did the funeral service affect how you felt?

Class Activity

Pick a particular culture, subculture, society, or country from a list provided by your instructor and research its funeral practices and attitudes toward the dead. If necessary, form teams so that there are enough choices to go around. Write a report wherein you detail these beliefs and practices.

References

Aries, P. (1974). *Western attitudes toward death: From the middle ages to the present.* Baltimore: Johns Hopkins University Press.

Bloch, M., & Parry, P. (1982). *Death and the regeneration of life.* Cambridge, UK: Cambridge University Press.

Braun, K. L., Tanji, V. M., & Heck, R. (2001). Support for physician-assisted suicide: Exploring the impact of ethnicity and attitudes toward planning for death. *Gerontology*, *41*(1), 51–60.

Brennan, M. (2005). Death and dying: Death is a biological certainty but the practices surrounding death and mourning are socially constructed. *Sociology Review*, *14*(3), 26–28.

Brosnius, J. P. (1995–1996). Father dead, mother dead: Bereavement and fictive death in Penan Geng society. *Omega: Journal of Death and Dying, 32*(3), 197–226.

Catlin, G. (1993). The role of culture in grief. *Journal of Social Psychology*, *133*(2), 173–184.

Clements, P. T., Vigil, G. J., Manno, M. S., Henry, G. C., Wilks, J., Das Sarthak, et al. (2003). Cultural perspectives of death, grief, and bereavement. *Journal of Psychosocial Nursing, 41*(7), 18–26.

Cox, G. R., & Fundis, R. J. (1992). Native American burial practices. In J. Morgan (Ed.), *Personal care in an impersonal world* (pp. 23–250). Amityville, NY: Baywood Publishing.

Crowder, L. (2000). Chinese funerals in San Francisco Chinatown. *Journal of American Folklore, 113*(450), 451–463.

Deloria, V. (1994). *God is red: A native view of religion*. Golden, CO: Fulcrum. (Original work published 1973)

Durkheim, E. (1976). *The elementary forms of the religious life.* Translated by J. W. Swain. Boston: George Allen & Unwin. (Original work published 1915)

Folte, T. R., & Deck, S. (1988). The impact of children's death on Shona mothers and families. *Journal of Comparative Family Studies, 19*, 432–451.

Gennep, A. V. (1960). *The rites of passage.* Chicago: University of Chicago Press.

Gijana, E. W. M., Louw, J., & Mangani, N. C. (1989). Thoughts about death and dying in an African sample. *Omega, 20*, 245–258.

Grabowski, J. A., & Frantz, T. (1993). Latinos and Anglos: Cultural experiences of grief intensity. *Omega, Journal of Death and Dying, 26*(4), 273–275.

Griener, K. A., Perera, S., & Ahluwalia, J. S. (2003). Hospice usage by minorities in the last year of life. *Journal American Geriatrics Society, 51*(7), 970–978.

Handy, E. S. C., & Pukui, M. K. (1972). *The Polynesian family system in Ka-'u, Hawai'i.* Rutland, VT: Charles E. Tuttle.

Harder, B. (2001, December 15). Evolving in their graves: Early burials hold clues to human origins. *Science News, 160*, 380–381.

Hayslip, B., & Peveto, C. A. (2004). *Shifts in attitude toward death, dying, and bereavement.* New York: Springer.

Hertz, R. (1960). A contribution to the study of the collective representation of death. In R. C. Needham (Trans.), *Death and the right hand* (pp. 197–216). London: Cohen & West.

Hirayama, K. K. (1990). Death and dying in Japanese culture. In K. Parry (Ed.), *Social work practice with the terminally ill* (pp. 159–174). Springfield, IL: Charles C. Thomas.

Holloway, K. F. C. (2003). *Passed on: African American mourning stories, a memorial.* Durham, NC: Duke University Press.

Hultkrantz, A. (1979). *The religions of the American Indians.* Berkeley: University of California Press.

Kalish, R. A., & Reynolds, D. K. (1981). *Death and ethnicity: A psychocultural study.* Farmingdale, NY: Baywood.

Kristof, N. D. (1996, September 29). For rural Japanese, death doesn't break family ties. *New York Times,* p. A1.

Kübler-Ross, E. (1969). *On death and dying.* New York: Touchstone.

Lama, U. (2007). *Funeral rites of the Hindus and the Buddhists.* Retrieved January 2007, from www.webhealing.com/articles/lama.html

LaMont, C. (1994). The Romantic period. In P. Rogers (Ed.), *The Oxford illustrated history of English literature* (pp. 274–324). New York: Oxford University Press.

Mandelbaum, D. (1959). Social uses of funeral rites. In H. Feifel (Ed.), *The meaning of death* (pp. 189–217). New York: McGraw-Hill.

Margolin, M. (1978). *The Ohlone way: Indian life in the San Francisco Monterey Bay area.* Berkeley, CA: Heyday Books.

McLennan, J., Akande, A., & Bates, G. W. (1976). Death anxiety and death denial: Nigerian and Australian students' metaphors of personal death. *Journal of Psychology, 127*(4), 399–407.

Moore, D. W. (2005, June 16). *Three in four Americans believe in paranormal.* Princeton, NJ: Gallup Poll News Service.

Munet-Vilaro, F. (1998). Grieving and death rituals of Latinos. *Oncology Nursing Forum, 25*(10), 1761–1763.

Nyamiti, C. (2007). *Ancestor veneration in Africa.* Retrieved January 2007, from www.afrikaworld.net/afrel/index.html

Oswalt, W. H. (1986). *Life cycles and lifeways.* Palo Alto, CA: Mayfield Publishing.

Peil, M. (1991). Family support for the Nigerian elderly. *Journal of Comparative Family Studies, 22,* 85–100.

Reincarnation. (2007). Retrieved January 2007, from www.allaboutspirituality.org/reincarnation.htm

Rodgers, L. S. (2004). Meaning of bereavement among older African American widows. *Geriatic Nursing, 25*(1), 10–16.

Rösch-Rhomberg, I. (1994). Hierarchical opposition and the concept of um-yang. *Anthropos, 89,* 471–491.

Salvador, R. J. (2003). What do Mexicans celebrate on the Day of the Dead? In J. D. Morgan & P. Laungani (Eds.), *Death and bereavement in the Americas: Death, value, and meaning series,* Vol. II (pp. 75–76). Amityville: Baywood.

Stannard, D. E. (1977). *The Puritan way of death.* New York: Oxford University Press.

Steiger, B. (1974). *Medicine power: The American Indian's revival of his spiritual heritage.* Garden City, NY: Doubleday.

Tanner, J. G. (1995). Death, dying and grief in the Chinese American culture. In J. K. Parry & A. S. Ryan (Eds.), *A cross-cultural look at death, dying, and religion* (pp. 183–192). Chicago: Nelson-Hall.

Thomas, N. (2001). The importance of culture throughout all of life and beyond. *Holistic Nursing Practice, 15*(2), 40–46.

Tschann, J., Kaufmann, S., & Micco, G. (2003). Family involvement in end-of-life hospital care. *Journal of the American Geriatrics Society, 51*(6), 835–840.

Warren, C. (1993). Disrupted death ceremonies: Popular culture and the ethnography of Bali. *Oceana, 64*(1), 36–56.

Waters, C. M. (2001). Understanding and supporting African Americans' perspectives of end-of-life care planning and decision making. *Qualitative Health Research, 11*(3), 385–398.

Watson, J. L., & Rawski, E. S. (1988). *Death ritual in late imperial and modern China.* Berkeley: University of California Press.

Wikan, U. (1988). Bereavement and loss in two Muslim communities: Egypt and Bali compared. *Social Sciences and Medicine, 27*(5), 451–460.

Witthoft, J. (1983). Cherokee beliefs concerning death. *Journal of Cherokee Studies, 8*(2), 68–72.

The American Healthcare System

It may seem a strange principle
to enunciate as the very first
requrement in a Hospital that
it should do the sick no harm.
—Florence Nightingale

Objectives

After reading this chapter, you will be able to answer the following questions:

- In the United States, how do medical professionals approach death and dying?
- What are hospice and palliative care?
- How much is spent on health care in the United States, and how many citizens are covered?

The Medical Approach to Dying

Paradoxically, remarkable technological advances in health care and medical treatment in the United States since World War II have created difficulties for terminally ill patients. Doctors are trained to save lives, and they try very hard (in some cases, too hard) to keep people alive who die anyway, but who die painfully and over a long period of time.

When people get sick in the United States, they typically go to a doctor to get treatment to become well. A terminally ill patient, however, cannot be made well. Such a patient does not fit into the concept of medicine as a healing art. Rather than see death as an inevitable and normal part of life, modern medical professionals view death as an unacceptable deviance from normality. Death is embarrassing, disruptive, and emotionally upsetting to many people in the medical world, because it violates physicians' sense of clinical objectivity and their goal of preserving life at all costs (Chambliss, 1966).

Typically, in the United States, a physician regards an ill patient as a person who needs to be cured. The goal is an instrumental one; that is, to return the person to health and social function. To be ill is to reject society's view that everyone should be well (Parsons, 1958). This view likely accounts for the reluctance of many people who have cancer to admit that they are ill, because they believe that they will be ostracized and dehumanized if their condition is known.

The stigma assigned to the dying oftentimes is intensified when a person is dying from AIDS.

The focus on the person dying from AIDS is usually about how the disease was contracted, not on the disease or its progression, because homosexual activity or needle sharing by drug users, the most highly publicized ways of contracting AIDS, are seen as socially deviant by people who are more upset by the behavior than by the disease (Earl, Martindale, & Cohen, 1992). This focus leads to aversive discrimination and a lack of assistance to the dying patient, who has enough to deal with already.

Death in Medical Education

Medical school professors historically have not taught their students how to deal with the dying and with death. This lack of instruction is improving, but only slowly (Dickinson, 2002). Changes in gross anatomy classes, such as holding memorial services for dissected cadavers, have ameliorated the tendency of medical students to become desensitized to the fact that cadavers were once living persons (Marks & Bertman, 1980).

Administrators in some medical schools now ensure that courses are offered on communicating with terminally ill patients, exposing students to the psychological and emotional aspects of dying, not just the physical aspects (Mermann, Gunn, & Dickinson, 1991). As of 2004, all medical students in the United States are examined not only on clinical skills, but also on how well they communicate with patients, including those who are dying. Also, the American Medical Association (AMA) is emphasizing the training of doctors to provide ways to lessen suffering, to treat the mental states of dying patients, and to help the dying and their families plan for death.

Dying in a Hospital

Where do people typically die? Most want to die at home (Hays, Gold, Flint, & Winer, 1999), but in the West, although many die in nursing homes, their homes, or hospice, the majority die in a hospital. The hospital saves society in general from disruption, and a family specifically from inconvenience, by taking over the dying process of the dying person. However, a hospital is a bureaucracy, and bureaucracies become dehumanized (Weber, 1958), thereby removing personal and emotional elements from the process of dying (Moller, 1996). Doctors and other medical professionals are trained and socialized to be impersonal toward the dying and to fight death as an unnatural thing to be defeated. People know that they will die, but they are socialized to see death as a thief taking life, rather than death being a part of life.

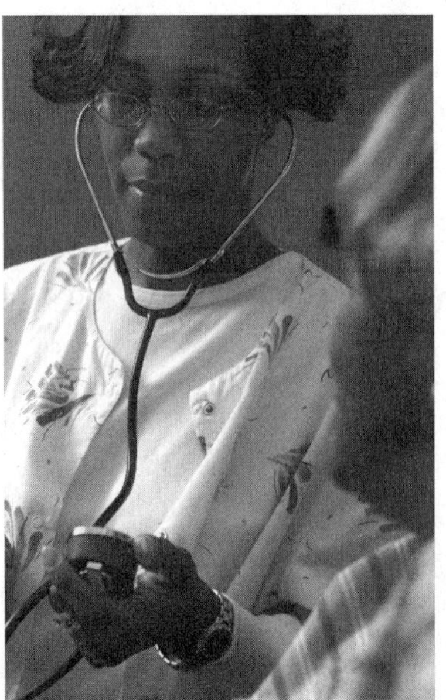

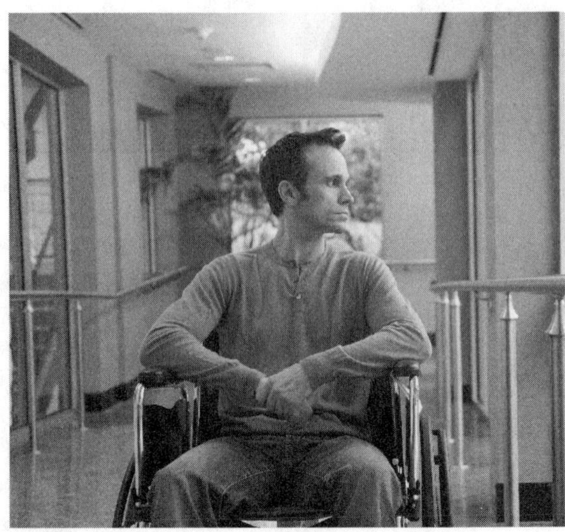

The *technological imperative* (what is new and can be used and, therefore, must be used) is another roadblock to caring for the dying. Every new development in medical machinery rapidly becomes the norm in practice, dedicated to the goal of keeping a patient alive and managing disease (Koenig, 1988). There is no room for death in this model.

Dying is something that can be a normal part of a hospital routine (van Eys, 1988), wherein a patient is allowed to hold on to self-esteem and do what is necessary to abate the loneliness of death. As part of this normal process, the patient and the patient's family must revise their current relationships, roles, and identities, while at the same time being as useful as possible. When the patient cannot live as he or she did outside the hospital and is essentially powerless and subject to the control of medical professionals who decide what is done and when, this process can be difficult.

Nursing Homes

Nursing homes are a common place for the infirm elderly. (Many nursing homes also are used as rehabilitation centers for those recovering from operations, injury, and illness.) Two-thirds of people living long term in a nursing home die there. Nursing homes must be licensed by the state and meet federal standards to receive Medicare and Medicaid payments. As such, nursing homes are as regimented as are hospitals, and they can be a very dispiriting experience for those who live there. Most nursing homes are understaffed (U.S. Department of Health and Human Services, 2001) because of low pay and difficult working conditions. The result is that even though some nursing homes are quite good, many people dread going there, and when they become old and infirm, plead with family members not to be put there.

Hospice and Palliative Care

Palliative care refers to pain management as well as to emotional and spiritual support for someone who is ill. Hospice care usually focuses on the terminally ill patient. Medical personnel are reluctant to use the term *palliative care*, because many

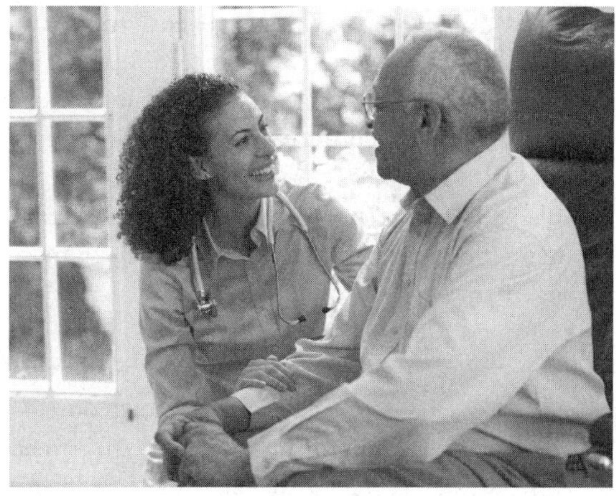

patients and families think it means "abandon all hope." The term *palliative*, however, comes from the Latin word *pallium*, or "cloak," meaning to protect people from discomfort. The word *palliate* means to ease symptoms without curing the disease. Palliative care does not necessarily mean, however, that a cure is no longer possible. Palliative care and curative care can go hand in hand.

Pain Management

Many patients suffer severe pain near death, and doctors do not always know how to ease it. Some doctors are afraid to administer certain drugs because of harsh antidrug laws, which require physicians to fill out forms in triplicate if they dispense powerful drugs that can kill a person. Although these laws are in place to ensure that physicians handle these drugs appropriately, results from a survey of New York State physicians revealed that 71% chose a weaker medication than needed to ease a patient's pain because they feared that they would be scrutinized by drug enforcement personnel. Some of these doctors also were mistakenly afraid that they would addict their patients. However, less than 1% of terminal patients treated with strong drugs become addicted—they usually do not live long enough to become addicted (Foley & Hendin, 1999).

From the Foley and Hendin (1999) study, physicians also reported being afraid that they would accidentally kill a patient. Of the physicians surveyed, 40% wrongly believed that using a dose of morphine big enough to control breathlessness would kill the patient. In truth, as long as a patient is given time to adjust, no dose that strong can kill a person. Out of fear, many doctors who could ease the pain of dying patients do not. Only recently have medical schools begun to introduce courses in pain management for physicians-in-training. Better pain management could allow patients more comfortable, if not easier, deaths.

Patients and their families have similar false beliefs. Many people, including doctors, do not realize that drugs bought and used on the street by addicts can be beneficial when used properly by people who need them.

Questions & Answers

Question: Is "home" the only place hospice care can take place?

Answer: No. Although most hospice services are delivered in a patient's residence, some patients receive hospice care in a nursing home or hospice center.

Question: Do hospice people make death come sooner?

Answer: Hospice workers do nothing to speed or slow the dying process. They simply offer support and comfort during the process of dying.

Hospice Care

The term *hospice* can be traced back to medieval times. The term originally referred to a place of shelter and rest for weary or ill travelers on a long journey. Today, **hospice** involves making terminally ill patients comfortable by providing them with pain medication but not providing further medical treatment. Hospice care allows a dying person to remain at home during the final days of life if he or she wishes. The goal of hospice is to make the person comfortable and pain-free, and able to make the best use of his or her remaining time.

The usual term of hospice care, as measured by Medicare (governmental "insurance" for persons 65 and older), is 60 days, which can be renewed. Four of five hospice patients are 65 years of age or older. In the 1970s, cancer patients made up the largest percentage of hospice patients, but today fewer than half (44.1%) of hospice admissions have cancer. The other 55.9% of patients have non-cancer diagnoses such as heart disease, dementia, or lung disease (National Hospice and Palliative Care Organization, 2007).

Hospice staff, nurses, and nonmedical volunteers make regular visits to assess the hospice patient's needs. Hospice workers are on call 24/7. When a patient is sick, upset, or needs help in any way, hospice workers are available. Hospice staff members are responsible for the following:

- Managing the patient's pain
- Assisting the patient with the emotional and spiritual aspects of dying
- Providing needed medicines
- Running errands
- Coaching the family on how to care for the dying person

Results from a study of psychosocial and spiritual issues among hospice patients (Kutner et al., 2003), revealed that 90% believed that life has value and worth, 87% believed that each day has

ORIGIN OF THE HOSPICE MOVEMENT

In 1967, Dame Cicely Saunders founded the first modern hospice in London. Dame Saunders is reported to have told her first patient, "You matter to the last moment of your life, and we will do all we can, not only to help you die peacefully, but to live until you die."

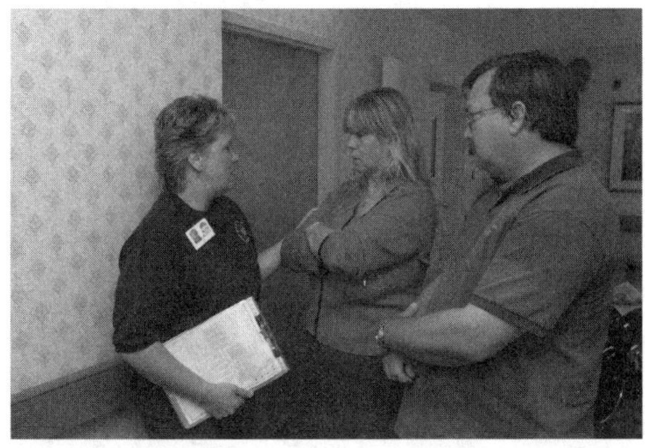

potential, and 82% had a positive outlook on life. Contrary to what some people might believe, for most hospice patients hope actually increases rather than decreases as they move closer to death. Possibly, the renewed hope is due to the fact that many hospice patients are encouraged to talk about what they are experiencing. Obviously, nothing can be more lethal to hope than silence.

Hospice Care Away from Home

For various reasons, a dying person might need to go from home to a hospice facility, permanently or for a short time. The family caretakers might need a break, the person might need more help with pain control than home care can handle, or the person's condition might have deteriorated to the point that home care is no longer workable. Even in hospice, the emphasis continues to be on family presence and involvement in tending to the patient and his or her needs, as well as on a pleasant ambience in the facility itself.

Cost and Coverage of the U.S. Healthcare System

In 2003, the United States spent 15.3% of its gross domestic product (GDP) on health care to cover only some of its citizens. This amount is more than many other developed countries in the West spend on providing health care for all of their citizens. In the United States, 44 million people are without any health insurance, and tens of millions more are underinsured (Bartlett & Steele, 2004).

Hospitals typically charge noninsured people 5 to 10 times what an insured person pays and discharge them from the hospital sooner than the insured, often before doctors think they should be released (Bartlett & Steele, 2004). When such people cannot pay a large bill, hospitals have been known to sue for payment, garnishee the person's wages, and take the person's assets, such as a house. A catastrophic accident or illness can bankrupt even the insured.

Over the last few decades, American health care has changed from a largely nonprofit system to a for-profit one. Today, profits and market forces affect every healthcare decision. Unfortunately, though, managing health care as a business has not reined in costs. Government is widely perceived as inefficient; however, Medicare's overhead averages about 2% a year, whereas private insurers' administrative costs are about 33% (Bartlett & Steele, 2004).

One reason for increasing healthcare costs is the development of expensive medical technology, which kicks the technological imperative into action. Better technology does mean better care, but the expense collides with the economic problem of scarcity of resources. Can Americans continue to pay for what they want? A more efficient method of financing health care seems more important as time goes on and costs continue to rise.

Change seems inevitable. Working Americans are dissatisfied with ever-rising healthcare costs, and even doctors, insurers, and other professionals, who traditionally have been against what they label "socialized medicine," have shown a definite shift in opinion.

The Cost of Drugs

A significant part of the rising cost of health care is the cost of drug therapy. Each year, $200 billion is spent in the United States on prescription drugs, and that amount is growing by 12% a year (Angell, 2004). This amount does not include money spent on drugs by hospitals and other healthcare facilities.

Until recently, the drug industry has been the most profitable industry in the United States.

A HEALTHCARE MANAGEMENT PROPOSAL

One healthcare management proposal, as explained by Bartlett and Steele (2004), is one in which a taxpayer-supported independent agency is created, similar in structure to the Federal Reserve System. The authors prescribe that the agency would be run by 14 board members appointed by the president with the consent of the Senate. The agency would set an overall policy for health care and influence its direction by controlling federal spending. The agency would be responsible for everything from research grants to providing basic care and catastrophic care for every American. Financing would stem from a tax on the total earnings of all businesses and a flat tax (like the Medicare tax) on all income—not just wages. Bartlett and Steele reported that this proposed agency would radically reduce medical errors with the establishment of a single information technology system that would link all hospitals, doctors' offices, pharmacies, and nursing homes.

How does it manage to keep its prices high? No competition! Patent rights guarantee exclusive rights to the patentee to sell brand-name drugs for up to 14 years before they become generic. Prices then drop to as little as 20% of the original price.

In response to the growing burden of drug costs, employers, health insurers, and states have begun to work to reduce these costs by negotiating discounts from pharmaceutical companies or instituting tiered formularies for insurance reimbursement (i.e., full coverage for generic drugs and partial or no coverage for brand-name drugs). Individuals have tried to control their drug expenditures by buying drugs more cheaply from Canada, until Congress passed a law making it illegal to do so.

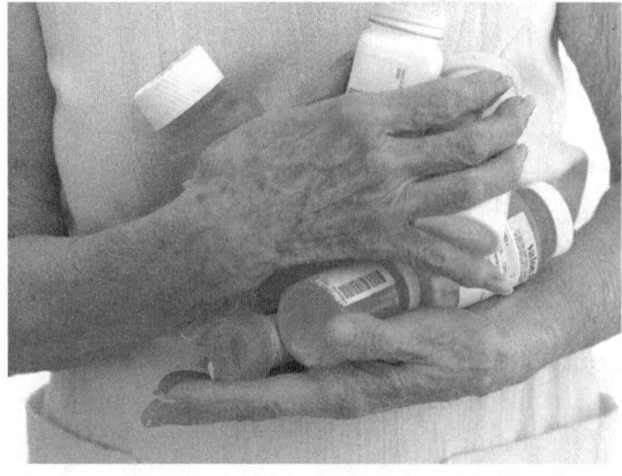

SUMMARY

- Currently, many physicians try to keep people alive who die anyway, and many of them die painfully and over a long period of time.
- Rather than viewing death as an inevitable and normal part of life, it is often viewed as an unacceptable deviance from normality.
- Medical school professors historically have not taught medical students how to deal with the dying and with death. Today, all medical students in the United States are examined not only on clinical skills, but also on how well they communicate with patients, including those who are dying.
- In the West, most people die in a hospital. Dying in a hospital can become a normal part of the hospital routine, in part, by helping patients hold on to self-esteem and abating loneliness.
- Nursing homes are a placement for the infirm elderly; also, they serve as rehabilitation centers for those recovering from operations, injury, and illness. Two-thirds of people who live long-term in a nursing home die there.
- Palliative care is pain management and emotional and spiritual support for someone who is ill. Hospice palliative care focuses on the terminally ill patient. Palliative care and curative care can go hand in hand. Hospice

workers make terminal patients comfortable and give them pain medication without medical treatment.

- In 2003, the United States spent 15.3% of its gross domestic product (GDP) on health care. A significant part of the rising cost of health care is the cost of drug therapy. Many Americans are dissatisfied with ever-rising healthcare costs.

Additional Resources

Books

Beresford, L. (1993). *The hospice handbook.* New York: Little, Brown, & Co. The terminally ill do have choices, and they can control the quality of their lives. This guide is useful in describing what hospice is, how to find the right one, and how to make an informed decision.

Walter, T. (1994). *The revival of death.* London: Routledge. A sociological look at the hospice movement and bereavement counseling. In this book, the following questions are poised: Who should people pay attention to regarding death issues—priests, doctors, counselors, or ourselves? Has psychology replaced religion in telling people how to die?

Worswick, J. A. (2000). *House called Helen: The development of hospice care for children.* New York: Oxford University Press. This book presents an authoritative account of how Helen House, the first children's hospice, in Oxford, England, came into being. Through the book, insight is offered regarding the needs of families and the difficulties they face caring for a child with a terminal illness.

Movie

Nothing in Common. (1986). Tom Hanks is David Basner, a successful advertising executive who must deal with his father (Jackie Gleason), who can no longer take care of himself and requires that his son take care of him.

Critical Thinking

1. How could you help someone who is dying enjoy a dignified end of life?
2. If you could no longer take care of yourself and could no longer live at home, in which "home away from home" would you want to live?

Class Activities

1. Invite a hospice worker to come to your class and ask about his or her work and what he or she witnesses when attending to dying patients.
2. Take a trip to a nursing home. While there, speak with one elder. Some questions you might ask the elder include: If you could change one thing in your life, what would it be? If you could be one age today, what age would that be and why? If you could get anything you wanted, what would it be? Discuss your interview with your classmates. In your discussion, include how your interviewee is similar/different from you. Also, explain the best and worst part of the experience.

References

Angell, M. (2004, July 15). The truth about the drug companies. *New York Review of Books, 51*(12).

Bartlett, D. L., & Steele, J. B. (2004). *Critical condition: How health care in America became big business and bad medicine.* New York: Doubleday.

Chambliss, D. F. (1966). *Beyond caring: Hospitals, nurses, and the social organization of ethics.* Chicago: University of Chicago Press.

Dickinson, G. E. (2002). A quarter-century of end of life issues in U.S. medical schools. *Death Studies,* 26(8), 635–646.

Earl, W. L., Martindale, C. J., & Cohen, D. (1992). Adjustment: Denial in the styles of coping with HIV infection. *Omega: Journal of Death and Dying, 24,* 35–47.

Foley, K., & Hendin, H. (1999). The Oregon report: Don't ask, don't tell. *Hastings Center, 29,* 37–42.

Hays, J. C., Gold, D. T., Flint, E. P., & Winer, E. P. (1999). Patient preference for place of death. In B. de Vries (Ed.), *End of life issues.* New York: Springer.

Koenig, B. A. (1988). The technological imperative in medical practice. In M. Lock & D. Gordon (Eds.), *Biomedicine examined* (pp. 465–497). Boston: Kluwer.

Kutner, J. S., Nowels, D. E., Kassner, C. T., Houser, J., Bryant, J. J., & Main, D. S. (2003). Confirmation of the "disability paradox" among hospice patients: Preservation of quality of life despite physical ailments and psychosocial concerns. *Palliative and Supportive Care, 1*(3), 231–237.

Marks, S. C., & Bertman, S. L. (1980). Experiences with learning about death and dying in the undergraduate anatomy curriculum. *Journal of Medical Education, 55*(1), 48–52.

Mermann, A. C., Gunn, D. B., & Dickinson, G. E. (1991). Learning to care for the dying: A survey of medical schools and a model course. *Academic Medicine,* 66(1), 35–38.

Moller, D. W. (1996). *Confronting death: Values, institutions, and human mortality.* New York: Oxford University Press.

National Hospice and Palliative Care Organization. (2007). *NHPCO facts and figures: Hospice care in America*. Retrieved April, 2008 from www.nhpco.org/research

Parsons, T. (1958). The definitions of health and illness in light of American values and social structure. In E. E. Jaco (Ed.), *Patients, physicians, and illness* (pp. 165–187). New York: Free Press.

U.S. Department of Health and Human Services. (2001). *Appropriateness of minimum nurse staffing ratios in nursing homes.* Report to Congress. Washington, DC: Health Care Financing Administration.

van Eys, J. (1988). In my opinion . . . normalization while dying. *Children's Health Care, 17*(1), 18–21.

Weber, M. (1958). Bureaucracy. In H. Gerth & C. C. Mills. (Trans.), *Max Weber* (pp. 196–244). New York: Free Press.

Chapter 5

Bioethics, Euthanasia, and Physician-Assisted Suicide

We all labor against our own cure;
for death is the cure of all diseases.
—Sir Thomas Browne

Objectives

After reading this chapter, you will be able to answer the following questions:

- How do ethics and morality differ?
- What is bioethics, and what is the role of a bioethicist?
- How do active and passive euthanasia differ?
- What are the religious, legal, and social views toward euthanasia?
- What is physician-assisted suicide?
- What is the current legal environment regarding physician-assisted suicide?
- How do issues of gender bias, pain relief, and the voluntary nature of physician-assisted suicide factor into arguments for and against the practice?

Controversy continues to swirl around the issues of legalized euthanasia and physician-assisted suicide (PAS). The controversy rests on differing views of the ethics and practical morality of such legislation, what effect it would have on the practice of euthanasia and PAS, who typically asks for it, and on whether improving pain management and palliative care would be a better first step.

What Is Medically Ethical Behavior?

Ethical behavior is defined by moral principles or values based on concepts of whether something is good or bad. **Moral behavior** is based on socially accepted codes or notions of right and wrong. Thus, ethics and morality are similar but not identical.

Ethical decision making must balance the rights of an individual to decide for himself or herself, the views of society as a whole, and the desires and wishes of a family and others close to the individual. **Justice** involves making decisions to balance contending interests so that everyone is treated fairly.

These definitions are, perhaps unfortunately, hypothetical. They address the question, "What should be done?" In reality, and in the bureaucratic setting of a hospital or other healthcare institution, the question more often is "What can be done?" and the answer is "Do everything possible, even if it is not always appropriate." In times past, when not much could be done to prolong death, sympathy and efforts to manage pain were the norm. Now, with the enormous advances in techniques, equipment, and drugs, the imperative to treat and cure at all costs sometimes overwhelms compassion.

Bioethics

The growing difficulty and complexity (as well as the dangers) of medical decision making have created the role of the **bioethicist**. A bioethicist is a hospital staff person who is educated in philosophy, psychology, religion, law, humanities, and the social sciences (Guyer, 1998). This person's role is to help the medical professionals, the family, and the patient make difficult medical decisions, especially for those patients at the end of their lives. The bioethicist meets with the patient, his or her family, and medical staff, collecting the facts and surveying the various views involved before offering a recommendation regarding next steps for the patient. If one or more parties balk at the bioethicist's decision, meetings are held so that all parties can talk over things. If these meetings fail to produce an agreed-upon path of action, the hospital's ethics committee reviews the case and makes a ruling.

In principle, the bioethicist represents the interests of the patient above all others. But the inevitable influence of the institutional setting and interaction with hospital medical professionals can erode the best of good intentions, and the bioethicist often comes to ally with the professionals and their views on patient care (DeVries & Subedi, 1998)—or even subvert his of her role by selling cover-ups for cost-cutting measures to managed-care insurance companies (Shalit, 1997).

The Doctor's Oath of Practice

All cultures have had guidelines in the form of codes, prayers, creeds, or oaths to guide their healers. One of the earliest oaths comes from the *Chareka Samhita* of ancient India. This oath calls for the medical student to "follow a path of personal sacrifice and commitment to duty." In China, ethical codes of conduct for physicians appear from the Taoist writer, Sun Szu-Miao. His writings stress the importance of "preserving life and serving the interest of the patient." A widely known Judaic text is the Daily Prayer of a Physician, attributed to Moses Maimonides, a twelfth-century Jewish physician in Egypt, but probably written by Marcus Herz, a German physician. This text first appeared in print in 1793 (see box).

Codes from other cultures are similar to the Hippocratic oath. Hippocrates, a Greek physician who lived from 466 BC to 377 BC, is known as the father of medicine. Even though not specifically spelled out in the oath, the implied message

DAILY PRAYER OF A PHYSICIAN

Almighty God, grant that my patients have confidence in me and my art and follow my directions and my counsel. Remove from their midst all charlatans and the whole host of officious relatives and know-all nurses, cruel people who arrogantly frustrate the wisest purposes of our art and often lead Thy creatures to their death. Should those who are wiser than I wish to improve and instruct me, let my soul gratefully follow their guidance. Should conceited fools, however, censure me, then let love for my profession steel me against them. Imbue my soul with gentleness and calmness when older colleagues, proud of their age, wish to displace me or to scorn me or disdainfully to teach me. Let me be contented in everything except in the great science of my profession. Never allow the thought to arise in me that I have attained to sufficient knowledge, but vouchsafe to me the strength, the leisure and the ambition ever to extend my knowledge. (Excerpts, translated by H. Friedenwald, 1917.)

Hippocratic Oath (modern version)*

I will apply, for the benefit of the sick, all measures required.

I will remember that there is art to medicine as well as science, and that warmth, sympathy, and understanding may outweigh the surgeon's knife or the chemist's drug.

I will respect the privacy of my patients, for their problems are not disclosed to me that the world may know.

Most especially must I tread with care in matters of life and death.

I will remember that I treat a sick human being, whose illness may affect the person's family and economic stability.

I will prevent disease whenever I can, for prevention is preferable to cure.

*Written in 1964 by Louis Lasagna, Academic Dean of the School of Medicine at Tufts University, and used in many medical schools today.

for doctors is "Above all, do no harm." Members of the American Medical Association (AMA) are bound by the Hippocratic oath in its modern version (Lasagna, 1964), in which the ideal ethical behaviors for medical doctors are explained (see box).

Many physicians today believe that the Hippocratic oath is outdated, because some of today's issues were unheard of at the time the oath was created. For example, years ago, no one had heard of legalized abortion or test-tube babies.

Physicians' Perspectives on Life and Death

Caring for dying patients is part of every doctor's training and experience. Yet physicians' perspectives regarding death differ. For example, most doctors admit that patient deaths disturb them very little. Others, although not as many, say that their patients' deaths, even those they knew only for a short time, are very disturbing. The most commonly reported grief symptom is "feeling upset when thinking about the patient" (Redinbaugh et al., 2003).

Medical Ethics and Capital Punishment

In 1976, the U.S. Supreme Court legalized capital punishment. Because the Eighth Amendment to the Constitution forbids cruel and unusual punishment, the method of using lethal injections was introduced. To make sure the lethal injections were administered properly, courts required medical personnel to attend executions (Gawande, 2007). The American Medical Association balked at this

A Physician's First Encounter with Death

As a new doctor assigned to the first of his clinical rotations on the Internal Medicine service, Dr. Sherwin Nuland helped an intern by agreeing to complete the admission workup on a new coronary patient who had just arrived. Before Nuland got far into the routine admissions work, the patient died of a massive, and inevitable, heart attack. Alone in that room with the corpse, Nuland tried everything to save the dead man. Then the door to the room swung open and Nuland's friend rushed in to see Nuland crying, out of control and begging the patient to live. His friend said, "It's okay, buddy—it's okay. You did everything you could. . . . Shep, now you know what it's like to be a doctor." (Nuland, 1995, p. 8.)

practice, resolving that "A physician . . . should not be a participant in a legally authorized execution" (Article 2.06 of the *AMA Code of Medical Ethics*).

One doctor, a prison physician, has a different view about attending executions. He feels obliged to attend inmates when they are about to die. He views executions as an end-of-life issue, a time when a doctor should make sure the person about to die is comfortable and does not have pain or suffering. Anti–capital-punishment activists have challenged his medical license and AMA membership, but he believes that it is wrong to stop attending executions. He and his medical team are paid quite well for their services; he donates his share of it to a children's shelter (Gawande, 2007).

Euthanasia

The ability to keep a dying person alive has raised difficult questions for the terminal patient and his or her physician, as well as policymakers and the general public. Should a patient be allowed to die? Should the medical profession help a patient die? (Weir, 1997).

In **euthanasia**, the physician takes some sort of action to end a patient's life. When the physician takes direct action to do so, it is sometimes called **active euthanasia**, to distinguish it from **passive euthanasia**, which is simply withholding or withdrawing the treatment needed to sustain life and allowing the patient to die. **Physician-assisted suicide** involves the physician supplying the means, usually medication, to a patient who then decides and takes the necessary action to end his or her life.

When it comes to distinguishing between active and passive euthanasia, proponents of active euthanasia argue that there are no important moral distinctions between the two practices, so both should be allowed. Opponents of active euthanasia, but who support the passive form, argue that, when life support is withdrawn, the cause of death is the underlying disease—not action by the physician.

If it were legal, more than a one-third of U.S. physicians would be willing to offer active euthanasia with medication, and one-fourth would be willing to give a lethal injection (Meier et al., 1998). An increasing number of people in the United States support the painless euthanasia of incurably ill patients—if they and their families request it (Blendon, Szalay, & Knox, 1992; Caddell & Newton, 1995; Rogers, 1996). This increased acceptance is paralleled in other countries (Genuis, Genuis, & Chang, 1994; Singer, Choudhry, Armstrong, Meslin, & Lowy, 1995; Steinberg, Najman, Cartwright, MacDonald, & Williams, 1997; Suarez-Almazor, Belzile, & Bruera, 1997; Van der Maas, Pijnenborg, & van Delden, 1995).

Knowing what makes euthanasia acceptable likely would help guide those professionals—physicians, psychologists, lawyers, and medical ethicists—who help patients and their families make end-of-life decisions, as well as those who make healthcare policy. They then would know what issues to discuss with patients and families, and policymakers likely would know how to shape guidelines, rules, and laws (Cuperus-Bosma, van der Wal, Looman, & van der Maas, 1999).

But what, specifically, might make euthanasia acceptable? Acceptability, according to Frileux, Lelievre, Munoz, Mullet, and Sorum (2003), depends mainly upon:

- the level of patient suffering in spite of treatment;
- the extent to which the patient requested the life-ending procedure;
- the age of the patient; and
- the curability of the illness.

Karen Ann Quinlan and Terri Schiavo

Ethical questions about the "right to die" have become prominent since the landmark case involving Karen Ann Quinlan in 1975. Because Quinlan was in a *persistent vegetative state* (PVS), a coma state of wakefulness without detectable awareness, her parents asked for her respirator to be removed. After much controversy, the New Jersey Supreme Court ruled that her respirator could be discontinued. Quinlan died in 1985.

A more recent case is the one involving Terri Schiavo. In 1990, Schiavo, then age 26, collapsed at her home in St. Petersburg, Florida, and never recovered. She entered a coma and was kept alive by the tools of modern medicine. She had experienced respiratory and cardiac arrest and remained in a coma for 10 weeks. She did not have a living will. After 3 years, she was diagnosed as being in a PVS. This condition of wakefulness persuaded her parents, Robert and Mary Schindler, that she could recover.

In 1998, her husband, who was also her legal guardian, petitioned the state courts to remove her feeding tube, but her parents objected. The case generated intense media attention, involvement by politicians and interest groups, a series of state and federal court actions, and eventually attempted intervention by the U.S. Congress.

Despite these efforts, the state courts steadfastly held that she was in a PVS and ordered that she should cease to receive life support. Her gastric feeding tube was removed (for the third time), and she died 13 days later of dehydration, on March 31, 2005, at the age of 41, in a Pinellas Park hospice facility.

The Schiavo case resulted in 14 appeals and numerous motions, petitions, and hearings in the Florida courts, all of which were denied, and five suits in Federal District Court, all of which also were denied. Also noteworthy is that a subpoena by a congressional committee was filed in an attempt to qualify Schiavo for witness protection, as was federal legislation (the Palm Sunday Compromise) and four denials of the Supreme Court of the United States to review the appeals courts' decisions.

The Palm Sunday Compromise, formally known as the Act for the Relief of the Parents of Theresa Marie Schiavo, was an act of Congress to allow the case to be moved to a federal court. The name "Palm Sunday Compromise" was invented by House Majority Leader Tom DeLay, highlighting the mixture of religion and politics that overshadowed the Schiavo case.

Religious Perspectives on Euthanasia

In this age of life-prolonging medicine, the deliberate decision to end a life generates a significant amount of religious discussion (O'Connell, 1995). Ethical concerns from a religious perspective likely will become even more central when or if euthanasia enters the mainstream of medical practice, and society struggles to achieve consensus on this issue.

The futility of medical treatment to sustain life has collided with religious ethics. In the case of Baby K, an anencephalic infant, physicians concluded that Baby K's life could not be sustained and that continued treatment would be futile. The infant's mother insisted that Baby K should be kept alive because God might choose to perform a miracle (Post, 1995).

In the mother's defense, Post (1995) insisted that religious beliefs should be taken seriously by medical personnel and included in medical or social policies concerning futile treatment. Others argued, however, that physicians should not be compelled to violate their own moral convictions and professional standards to accommodate the religious beliefs of others (Paris & Reardon, 1992). Refusal to continue futile treatment "is not abandonment of the patient; it is an assertion of professional responsibility" (Paris & Reardon, 1992, p. 133). Before refusing to provide treatment, the physician should explain why the proposed treatment is futile, and, if possible, arrange a conference with the hospital ethics committee or the pastoral care department. Often a consensus does emerge, thereby averting a break in the physician–patient relationship.

Is Legal Availability of Euthanasia Justified?

People, in general, are becoming more receptive to euthanasia. Advances in medical technology often cause people to worry about lingering, nasty deaths while hooked to machines, unable to communicate, the modern equivalent of the seventeenth- and eighteenth-century fear of being buried alive (Daniel, 1997). But what are the arguments and justifications, pro and con, for euthanasia?

Proponents of legalized euthanasia argue that the right to self-determination encompasses the right to choose how and when to die. They believe that keeping a person alive who wishes to die is not only an infringement of that person's rights, but an irresponsible use of resources (McLean & Britton, 1996). Treatment costs are high, for example, for AIDS and cancer, but very low for lethal injection. These proponents also argue that because euthanasia is already taking place, it should be made legal so that it can be regulated. For instance, a doctor can administer drugs to relieve pain knowing that he or she might kill the patient (known as **double effect**). As long as the doctor's intention is to relieve pain, this practice should be acceptable, and the death that ensues should be ruled accidental.

Many opponents to legalize euthanasia, however, worry about an inevitable "slippery slope," as demonstrated by the case of a healthy 50-year-old woman who, distressed after her two sons died, was helped to die by her doctor. The doctor was censured but not convicted of wrongdoing, thus establishing mental suffering as a valid reason for euthanasia (Keown, 1995). The decision to help a person end his or her life might be difficult at first, but the more it is done the easier it might become. In other words, the line between what is and is not acceptable might become blurred (Daniel, 1997).

Many argue that *palliative care*—pain management, symptom control, and psychological and spiritual support—is the acceptable alternative to euthanasia (George, 1997). Most doctors, however, are in need of training in both palliative care and medical ethics (Keown, 1995). Also, a shortage of available beds and funds makes extensive use of palliative care difficult. Perhaps, rather than campaigning for legal euthanasia, doctors and families of the terminally ill should be demanding adequate palliative care (Nathanson, as cited in Daniel, 1997).

How Patients View Euthanasia

What might lie behind a patient's requests for euthanasia? Mak, Elwyn, and Finlay (2003) revealed that concerns are not always confined to physical and functional decline. They also stated that many patients experience hidden psychosocial and existential issues embedded in life experience, fears about the future, and yearnings for care and social connection. Many patients express fears of pain or a painful death, lack of quality of life, and lack of hope (Johansen, Hølen, Kaasa, Loge, & Materstvedt, 2005). Furthermore, they might fear physical disintegration and loss of function and loss of personal relationships, which leads to a perceived loss of self and wholeness (Lavery, Boyle, Dickens, Maclean, & Singer, 2001) that gradually diminishes until they often-

MY STORY: "STOP! LET HER DIE"

I always have believed that doctors should do everything in their power to keep everybody alive. That was especially true for my grandmother. That was very clear for me.

Suddenly, my grandmother had a stroke. We were told that her stroke was too severe and that she probably would soon die. While she was in the hospital, only one family member at a time could visit her—and then for only five minutes. I thought my turn would never arrive to get one last visit. But it did.

I walked back to the intensive care ward to find two nurses working to get my grandmother to breathe. Apparently, she had just quit breathing. When I saw them working so hard, I thought, "How cruel!" Just as I thought it, I also was shocked at my reaction. What had changed the way I previously had believed?

Then, I knew. I changed my beliefs when reality for me changed. I think I understood that a dignified death isn't about force; it's about letting death take its course. I feel like I grew up a lot that day.

times see a future worse than death itself (Mak et al., 2003).

The prospect of good quality end-of-life care and social connectedness might help patients see their reality differently and lead them to reevaluate the desire for death (Mak et al., 2003). This reevaluation suggests that improvements in palliative care should precede consideration of legalized euthanasia.

Beyond assessing mental competence or determining legal guidelines, physicians and other healthcare professionals must acquire the skills for providing good end-of-life care, which includes the ability to connect with patients, to diagnose suffering, and to understand patients' hidden agendas through in-depth exploration. These skills are especially important for encouraging patients' feelings of hope and personal worth. Thus, to give physicians better communication skills and attitudes, medical education should include medical humanities, experiential learning, and reflective practice (Bolton, 2001; Vass, 2002).

Physician-Assisted Suicide

Most people judge euthanasia to be less acceptable than physician-assisted suicide (PAS), the process in which the physician simply gives the patient the means to end his or her life. With PAS, the patient takes the action and can until the last minute decide not to go ahead with the act (Rogers, 1996).

In the past, most people died relatively quickly as a result of accident or illness. Today, despite advances in palliative care, death is too often protracted, painful, and undignified. In the United States, 80% to 85% of people die in institutions, 70% of those after a decision to withdraw or withhold treatment, and the great majority are elderly (Fraser & Walters, 2000).

Results from public opinion polls consistently support PAS. In one poll, even 50% of Catholic voters answered "yes" to the question, "Shall the law allow terminally ill adult patients obtain a physician's prescription for drugs to end life?" (Dietz, 1997). Some recent report results suggest that attitudes toward PAS become more positive with age (Littlejohn & Burrows-Johnson, 1996; Sedlitz, Duberstein, Cox, & Conwell, 1995).

In 2005, a majority (70%) of 1,010 Americans polled favored allowing some form of PAS. This percentage is up from previous years, but less than the peak of 73% approving in 1993 (Taylor, 2005).

PAS is controversial. This controversy, however, is not new. Beginning in 1870 and continuing until the 1930s, there was widespread public debate in the United States over legalization of PAS. World War II and the reactions to the Nazi death camps suspended further discussion until 1971, when, in the Netherlands, a doctor who admitted administering a lethal dose of morphine was given a one-year suspended sentence. The leniency of the sentence prompted a public debate, and in 1984, the Royal Dutch Medical Association offered guidelines to help the courts

Dr. Death

The most publicized advocate of PAS has been Dr. Jack Kevorkian ("Dr. Death"), a retired Michigan pathologist. Despite arrests, imprisonment, and loss of his medical license, he helped 130 people commit suicide.

Before finally being convicted of second-degree murder in 1999, he was tried four times, resulting in three acquittals and one mistrial. Kevorkian's conviction came after he was shown in a videotape on the TV program *60 Minutes,* helping 52-year-old Thomas York, who had Lou Gehrig's disease, commit suicide. The judge sentenced Dr. Kevorkian to 10 to 25 years in prison. He was released in 2007, after serving 8 years.

decide at what point euthanasia was a crime. In 1990, the Ministry of Justice accepted these criteria, and in 1993, the Dutch parliament voted in favor of this reporting system (Daniel, 1997). PAS has strong public support in the Netherlands, where it is monitored by the government. In 2001, about 0.2% of all deaths in the Netherlands were the result of PAS (van der Heide et al., 2007). Because people are living longer, the practice of PAS is likely to increase.

One state, Oregon, as the result of a citizen initiative ballot (Measure 16), passed the Death with Dignity Act, permitting PAS death under very restricted conditions. It is the only U.S. state that allows PAS. In Oregon, a physician must sign an Attending Physician's Compliance Form (Oregon State Public Health Division, Center for Health Science, 2006), which is sent to the Oregon Public Health Department to ensure that the physician has complied with the law. On this form, the physician must attest to the following:

- The patient has requested three times the physician's assistance in committing suicide, the last in writing, with the statement dated and signed by the patient in the presence of two witnesses.
- The physician must wait at least 15 days after the initial oral request to the second oral request and at least 2 days after the final written request before writing the prescription for the lethal drug. The patient's written request for medication to end his or her life is attached to the compliance form.
- Two physicians have determined that the patient has a life expectancy of 6 months or less.
- The patient is not suffering from a psychiatric or psychological disorder or depression causing impaired judgment.
- At least one of the two witnesses to the patient's written request for the lethal prescription is a person who is not a relative of the patient, does not stand to benefit from the estate of the patient, and is not an employee of the institution where the patient is being treated.

The physician also must indicate on the form that the patient was fully informed about:

- his or her medical diagnosis;
- his or her prognosis;
- the potential risks associated with taking the medication;
- the probable result of taking the medication; and
- the feasible alternatives, including but not limited to comfort care, hospice care, and pain control.

The patient has the right to rescind the request for medication to end his or her life at any time.

In 2003, 38 people (one-tenth of 1% of all Oregon deaths) committed PAS. Twenty-one PAS deaths occurred in 2001, and fewer than half that in 1998 (Lee, 2003). Most of those selecting PAS people had cancer and were well-educated white males. The top three reasons they cited for wanting to end their lives were:

- loss of the ability to make their own decisions (84%);
- decreasing ability to participate in activities they enjoyed (84%); and
- loss of control of their bodily functions (47%) (Lee, 2003).

Physician-Assisted Suicide and the Law

In the United States, the "liberty interest"—an individual's right of choice—is guaranteed by the

Questions & Answers

Question: Are any other states besides Oregon trying to legalize PAS?

Answer: In 2004, Arizona, Hawaii, and Vermont introduced state bills to allow PAS. At the same time, John Ashcroft, then United States Attorney General, issued a directive making it illegal for doctors to prescribe controlled narcotics to help terminally ill patients die. In 2006, the Supreme Court ruled (6–3 in *Gonzales vs. Oregon*) that Ashcroft had overstepped his authority.

Fourteenth Amendment. Thus, the issue of PAS is as much about control as about dying, and patients, and possibly family, should have the right to participate in all end-of-life decisions. However, 34 states have statutes explicitly making it illegal for anyone to assist in a suicide.

Shortly after passage of Oregon's Death with Dignity Act, opponents of the law persuaded the lower house of the Oregon legislature to return Measure 16 to the voters for repeal.

Some months earlier, the ninth circuit federal appeals court upheld Measure 16 but allowed a stay until the Supreme Court ruled that Americans did not have a constitutional "right to die." The Supreme Court, however, did not preclude states from passing laws establishing such a right (Savage, 1997).

In their decision to uphold Measure 16, the ninth circuit judges said that the "liberty interest" should allow competent, terminally ill patients the right to choose the time and manner of their death. They considered that adequately rigorous safeguards could be implemented in the decision process to prevent abuse: "We believe that the possibility of abuse . . . does not outweigh the liberty interest at issue" (*Compassion in Dying v. State of Wash,* 79 F. 3d 790, p. 837).

Addressing the issue of physician-assisted suicide, the judges stated:

> We see no ethical or constitutionally recognizable difference between a doctor's pulling the plug on a respirator and his prescribing drugs which will permit a terminally ill patient to end his own life. . . . To the extent that a difference exists, we conclude that it is one of degree and not one of kind. (*Compassion in Dying v. State of Wash,* 79 F. 3d 790, p. 824)

The judges also observed that "today, doctors are generally permitted to administer death-inducing medication, as long as they can point to a concomitant pain-relieving purpose" (p. 822). Physicians are aware of this *double effect,* a term that "originates in Roman Catholic moral theology, which holds that it is sometimes morally justifiable to cause evil in the pursuit of good" (May, 1978, p. 316).

Specifically, in medical usage, *double effect* can be described as follows: The intent of palliative treatment of the terminally ill is to relieve pain and suffering, but the patient's death is a possible side effect of the treatment. It is, therefore, ethically acceptable for a physician to increase pain-relieving medication gradually, being aware that the medication may depress respiration and cause death.

In November 1997, 60% of Oregon voters rejected the repeal of Measure 16. The appeals court then lifted the stay. Both proponents and opponents of Measure 16 predict the adoption of similar measures in other states (Murphy, 1997).

In Australia, The Rights of the Terminally Ill Act went into effect July 1, 1996, in the Northern Territory, but the legislation was short-lived. In March 1997, the federal parliament effectively repealed it by passing the Euthanasia Laws Bill (Gordon, 1997). Draft legislation in the state of South Australia, however, if passed, will challenge it. Both the Oregon and Northern Territory laws had exhaustive provisions designed to safeguard the integrity of the legislation and to prevent abuse (Oregon Revised Statute 127; Cordner, 1995).

Has all the legal maneuvering about PAS resulted in justice? To most people, medical justice means the fair and equal treatment of patients. But the current situation seems unjust. For instance, terminally ill patients often are too debilitated to take active steps to end their suffering should they choose to do so.

Because it is illegal in most states for a person to assist a suicide, many terminal patients are denied choices available to the more privileged in society, because they are much more likely to have a relationship of trust with a medical practitioner who will discreetly help to alleviate their suffering. When commenting on the demise of his legislation, the former Northern Territory chief minister observed that the senators who voted for repeal belonged to a privileged, wealthy group who, themselves, have access to voluntary euthanasia (Ceresa, 1997).

Religion is another factor inhibiting beliefs about the suitability of PAS. In Michigan, approximately 30% of physicians who opposed assisted suicide did so primarily because of religious conviction (Bachman, 1996). The principal opponents of both the Oregon and Northern Territory legislations held strong religious views. Results from a number of other studies suggest that among the general population, fervent religious belief is an important predictor of opposition to PAS (Bachman, 1996; Suarez-Almazor, Belzile, & Bruera, 1997; Ward, 1980). As the ninth circuit judges stated:

> Those who believe strongly that death must come without physician assistance are free to follow that creed, be they doctors or patients. They are not free, however, to force their views, their religious convictions, or their philosophies on all other members of a democratic society, and to compel those whose values differ from theirs to die painful, protracted, and agonizing deaths. (*Compassion in Dying v. State of Wash,* 79 F. 3d 790, p. 839)

If both patients and physicians were free to choose, patients could select a physician holding views on PAS or euthanasia similar to their own.

Another important matter is the impact of terminal illness on patients' families. Currently, it is illegal to assist a person in committing suicide in two-thirds of the United States. Consequently, people who are in unbearable pain often die alone (if they commit suicide), because they do not want to put loved ones at legal risk. When considering the possibility of this kind of risk, the ninth circuit judges observed that almost all who had agreed to assist the dying avoided prosecution, but would "likely suffer pain and guilt for the rest of their lives. This burden would be substantially alleviated if doctors were authorized to assist terminally ill persons to end their lives and to supervise and direct others in the implementation of that process" (p. 836). According to Fraser and Walters (2000), it seems that a democratic society that observes justice and liberty should permit differing opinions and allow terminally ill people some freedom to decide for themselves when and how they die.

Gender Bias and Physician-Assisted Suicide

Proponents of PAS often offer a story or case study to convince the reader or listener. One such story (Vorenberg and Wanzer, 1997) is the case of "Uncle Louis," who is in constant pain because there is supposedly no good pain management for his type of cancer. After many therapies and surgery, he is definitely terminal. He has discussed PAS with his physician, and he now wants it. Proponents then ask if Uncle Louis should be left to suffer.

The implication is that Uncle Louis has a right to die. But, as Keenan (1998) asks, how common is the case of Uncle Louis? Is he really representative of the people asking for PAS? In most cases, the person asking for PAS is usually a woman, not a man (Vorenberg & Wanzer, 1997). What might the reasons be? Many more elderly poor are women, and women are twice as likely to suffer from depression as men. Age, poverty, and depression are among the leading reasons why people ask for PAS. The female patient also is more likely to be worried about her condition's impact on others. And a certain type of woman—depressive, self-effacing, and near the end of a life largely spent serving others—might be particularly vulnerable to the offer of PAS.

The case of Uncle Louis is about one man who has tried every possible option, consulted physician and family, and apparently faces unmanageable pain. He has considered his decision, but he is unable to carry it out because laws prohibit it. According to Keenan (1998), the more likely case is that of a woman who, if she fears pain, fears it because her healthcare providers do not properly manage it. She chooses PAS because she does not want to burden her family.

Gender inequality involving the wishes of the dying is found in the courts as well. After hearing families testify about an incompetent patient's wishes to be removed from life support, judges rule in favor of a male patient in 75% of cases, but only 15% for females. In their opinions, it appears that most judges treat men's decisions as rational but women's as emotional and immature (Miles & August, 1990).

For Keenan (1998), the irony of a case like Uncle Louis's is that it is an attempt to persuade people to change the law for a rather small number of empowered persons. The cost of this persuasion is doing away with those persons who already find themselves isolated from society, family, and the healthcare industry.

Pain and PAS

A second questionable aspect of the Uncle Louis case is the absence of pain relief medication (Keenan, 1998). In 1994, the New York State Task Force on Life and the Law reported, "Taken together, modern pain relief techniques can alleviate pain in all but extremely rare cases. Effective techniques have been developed to treat pain for patients in diverse conditions" (Martyn & Bourguignon, 1997). Yet, all too often, pain relief is not provided.

Actually, pain relief is a minor factor in the motivation of people who seek PAS, according to the medical ethicist Ezekiel Emanuel (1997). According to Emanuel, "No study has ever shown that pain plays a major role in motivating patient requests for physician-assisted suicide or euthanasia" (p. 75). Distress and dependency are the primary concerns of PAS candidates.

How Voluntary Is PAS?

How likely is it that most PAS candidates would enjoy the choice that Uncle Louis has? Of 3600 Dutch deaths reported as PAS in 1994, about 1000 were cases wherein the physician took the patient's life without an explicit request from the family or the patient (Keenan, 1998). Dutch statistics on PAS, however, leveled off and then declined in the period from 1995 to 2001 (Onwuteaka-Philipsen et al., 2007).

Even more unsettling about the possibility of involuntary PAS is that the Royal Dutch Medical Society and the Dutch courts have extended mercy killing to infants and to psychiatric patients. Regarding these developments, two Dutch lawyers commented that the increase in involuntary euthanasia and mercy killing in the Netherlands has gone unchecked, despite legal conditions that were designed to guarantee volunteerism (Keown, 1995). In response to these concerns, in the Netherlands euthanasia requests are assessed by the public prosecutor only after being advised by a multidisciplinary committee of medical, ethics, and legal specialists. Dutch statistics on PAS, however, leveled off and then declined in the period 1995–2001, accompanied by an increase in effective pain management (Onwuteaka-Philipsen et al., 2007).

Could a similar creep toward involuntary PAS happen in the United States? The Dutch are a more homogenous society, with universal health care. U.S. society is fragmented and economically stratified, with a patchwork healthcare system. The likelihood of creep toward involuntary PAS, therefore, might be greater in the United States (Kaveny, 1997).

Hard Cases and Representative Cases

Real cases like Uncle Louis's exist (Keenan, 1998). Ethicists call them "hard cases," meaning they raise the question of whether a particular law should be absolute. For instance, an abused wife who kills her husband might be morally excused or even morally right, and therefore, a judge and jury might be persuaded to "let her off." Legalizing her action, though, might make it an acceptable alternative and jeopardize other, more civil, methods for resolving domestic conflict. A hard case like the abused wife as an exception to the law does not justify creating a new law—nor should it be used to nullify an existing law.

Thus, in debating PAS legislation, it seems more important to ask whether cases cited in defense or rebuke are representative cases or hard cases. Does Uncle Louis represent a large group for whom the law should be changed? If he is not representative, then it is exactly like the case of the abused wife. Hard cases depend not on legislators making new laws, but on judges and juries interpreting existing laws and precedents for a particular case.

If the one case of Uncle Louis is not representative, what might be a representative case (Keenan, 1998)? More likely, it might be an isolated and depressed woman who does not want to be a burden, who has, at best, uncertain access to adequate health care, and whose own wishes are rarely solicited or heeded. When this case is taken into account, it seems that the critical issue facing Americans in caring for the dying is not lack of autonomy, but the inability to care properly for the dying. In short, the typical case is a reminder of a society's failure to the aging, to women, and to the poor.

What, then, would be the social effect of a law that permits PAS? Proponents for the case of Uncle Louis are only interested in the autonomous person. But opponents of legalization try to persuade others that the law that the friends of "Uncle Louis" want invalidated is the same law that keeps the person of more common instance from being marginalized to death.

SUMMARY

- Ethical behavior is defined by moral principles or values based on concepts of good or bad.
- The growing difficulty and complexity (as well as the dangers) of medical decision-making have created the role of the *bioethicist,* whose job it is to help medical professionals and families make difficult medical decisions, especially for people at the end of life.
- All cultures have guidelines—codes, prayers, creeds, or oaths—to guide their healers. Members of the AMA are bound by the Hippocratic Oath. Even though not specifically spelled out in the oath, the implied message for doctors is "do no harm."
- In euthanasia, the physician takes an action to end the patient's life. When the physician takes direct action to do so, it is called *active euthanasia,* distinguishing it from *passive euthanasia*, which is simply withholding or withdrawing the treatment needed to sustain life and allowing the patient to die. *Physician-assisted suicide* (PAS) involves the physician supplying the means, usually medication, to a patient who then decides and takes the necessary action.
- If it were legal, more than one-third of U.S. physicians would be willing to offer active euthanasia with medication. One-quarter would be willing to give a lethal injection. An increasing number of people in the United States support painless euthanasia of incurably ill patients—if they and their families request it.
- Proponents of legalized euthanasia argue that rights to self-determination include the right to choose how and when to die.
- Opponents of legalized euthanasia worry about a "slippery slope" wherein ending a life might be a difficult decision at first, but then become easier the more it is done.
- Most people are more supportive of physician-assisted suicide. In 2005, a majority (70%) of 1,010 Americans polled favored allowing some form of PAS.
- In the United States, 34 states have statutes explicitly making it illegal for anyone to assist in a suicide.
- Currently, Oregon is the only state that allows PAS. In 2003, 38 people (one-tenth of 1% of all Oregon deaths) were attributed to PAS.
- In Australia, the Rights of the Terminally Ill Act went into effect July 1, 1996, in the Northern Territory, but in March 1997 the federal parliament effectively repealed it by passing the Euthanasia Laws Bill.
- Women ask for PAS more often than men.
- When debating PAS legislation, it is important to ask whether cases cited in defense or rebuke are representative cases or hard cases.

ADDITIONAL RESOURCES

Books

Shavelson, L. (1995). *A chosen death: The dying confront assisted suicide.* New York: Simon & Schuster. An argument for assisted suicide, this book is a portrait of five dying people who chose euthanasia.

Smith, W. J. (1997). *Forced exit: The slippery slope from assisted suicide to legalized murder*. New York: Crown. A well-written argument against physician-assisted suicide is presented in this book.

Woodman, S. (1998). *Last rights: The struggle over the right to die.* New York: Plenum Press. An examination of the right-to-die movement and the medical, ethical, legal, and social issues surrounding euthanasia are addressed in this book.

Movie

Million Dollar Baby. (2005). Story of a fighter who fought both to live and die—her way.

Critical Thinking

1. Was the removal of Terri Schiavo's feeding tube active or passive euthanasia? Explain.
2. If you have a terminal illness, with a paralyzed body but active mind, describe three good reasons for continuing to live.

Class Activities

1. Interview a person who deals with terminal illness on a daily basis (e.g., a physician or nurse) and report findings to the class.
2. As a class, debate whether PAS should be legalized.

References

American Medical Association (AMA), Council on Ethical and Judicial Affairs (CEJA). (2006–2007). *AMA Code of Medical Ethics*. Chicago: AMA.

Bachman, J. (1996). Attitudes of Michigan physicians and the public toward legalizing physician-assisted suicide. *New England Journal of Medicine, 334*, 303–308.

Blendon, R. J., Szalay, U. S., & Knox, R. A. (1992). Should physicians aid their patients in dying? The public perspective. *Journal of the American Medical Association, 267*, 2658–2662.

Bolton, G. (2001). *Reflective practice writing for professional development.* London: Sage.

Caddell, D. P., & Newton, R. R. (1995). Euthanasia: American attitudes toward the physician's role. *Social Science and Medicine, 40*(12), 1671–1681.

Ceresa, M. (1997, March 24). Others will follow. *The Australian*, p. 2.

Cordner, S. (1995). Reactions to Australian state's euthanasia law. *Lancet, 345*, 1561–1562.

Cuperus-Bosma, J. M., van der Wal, G., Looman, C. W. N., & van der Maas, P. J. (1999). Assessment of physician assisted death by members of the public prosecution in the Netherlands. *Journal of Medical Ethics, 25*, 8–15.

Daniel, C. (1997). Killing with kindness. *New Statesman, 126*(4347), 16–18.

DeVries, R., & Subedi, J. (1998). *Of bioethics and society: Constructing the ethical enterprise*. Upper Saddle River, NJ: Prentice Hall.

Dietz, D. (1997, March 11). Assisted-suicide debate splits Catholics. *The Statesman-Journal* (Salem, OR), p. 2A.

Emanuel, E. (1997, March). Whose right to die? *The Atlantic Monthly*, pp. 73–79.

Fraser, S. I., & Walters, J. W. (2000). Death—whose decision? Euthanasia and the terminally ill. *Journal of Medical Ethics, 26*(2), 121.

Friedenwald, H. (translator). (1917). Daily prayer of a physician. *Bulletin of the Johns Hopkins Hospital, 28*, 260–261.

Frileux, S. C., Lelievre, M. T., Munoz, S., Mullet, E., & Sorum, P. C. (2003). When is physician assisted suicide or euthanasia acceptable? *Journal of Medical Ethics, 29*(6), 330–336.

Gawande, A. (2007). *Better: A surgeon's notes on performance.* Metropolitan Books: Henry Holt and Company.

Genuis, S. J., Genuis, S. K., & Chang, W. C. (1994). Public attitudes toward the right to die. *Canadian Medical Association Journal, 150*, 701–708.

George, R. MD. (1997). Senior lecturer in palliative care at University College London. Quoted in Daniel, 1997.

Gordon, M. (1997, March 29). How euthanasia law was sunk. *The Australian*, Focus, 20.

Guyer, R. L. (1998, February 6–8). When decisions are life-and-death. *USA Weekend, 26*.

Johansen, S., Hølen, J. C., Kaasa, S., Loge, J. H., & Materstvedt, L. J. (2005). Attitudes towards, and wishes for, euthanasia in advanced cancer patients at a palliative medicine unit. *Palliative Medicine, 19*(6), 454–460.

Kaveny, M. C. (1997). Assisted suicide, euthanasia, and the law. *Theological Studies, 58*, 124–148.

Keenan, J. F. (1998, November 14). The case for physician-assisted suicide? *America,* 14.

Keown, J. (Ed.). (1995). *Euthanasia examined.* New York: Cambridge University Press.

Lasagna, L. (1964). Hippocratic Oath, modern version. Tufts University.

Lavery, J., Boyle, J., Dickens, B., Maclean, H., & Singer, P. (2001). Origins of the desire for euthanasia and assisted suicide in people with HIV-1 or AIDS: A qualitative study. *Lancet, 358*, 362–367.

Lee, D. (2003). Physician-assisted suicide: A critique of intervention. *Hastings Center Report.* Retrieved October 1, 2008, from http://findarticles.com/p/articles/mi_go2103?is_200301/ai_n7361257

Littlejohn, T., & Burrows-Johnson, J. (1996). An attitudinal survey of euthanasia in Windward Oahu. *Hawaii Medical Journal, 55*, 265–269.

Mak, Y. W., Elwyn, G., & Finlay, I. G. (2003). Patients' voices are needed in debates on euthanasia. *British Medical Journal, 327*(7408), 213–215.

Martyn, S., & Bourguignon, H. (1997). Physician-assisted suicide: The lethal flaws of the ninth and second circuit decisions. *California Law Review, 85*(2), 400.

May, W. (1978). Double effect. In W. Reich (Ed.), *Encyclopedia of bioethics* (p. 316). New York: The Free Press.

McLean, S., & Britton, A. (1996). *Sometimes a small victory.* Glasgow, Scotland: Institute of Law & Ethics in Medicine, Glasgow University.

Meier, D. E., Emmons, C. A., Wallenstein, S., Quill, T., Morrison, R. S., & Cassel, C. K. (1998). National survey of physician-assisted suicide and euthanasia in the United States. *New England Journal of Medicine, 338*, 1193–1201.

Miles, S., & August, A. (1990). Courts, gender, and the right to die. *Law, Medicine, and Health Care, 18*, 85–95.

Murphy, K. (1997, November 5). Voters in Oregon soundly endorse assisted suicide. *Los Angeles Times*, p. A1.

Nuland, S. B. (1995). *How we die.* New York: Vintage Books.

O'Connell, L. J. (1995). Religious dimensions of dying and death. *The Western Journal of Medicine, 163*(3), 231.

Onwuteaka-Philipsen, B. D., van der Heide, A., Koper, D., Keij-Deerenbergm, I., Rietjens, J. A., Rurup, M. L., et al. (2007). Euthanasia and other end-of-life decisions in the Netherlands in 1990, 1995, and 2001. *Lancet* online. Retrieved March 2007 from http://image.thelancet.com/extras/03art3297web.pdf

Oregon State Public Health Division, Center for Health Science. (2006). Attending Physician's Compliance Form (ORS 127.800-ORS 127.897). Retrieved March 2007 from http://egov.oregon.gov/DHS/ph/pas/index.shtml

Paris, J. J., & Reardon, F. E. (1992). Physician refusal of requests for futile or ineffective interventions. *Cambridge Quarterly of Healthcare Ethics, 1*, 127–134.

Post, S. G. (1995). Baby K: Medical futility and the free exercise of religion. *Journal of Law and Medical Ethics, 23*, 20–26.

Redinbaugh, E. M., Sullivan, A. M., Block, S. D., Gadmer, N. M., Lakoma, M., Mitchell, A. M., et al. (2003). Doctors' emotional reactions to recent death of a patient: Cross sectional study of hospital doctors [Electronic version]. *British Medical Journal, 327*(185). Retrieved April 21, 2008, from http://www.bmj.com/cgi/content/full/327/7408/185

Rogers, J. R. (1996). Assessing right to die attitudes: A conceptually guided measurement model. *Journal of Social Issues, 52*, 63–84.

Savage, D. (1997, June 27). High Court refuses to grant constitutional "right to die." *Los Angeles Times*, p. A1.

Sedlitz, L., Duberstein, R., Cox, C., & Conwell, Y. (1995). Attitudes of older people towards suicide and assisted suicide: Analysis of Gallup poll findings. *Journal of the American Geriatrics Society, 43*, 993–998.

Shalit, R. (1997). When we were philosopher kings. *The New Republic, 216*(17), 24–28.

Singer, P. A., Choudhry, S., Armstrong, J., Meslin, E. M., & Lowy, F. H. (1995). Public opinion regarding end-of-life decisions: Influence of prognosis, practice, and process. *Social Science and Medicine, 41*, 1517–1521.

Steinberg, M. A., Najman, J. M., Cartwright, C. M., MacDonald, S. M., & Williams, G. M. (1997). End of life decision making: Community and medical practitioners' perspectives. *Medical Journal of Australia, 166*, 131–135.

Suarez-Almazor, M., Belzile, M., & Bruera, E. (1997). Euthanasia and physician-assisted suicide: A comparative survey of physicians, terminally ill cancer patients, and the general population. *Journal of Clinical Oncology, 15*, 418–427.

Taylor, H. (2005, May 27). Poll: U.S. adults favor euthanasia and physician-assisted suicide. Harris Interactive Inc. Retrieved March 2007 from www.deathwithdignity.org/fss/opinion/harrispoll04.27.05.asp

Van der Heide, A., Onwuteaka-Phillipsen, B. D., Rurup, M. L., Buiting, H. M., van Delden, J., Hanssen-deWolf, J. E., et al. (2007). End-of-life practices in the Netherlands under the Euthanasia Act. *New England Journal of Medicine, 356*(19), 1957–1965.

Van der Maas, P. J., Pijnenborg, L., & van Delden, J. J. M. (1995). Changes in Dutch opinions on active euthanasia, 1966 through 1991. *Journal of the American Medical Association, 273*, 1411–1414.

Vass, A. (2002). What's a good doctor, and how can we make one? *British Medical Journal, 325*, 667–668.

Vorenberg, J., & Wanzer, S. (1997, March–April). Assisting suicide. *Harvard Magazine*, p. 30.

Ward, A. (1980). Age and acceptance of euthanasia. *Journal of Gerontology, 35*, 421–431.

Weir, R. F. (Ed.). (1997). *Physician-assisted suicide.* Bloomington: Indiana University Press.

Chapter 6

Terminal Diseases and Conditions

It has been often said, that it is not death,
but dying which is terrible.
—Henry Fielding

Objectives

After reading this chapter, you will be able to answer the following questions:

- What are the leading causes of death in the United States each year?
- What terminal diseases are most common in women and children?
- How do drug, alcohol, and tobacco abuse contribute to premature death?
- How have treatments affected the life span of people with HIV/AIDS?
- What terminal illnesses/conditions affect the elderly?

Today, most deaths in the United States are due to progressive, chronic, terminal diseases, such as heart disease, cancer, and Alzheimer's disease (Hoyert, Kung, & Smith, 2003). Chronic conditions such as drug and alcohol abuse and addiction also are responsible for a significant number of deaths, as are accidents, homicides, and suicides. Many people think that only the elderly are affected by chronic, terminal diseases. Approximately 1 million children in the United States, however, are seriously ill with a life-threatening condition (Field & Behrman, 2003). Thus, people of all ages die due to terminal diseases and conditions (see Table 6.1).

Terminal Diseases of Women

The top six causes of death from disease (heart, cancer, stroke, lung, diabetes, Alzheimer's) are similar for males and females, but some differences exist (Jemal et al., 2008). Heart disease causes more deaths among women than all forms of cancer combined. More women than men die from heart disease, with heart disease accounting for one-third of all women's deaths in the United States. Yet, according to the American Heart Association (2007), only 8% of women know that heart disease is a threat to their health.

Table 6.1 LEADING CAUSES OF DEATH IN THE UNITED STATES BY AGE (YEARS)

Rank	1 to 4	5 to 14	15 to 24	25 to 44	45 to 65	65+
1	Accidents	Accidents	Accidents	Accidents	Cancer	Heart
2	Birth defects	Cancer	Homicide	Cancer	Heart	Cancer
3	Homicide	Homicide	Suicide	Heart	Accidents	Stroke
4	Cancer	Birth defects	Cancer	Suicide	Stroke	Lung disease

Source: CDC (2000).

A woman is more likely to survive a heart attack than a man, but women who have invasive heart surgeries (such as a coronary bypass) are more likely to die (Swahn, 2007). Doctors are not sure why. One possibility is that women tend to have smaller hearts and blood vessels, which could complicate a surgical procedure. Women also tend to experience more side effects from medicines. In addition, women are usually older than men by the time they develop heart problems, so the effects of old age also might worsen their chances of surviving heart surgery.

The second leading cause of death for women is cancer. According to the American Cancer Society, lung cancer kills more women than any other type of cancer (Jemal et al., 2008), with 90% of these deaths linked to cigarette smoking. Breast cancer is the second leading cause of cancer deaths among women, but it is a distant second. An estimated one in every two women die from lung cancer compared to one in every nine from breast cancer (Jamal et al., 2008).

Terminal Diseases of Youth

Cancer, a leading cause of death among young people, encompasses many diseases that have one thing in common—cells in the body grow abnormally and out of control. Over time, these cells spread throughout the body and destroy normal tissue, making the person very sick.

Approximately 12,500 children and adolescents are diagnosed with cancer every year and approximately 2,500 die from it. Approximately 1 in 300 American boys and 1 in 333 American girls will develop cancer before reaching the age of 20 (CureSearch, 1996).

A young person is most likely to be diagnosed with cancer of the white blood cells, or **leukemia**, than other types of cancer. The rapid growth of white blood cells stops the production of normal blood cells, a condition that causes a person to be fatigued, have excessive bleeding, and lowered resistance to infection.

Skin cancer is another potentially deadly cancer for youth. One type of skin cancer, *melanoma*, is the most deadly. Excessive exposure to the sun can increase the risk of skin cancer, which can spread to other types of cancer, such as liver, lung, and brain. Yet, instead of spending less time in the sun, young people typically spend more time in the sun, visiting tanning parlors, and using sunscreen incorrectly or not at all.

Asthma is another potentially fatal illness that kills 5,000 people a year. Asthma is a long-term, chronic inflammatory disorder that blocks air flow in and out of the lungs. This illness usually appears in children between infancy and age 5. Symptoms of asthma include wheezing, difficulty in breathing, shortness of breath, and coughing spasms.

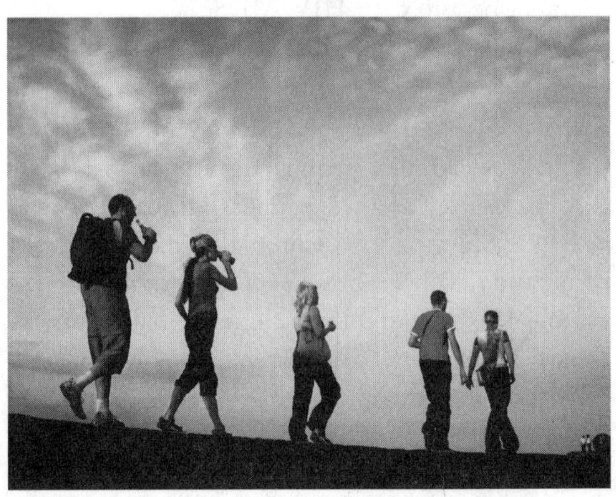

Most asthma attacks are not life-threatening. According to the Joint Council of Allergy, Asthma, and Immunology (1999), asthma has become the most common chronic disease of childhood, accounting for one-fourth of all school absences. Overall, 13% of all students ages 5 to 19 have asthma. In childhood, asthma strikes more boys than girls. In adulthood, more women than men have asthma.

Diabetes is a chronic disease characterized by the body's failure to properly use or make the hormone insulin, which is needed to store or use glucose (blood sugar). Diabetes is manifested as *type I diabetes*, referred to as juvenile or insulin-dependent diabetes, in which the body is unable to produce insulin. Type I diabetes mainly occurs in children and adolescents 18 years and younger. In *type II diabetes*, referred to as adult-onset or non-insulin-dependent diabetes, the body is unable to use the limited amount of insulin that it has. Type II diabetes usually occurs in adults over 30 years of age.

Approximately 800,000 new cases of diabetes are diagnosed each year, or 2,200 each day. Over half of the 10.5 million people with diabetes are undiagnosed because they do not yet have symptoms (U.S. Department of Health and Human Services [USDHHS], 2000).

Drug and Alcohol Abuse

Illegal drugs include marijuana, cocaine, heroin, acid, inhalants, methamphetamines, and a variety of other drugs, including alcohol if users are younger than 21 years of age. For all ages, any use of an illegal drug not prescribed for medical purposes is considered abuse (see Table 6.2). Alcohol and other drugs are abused more by males than females (USDHHS, 2000).

Although alcohol is legal for persons over 21 years of age, it can be abused if consumed in excessive quantities or continuously without control. Binge drinking (in one setting, drinking five or more drinks for males and four or more for females) is a serious problem for many college students, and a number of deaths from it have been recorded.

Table 6.2 Alcohol and Illegal Drug Use Among Americans (%)

Substance	18- to 25-year-olds	All Americans
Alcohol	61.4	50.1
Marijuana/hashish	17.0	6.2
Hallucinogens	1.7	0.4
Cocaine	2.2	1.0
Stimulants	1.3	0.5
Inhalants	0.4	0.2
Tranquilizers	1.7	0.8
Sedatives	0.2	0.1
Heroin	0.1	0.1

Source: Substance Abuse and Mental Health Services Administration (2005).

Frequently, college students are pictured drinking on TV, in magazine ads, and on billboards. They look happy. They are led to believe that only fun can come from drinking alcohol. But irresponsible drinking can be fatal, either directly or as a cause of death by other means (e.g., auto accidents or chronic diseases aggravated by alcohol).

Deaths Linked to Alcohol

In 2000, 85,000 deaths were attributed to alcohol (Mokdad, Marks, Stroup, & Gerberding, 2004). As many as 140,000 deaths could be attributed to alcohol if mortality among previous alcohol drinkers were included. These deaths occur in all age groups and are highest among college-age students (Substance Abuse and Mental Health Services Administration [SAMHSA], 2005).

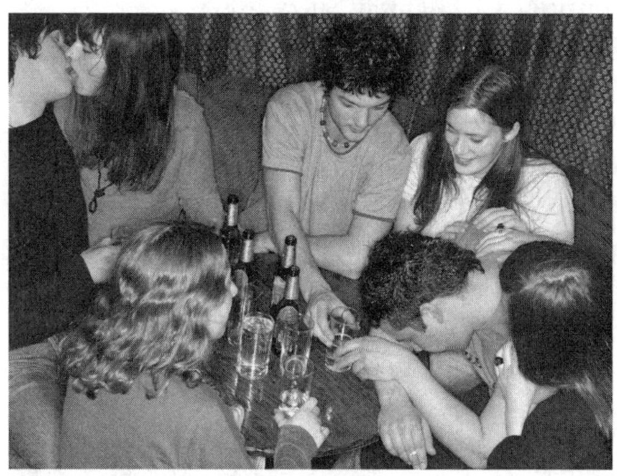

The leading cause of death for those aged 3 to 45 is traffic accidents. Alcohol is related to 38% of all traffic fatalities. Alcohol is linked not only to auto accidents, but also to falls, fires, and deaths from drowning. Alcoholism also is a factor in homicide, suicide, domestic violence, and child abuse (USDHHS, 2000).

Do you know at what time of day and day of the week you are most likely to be killed in an auto accident? The answer is: "Times when most people drink alcohol." Alcohol consumption is higher through the night (9 PM until 6 AM). Almost 75% of drivers in nighttime, single-vehicle fatal crashes had alcohol in their blood, and 52% of all fatal alcohol-related auto accidents occur on weekends, which are when most people drink too much and then drive (National Highway Traffic Safety Administration, 2005).

The effect that alcohol has on a person can be measured by Blood Alcohol Concentration, or BAC, the percentage of alcohol per volume of blood. Typically, one drink (one 12-ounce beer, one highball, or one glass of wine) gives a BAC of 0.02 to 0.03. After three drinks, a person is typically at or over 0.08, which is the legal intoxication point for adults.

Until recently, 0.10 was the legal definition for intoxication in most states. Before the reduction, almost 60% of car injuries were fatal when drivers aged 16 to 20 had BACs greater than or equal to 0.10. Since the legal level of BAC was lowered, there have been fewer car crashes, in general, and fewer crashes involving drivers aged 16 to 20 who had a BAC greater than or equal to 0.10 (Insurance Institute for Highway Safety, 2005).

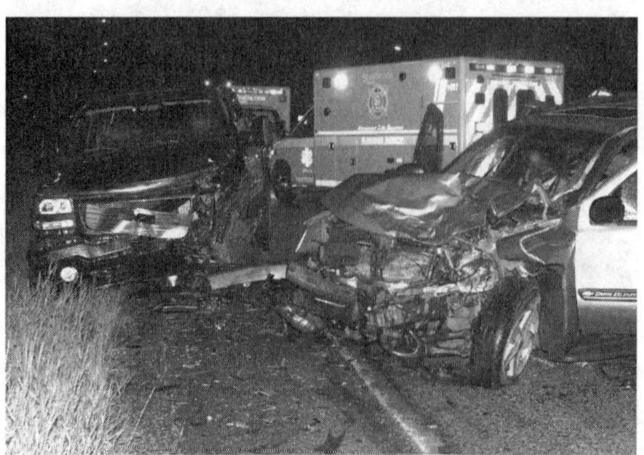

Reductions in fatal car crashes for people, in particular youth, are probably due to several factors:

- In most states, the legal drinking age was raised from 18 to 21, with stricter enforcement.
- An increased emphasis on zero-tolerance no-drinking-and-driving for those under age 21.
- Efforts to educate about the dangers of drinking and driving.
- Since the dramatic increase in gasoline price in 2008, fewer miles driven have led to fewer accidents and fatalities (Morrisey & Grabowski, 2008).

Deaths Linked to Illicit Drug Use

Many young people do not perceive illicit drug use to be risky, and the percentage of youth who perceive risk associated with illicit drug abuse is declining. For example, the percentage of youth who perceive risk in using cocaine decreased from 64% in 1994 to 54.3% in 1998 (USDHHS, 2000).

Death due to illicit drug use is considered a common occurrence. Causes of illicit drug-induced deaths include intentional injuries, such as suicide, as well as accidental poisoning. From 1990 to 2000, drug-related deaths increased 62%. Use of five major illicit drugs (e.g., marijuana, heroin, morphine, methamphetamine [speed], and cocaine) increased from 1990 to 2000 (Johnston, O'Malley, & Bachman, 2001). As with alcohol, more males than females abuse, and die from, the use of illicit drugs (USDHHS, 2000).

The message regarding alcohol and other drugs is an all too common one—they can kill. Many adolescents understand this message. Even with rising drug use among adolescents, almost 79% of them reported that they had not used alcohol or illicit drugs during the month prior to their being surveyed (USDHHS, 2000).

Deaths Due to Tobacco Use

Tobacco use is the single most preventable cause of death in the United States, and it is responsible for more than 430,000 deaths per year in this country.

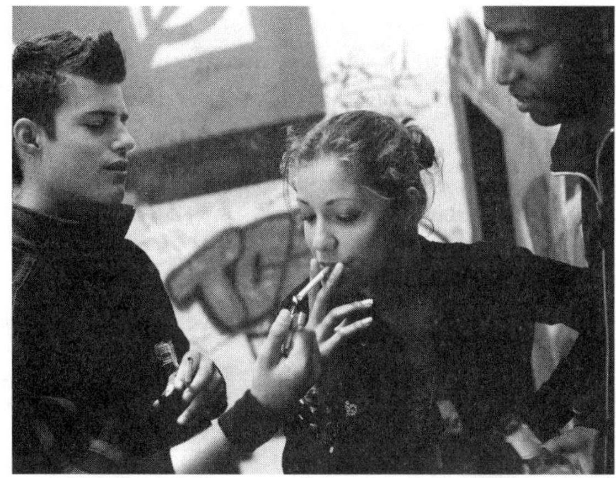

This number is more than the total number of people who died in World War II. Another way to look at tobacco deaths is that about four times more people die each year from tobacco-related illnesses than the total number of Americans who die each year from AIDS, murders, auto accidents, drugs, and war (see Table 6.3).

Table 6.3 TOBACCO USE IN THE UNITED STATES, 2005 (%)

Type	Ages 18 to 25	All Americans
All forms	44.3	29.4
Cigarettes	39.0	24.9
Cigars	12.0	5.6
Smokeless tobacco	5.1	3.2

Source: Substance Abuse and Mental Health Services Administration (2005).

Most tobacco smoking in the United States begins in early adolescence; the average age of initiation is 11.6 years. Approximately 34.8% of teens smoke. At least 50% of those who smoke as adolescents will continue to smoke for at least 16 to 20 years. The number of teenagers who become daily smokers before the age of 18 is believed to be more than 3,000 every day, with another 6,000 teens under the age of 18 smoking their first cigarette (CDC, 2003).

MY STORY: TAKING THE CHANCE

My attitude about smoking is that it's okay, at least for now, and it's not going to cause me to have a heart attack or to die early. All of the people I ever knew who died of a heart attack were old enough to die whether they smoked or not. Besides, many of my friends smoke cigarettes. We like the "look" smoking gives us. I'm going to become a scientist, so I believe in facts rather than the scare tactics about smoking. Well, at least this is the way I used to think.

One day when I was hanging out with Tyler, his dad told us that he wanted to talk with us about smoking (at first, I thought, another scare-tactic speech!). Tyler's dad told us that he had smoked cigarettes for 24 years—half of his life—and he wished that he had stopped smoking years ago rather than waiting until last year. You know, his talk made sense.

One of the things that Tyler's dad explained about smoking was that cigarettes gear you up rather than relax you. He said that the fact that you are getting what you want makes smoking seem relaxing. Well, that was a fact that this future scientist had not heard before!

Next, he told us that he started smoking because it made him feel like a "big man." I was beginning to see that myself. Finally, Tyler's dad asked us to quit smoking, explaining that if we stop smoking, we could reverse any risk for future heart attacks if irreversible damage had not already begun. We told him that we would think about it.

I guess the part that really caused me to consider quitting smoking, though, was that Tyler's dad, a smart man—a scientist—will not get to watch Tyler play another college soccer game or see him graduate. You see, Tyler's dad died last week of a heart attack. Maybe it was the smoking that killed him. Maybe it wasn't. I don't think I want to take that chance anymore.

HIV and AIDS

At the outset a scourge potentially as devastating as the Bubonic Plague of the Middle Ages, HIV/AIDS, which appeared only 15 years ago, is now treatable with a drug regimen that, although not a cure, has extended the life span of people with AIDS (Cates, Graham, Boeglin, & Tielker, 1990). However, the virus is notorious for its ability to mutate rapidly, and the race to keep up with new drugs never slows or stops.

One unfortunate side effect of the availability of effective treatment for AIDS has been a change in attitude on the part of some young gay men. These men ignore the risks of "barebacking," which refers to having sex without condoms (Johnson, 2008).

At first, HIV/AIDS seemed restricted to gay men. Now its reach extends to heterosexual men, women, and children. The result of AIDS in many parts of Africa, for instance, has been the creation of an entire generation of orphans.

The course of untreated or untreatable AIDS takes a terrible toll on the patient, loved ones, family, and caregivers. The patient goes from being HIV positive to having full-blown AIDS, typically cycling between periods of fairly good health and battles with opportunistic diseases (Walker, Pomeroy, McNeil, & Franklin, 1996).

The AIDS patient usually is devastated by a decline in physical appearance, stamina, memory, and coordination; extreme weight loss; lack of energy; and other physical changes. Even worse, many patients develop AIDS dementia, progressing from memory loss, inability to concentrate and confusion, to incontinence and total dependence (Moynihan, Christ, & Silver, 1988). Social and financial support also might diminish or disappear.

HIV/AIDS also has a social stigma attached to it (Pomeroy, Walker, McNeil, & Franklin, 1993). Because AIDS is typically associated with homosexual activity and illegal IV drug use, physical disfigurement, cognitive decline, lack of a cure, and fear of contagion, those with AIDS might feel less desirable, less valuable, and even less human (Dane, 1991; Saylor, 1990). At each stage of decline, stigma further isolates the patient (Pomeroy et al., 1993).

Social disapproval also might extend to those anticipating the loss of a loved one (O'Neil, 1989). "Losing a friend or lover to AIDS stigmatizes the survivor as probably gay, probably sexually promiscuous, perhaps a drug user, and probably a future victim of AIDS" (Biller & Rice, 1990, p. 288).

Terminal Conditions/ Diseases of the Elderly

Although chronic illnesses can occur at any age, they are more common in the middle and later years. More than 100 million Americans live with chronic conditions, and elders account for 40% of those in the United States with chronic illnesses, even though they comprise only about 13% of the population. With the exception of acute diseases, pneumonia/influenza, accidents, and blood poisoning, 7 of the top 10 causes of death of elders are chronic diseases, including heart disease, cancer, stroke, chronic obstructive pulmonary disease, diabetes mellitus, Alzheimer's disease, and kidney disease (USDHHS, 2000).

Alcohol and Drug Abuse by the Elderly

Just as alcohol can be a problem for youth, it likewise can become a cause for concern among the elderly, with elderly men five times more likely to abuse alcohol than elderly women. Alcohol abuse among the elderly is associated with car accidents, suicides, and homicides. Also, long-term heavy drinking shortens life expectancy and worsens chronic diseases such as diabetes and high blood pressure and increases the risk of heart attack, stroke, and cancers of the esophagus, mouth, throat, larynx, colon, and rectum (Valliant, 2002).

The main substance problem leading to death among the elderly is overuse of prescription tranquilizers. Elder substance abuse, however, is confined to about 2% to 4% of the elder population (Ferrini & Ferrini, 2000). This rate is considerably lower than the 10% quoted for the population as a whole.

Falls: A Serious Matter for the Elderly

Many old people die as a result of falling. Every year, 1.5 million elders break bones during falls. One in every two women, and one in every eight men, is expected to have a broken bone due to **osteoporosis** (Ferrini & Ferrini, 2000), fragility caused by a decrease in bone mass with decreased density and enlargement of bone spaces. Estimates indicate that osteoporosis contributes to 90% of hip fractures.

Hip fractures are more likely to lead to functional impairment and are associated with a high mortality risk, including death from heart attack, stroke, and cancer. This association is one reason that the elderly frequently die as a result of falls.

Cardiovascular Disease

Cardiovascular disease (atherosclerosis) is the leading cause of death among elders, causing almost half of all elder deaths, and its incidence increases with age (American Heart Association, 2007). **Atherosclerosis** is a disease of the blood vessels in which the arteries narrow, sometimes completely closing, which hampers or stops the cardiovascular system (see Figure 6.1 for a picture of a healthy cardiovascular system). Atherosclerosis is accelerated by inactivity, obesity, smoking, and high-fat diets. A major contributor to atherosclerosis is elevated cholesterol.

Atherosclerosis is a big contributor to heart attacks, the major killer of elders. Older people have more than two times as many the number of heart attacks as younger people. At any age, however, women are more likely to die of a heart attack, or **myocardial infarction**, than men (Legato, 1993).

When the heart muscle is damaged, from a heart attack, for example, and is no longer able to pump blood effectively, the person has a condition called **congestive heart failure (CHF)**. This condition affects more than 5 million people in the United States (Fuster, O'Rourke, Walsh, & Poole-Wilson, 2007).

Another condition of the cardiovascular system is **hypertension**, or high blood pressure.

Figure 6.1 THE CARDIOVASCULAR SYSTEM.

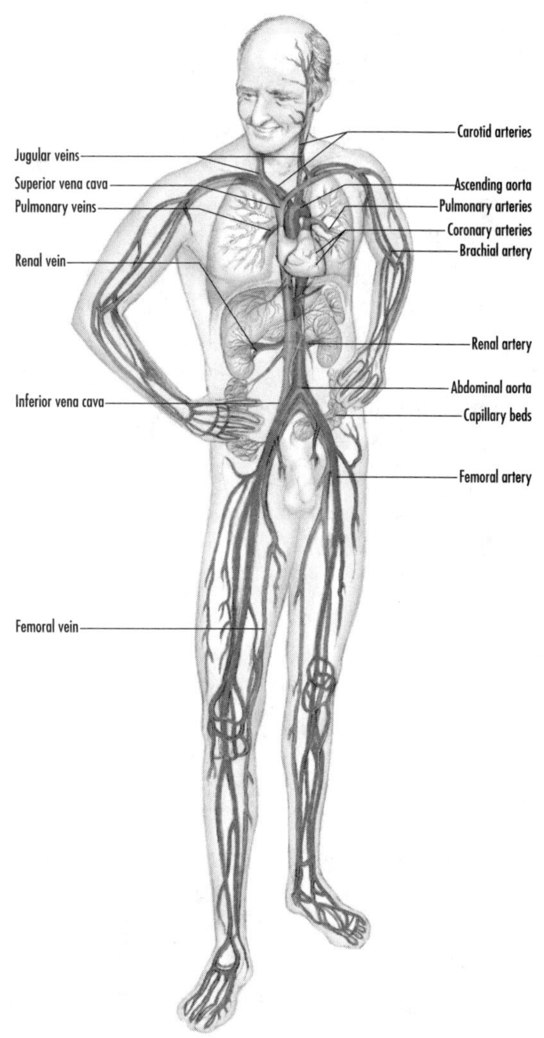

Hypertension is called the "silent killer," because most people with the disease have no symptoms. The measure for hypertension, measured by a sphygmomanometer, is either a systolic blood pressure reading (the upper number) greater than 140 or a diastolic blood pressure reading (the lower number) greater than 90. Hypertension is a risk factor for heart attacks and stroke, and the higher the blood pressure reading, the greater the risk. To reduce hypertension, it is suggested that people restrict salt, reduce alcohol, reduce dietary fat, reduce their weight, exercise, and quit smoking.

Cancer

Cancer, the number two killer among elders, is a general term used to describe any number of malignant tumors that can affect almost any body system. Some types of cancer are rapid and almost always fatal, such as pancreatic cancer. Other types of cancers grow more slowly, such as most prostate cancers. The risk of developing cancer increases with age; more than one-half of cancer victims are over age 65 (Jemal et al., 2008).

Typically, cancer is treated with surgery, chemotherapy, radiation, or a combination of the three. With radiation and chemotherapy, normal cells are damaged along with cancerous cells. Although it is difficult for elders' bodies to tolerate radiation and chemotherapy, elders also are usually less able to tolerate the anesthesia needed for long surgical treatments.

The single most effective way to prevent the likelihood of getting cancer is to quit smoking. Lung cancer is the most frequent type of cancer in both men and women. Ninety percent of all lung cancer is attributed to cigarette smoking, and the more a person smokes, the greater is his or her risk. (In women, breast cancer is the second most frequent cancer, and prostate cancer is second among men.)

People who smoke two or more packs of cigarettes a day have death rates as much as 25 times greater than nonsmokers. Cigarette smoking decreases life expectancy by as much as 8 years. By age 75, two-thirds of those who smoke are dead, compared to only one-third of nonsmokers. Interestingly, within one year after quitting smoking, a person's risk of getting lung cancer declines.

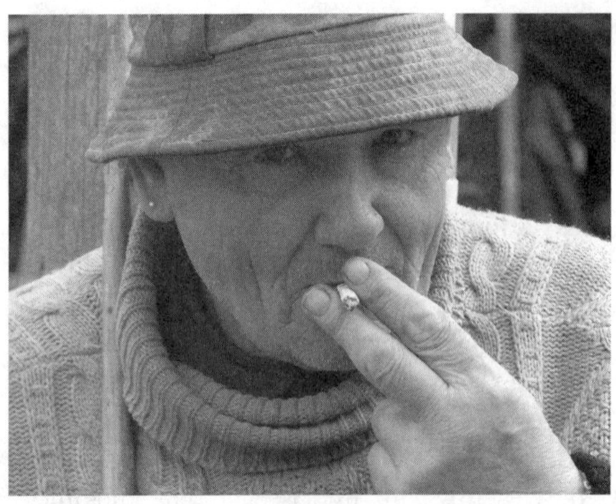

Stroke

The third leading cause of death among elders is stroke (American Heart Association, 2007). Most **strokes** are caused by blood clots or traveling cholesterol clumps that become lodged in blood vessels, cutting off blood supply to the brain. The main risk factor for a stroke is hypertension. Also, smokers have an increased risk for stroke.

Each year almost 700,000 people in the United States suffer a stroke, with men having an 8% higher risk of dying from it than women (American Heart Association, 2007). Sometimes, a mini-stroke, or **transient ischemic attack (TIA)**, which is a temporary blockage in brain arteries, serves as a warning sign of a real stroke to come.

Alzheimer's Disease

Alzheimer's disease was named for Alois Alzheimer, a German physician who, in 1907, described what he observed under the microscope in tissues obtained from patients who were believed to have died from **senile dementia**, the medical term for impairment or loss of mental functions in elderly persons. By definition, **Alzheimer's disease** is a disease of mental dysfunction in the elderly, an age-associated form of dementia, a gradual wasting of brain tissue and loss of memory for which there is no cure.

Alzheimer's is characterized by irreversible memory loss, reduced ability to use language, loss of problem-solving skills, and reduced mobility. Typically, Alzheimer's begins to attack the brain decades before the first symptoms of memory loss appear. In the end, this disease usually leads to death.

The onset of Alzheimer's usually occurs between ages 45 and 65. Cases have been observed in people as young as 38, but Alzheimer's is most commonly confined to the 65-and-over population. Nearly half of all people over 85 have Alzheimer's. More than 5 million people in the

United States have Alzheimer's. Given 400,000 new cases each year, this number is likely to increase as the baby boomers age. It is predicted that the number of people with Alzheimer's will increase to 7.7 million by 2030, unless a cure or a way to prevent the disease is found (Alzheimer's Association, 2007).

On average, people diagnosed with Alzheimer's live 6 to 8 years. However, the disease can cause its fatal harm in as short as 1 year or allow a person to linger for 16 or more years before death.

Alzheimer's is responsible for the death of 72,000 people each year, with almost twice as many women dying with it as men (Alzheimer's Association, 2008). Because the risk of Alzheimer's disease increases with age, one reason that more women are affected by Alzheimer's disease is that they usually outlive men.

Alzheimer's cases vary, but generally four phases have been identified:

- In the first phase, family members might notice that the person has less energy and has more difficulty learning things or understanding instructions.
- In the second phase of the illness, the person might have difficulty making plans or decisions. Forgetfulness is more frequent, and the person might repeat things.
- By the third phase, the person is obviously disabled, unaware of time, place, or events. The person might not even recognize loved ones.
- The fourth phase of the illness is characterized by aimless wandering, increasingly fading memory, depression, and weakness.

Results from research by Fackelmann (2005) revealed that active minds stay sharp, meaning that the best way to prevent Alzheimer's might be simply to have fun. The most active elders, both mentally and physically, reduced their risk of developing dementia by 63% compared with the least active elders. The best advice is to add a little more zest to life.

Interestingly, another activity was found to slow the progression of Alzheimer's (Kaufman, 2005). Among 68 subjects aged 49 to 94, it was found that Alzheimer's patients with higher levels of spirituality (i.e., meaning and purpose in life) or religiosity (i.e., practice of established dogma in places of worship) had a significantly slower progression of cognitive decline.

About 60% to 70% of people with Alzheimer's live in a family home (Kornblum, 2005). Thus, spouses, partners, and other family members must deal with the ravages of the illness. Although experiences vary from person to person, caregivers and professionals offer the following advice for caregivers:

- Do not take Alzheimer's behavior personally.
- Become educated about the progression of the disease.
- Prepare legal documents while the person with Alzheimer's is still lucid.
- Get help, including support groups.
- Take care of yourself.

> One man recounted how hard it is to take care of his wife but that he does it with love. He added, "I have so many men friends whose wives got cancer. They went through chemotherapy. And then they died. Don't feel sorry for me. My men friends lost their wives. They don't have their wives to hug and kiss. They'd give anything to have what I have." (Kornblum, 2005, p. 7D)

Summary

- In the United States, most deaths are due to progressive, chronic, or terminal diseases, such as heart, cancer, and Alzheimer's. Drug and alcohol abuse and addiction also are responsible for a significant number of deaths, along with accidents, homicides, and suicides.
- The top six causes of death from disease are heart, cancer, stroke, lung, diabetes, and Alzheimer's. More women than men die from heart disease.

- The second leading cause of death for men and women is cancer. Lung cancer kills more women than any other type of cancer, with 90% of these deaths linked to cigarette smoking. Approximately 12,500 children and adolescents are diagnosed with cancer every year, and 2,500 die.
- Type II diabetes usually occurs in adults over 30 years of age. Over half of the 10.5 million people with diabetes remain undiagnosed, because they do not yet have symptoms.
- Illegal drugs include marijuana, cocaine, heroin, acid, inhalants, methamphetamines, and a variety of other drugs, including alcohol if you are younger than 21 years of age or tobacco if you are younger than 18 years of age. For all ages, any use of an illegal drug not prescribed for medical purposes is considered abuse. Alcohol and drugs are abused by more males than females.
- Alcohol can be abused if consumed in excess quantities or continuously without control. Binge drinking (drinking in one setting 5 or more drinks for males and 4 or more for females) is a serious problem for many college students, and a number of deaths from it have been recorded. Irresponsible drinking can be fatal, either directly or as a cause of death by other means (e.g., auto accidents or chronic diseases aggravated by alcohol).The leading cause of death for those ages 3 to 45 is traffic accidents. Alcohol is related to 38% of all traffic fatalities.
- Tobacco use is the single most preventable cause of death in the United States. Most tobacco smoking in the United States begins in adolescence; the average age is 11.6 years.
- At first, HIV/AIDS seemed restricted to gay men. Now its reach extends to heterosexual men, women, and children. In many parts of Africa, AIDS has created an entire generation of orphans.
- The main substance problems leading to death among the elderly are overuse of prescription tranquilizers.
- Many old people die as a result of falling. Every year, 1.5 million elders break bones during falls.
- Cardiovascular disease (atherosclerosis) is the number one cause of death among elders, causing almost half of all elder deaths, and its incidence increases with age.
- Alzheimer's disease is a disease of mental dysfunction in the elderly, an age-associated form of dementia, a gradual wasting of brain tissue and loss of memory for which there is no cure. More than 5 million people in the United States have Alzheimer's, a number predicted to increase to 7.7 million by 2030.

ADDITIONAL RESOURCES

Books

Albom, M. (1997). *Tuesdays with Morrie.* New York: Doubleday. In this book, an account is offered from Mitch Albom about rediscovering Morrie Schwartz, a college professor of his from nearly 20 years earlier, in the last months of the older man's life. Mitch visited Morrie in his study every Tuesday, just as they did back in college. Their rekindled relationship turned into one final "class"—lessons in how to live.

Keizer, G. (2002). *God of Beer.* New York: HarperCollins. *God of Beer* is a novel about high schoolers in northeastern Vermont who engage in civil disobedience to lower the drinking age. On the road to success, they suffer a reverse, which teaches them about acceptance of change and facing reality. The book likely will resonate for those who remember their high school days.

Movies

Steel Magnolias. (1989). In this comedy-drama, the lives of several women from a small town are followed, particularly one woman (Sally Field) with a diabetic daughter (Julia Roberts), who decides to have a child despite having Type 1 diabetes and the complications that result from that decision.

Angels in the Dust. (2007). This movie offers a straightforward look at death from AIDS. The story is about a stubborn Dutchwoman, Marion Cloete, and her husband, Con, who run a school and orphanage in rural South Africa, caring for hundreds of children living with HIV/AIDS or whose parents have it or have died of it, and the battles they fight with stubborn parents and the obstinate South African health minister Manto Tshabalala-Msimang, who thinks garlic and beetroot will cure AIDS.

Critical Thinking

1. How can you prevent friends or family members from being killed in an automobile accident involving alcohol?
2. If your father had a heart attack and decided that he was not going to lose weight, exercise, or quit smoking, what convincing evidence would you use to convince him to change his mind?

Class Activity

Read *Tuesdays with Morrie.* With classmates, discuss what, if anything, was "good" about Morrie having a terminal illness.

References

Alzheimer's Association. (2007, March 20). *Alzheimer's disease prevalence rates rise to more than 5 million in the United States.* Retrieved April 29, 2008, from www.alz.org/news_and_events_in_the_news.asp

Alzheimer's Association. (2008). *Alzheimer's disease facts and figures.* Chicago: Author.

American Heart Association. (2007). *Heart disease and stroke statistics, 2007.* Retrieved June 2007 from www.americanheart.org

Biller, R., & Rice, S. (1990). Experiencing multiple loss of persons with AIDS: Grief and bereavement issues. *Health & Social Work, 15,* 283–290.

Cates, J. A., Graham, L. L., Boeglin, D., & Tielker, S. (1990). The effect of AIDS on the family system. *Families in Society, 71,* 195–201.

Centers for Disease Control and Prevention (CDC). (2000). *National vital statistics report, 48*(11), 1–120.

Centers for Disease Control and Prevention (CDC). (2003). *Youth risk behavior surveillance—United States, 2003.* Retrieved April 29, 2008, from www.cdc.gov/mmwr/PDF/SS/SS5302.pdf

CureSearch, National Childhood Cancer Foundation. (1996). *Childhood cancer statistics, 1995.* Retrieved April 29, 2008, from www.curesearch.org/our_research/index_sub.aspx?id=1475

Dane, B. O. (1991). Anticipatory mourning of middle-aged parents of adult children with AIDS. *Families in Society, 72,* 108–115.

Fackelmann, K. (2005, January 25). Minds in motion stay sharp. *USA Today*, pp. 1D–2D.

Ferrini, A. F., & Ferrini, R. L. (2000). *Health in the later years* (3rd ed.). New York: McGraw-Hill.

Field, M., & Behrman, R. E. (2003). *When children die.* New York: Robert Wood Johnson Foundation.

Fuster, V., O'Rourke, R. A., Walsh, R., & Poole-Wilson, P. (2007). *Hurst's the heart* (12th ed.). New York: McGraw-Hill.

Hoyert, D., Kung, H. C., & Smith, B. L. (2003). Deaths: Preliminary data for 2003. *National vital statistics report.* Retrieved April 29, 2008, from www.cdc.gov/nchs/data/nvsr/nvsr53/nvsr53_15.pdf

Insurance Institute for Highway Safety. (2005). Special issues: Alcohol-impaired driving. *Status Report, 40*(4), 1–8.

Jemal, A., Siegel, R., Ward, E., Murray, T., Xu, J., & Thun, M. J. (2008). Cancer statistics, 2007. *CA: A Cancer Journal for Clinicians, 58*(1), 71–96.

Johnson, R. (2008). Gay men and bareback sex. *Gay Life* Newsletter. About.com, Inc., a New York Times Company.

Johnston, L. D., O'Malley, P. M., & Bachman, J. G. (2001). *Monitoring the future: National survey results on drug use, 1975–2000. Volume II: College students and young adults ages 19–40.* Washington, DC: National Institute on Drug Abuse.

Joint Council of Allergy, Asthma, and Immunology. (1999). Stinging insect hypersensitivity: A practice parameter. *Journal of Allergy & Clinical Immunology, 103*(5), 963–980.

Kaufman, Y. (2005, June). *The effects of spirituality and religiosity on the rate of decline and quality of life in Alzheimer's disease.* Paper presented at the Annual Meeting of the American Academy of Neurology, Miami Beach, Florida.

Kornblum, J. (2005, July 14). Love guides in Alzheimer's care. *USA Today.* Retrieved April 29, 2008, from http://www.usatoday.com/news/health/2005-07-13-alzheimers-caregivers_x.htm

Legato, M. J. (1993). *The female heart: The truth about women and heart disease.* New York: Simon & Schuster.

Mokdad, A. H., Marks, J. S., Stroup, D. F., & Gerberding, J. L. (2004). Actual causes of death in the United States, 2000. *Journal of the American Medical Association, 291*(10), 1238–1244.

Morrisey, M., & Grabowski, D. (2008). As gas prices go up, auto deaths decline. Study reported by the Associated Press, July 11, 2008. See also *TIME Magazine,* July 14, 2008.

Moynihan, R., Christ, G., & Silver, L. G. (1988). AIDS and terminal illness. *Social Casework, 69,* 380–387.

National Highway Traffic Safety Administration. (2005). *Alcohol involvement in fatal motor vehicle traffic crashes, 2003.* Springfield, VA: National Center for Statistics and Analysis.

O'Neil, M. (1989). Grief and bereavement in AIDS and aging. *Generations, 13*(4), 80–82.

Pomeroy, E. C., Walker, R. J., McNeil, J. S., & Franklin, C. (1993). *The stigma of AIDS: An exploratory study.* Unpublished manuscript.

Saylor, C. (1990). Stigma. In I. M. Lubkin (Ed.), *Chronic illness: Impact and intervention* (pp. 65–85). Boston: Jones & Bartlett.

Substance Abuse and Mental Health Services Administration. (2005). Retrieved April 29, 2008, from www.samhsa.gov/nhsda/2k3tabs/toc.htm

Swahn, E. (2007). *Study of women heart-surgery patients.* Paper presented at European Society of Cardiology, Munich, Germany.

U.S. Department of Health and Human Services. (2000). *Healthy people 2010*. Washington, DC: Government Printing Office.

Valliant, G. E. (2002). *Aging well.* New York: Little, Brown and Co.

Walker, R. J., Pomeroy, E. C., McNeil, J. S., & Franklin, C. (1996). Anticipatory grief and AIDS: Strategies for intervening with caregivers. *Health and Social Work, 21*(1), 49–58.

Chapter 7

Processes of Dying

Do not go gentle into that good night,
Old age should burn and rave at close of day;
Rage, rage against the dying of the light.
—DYLAN THOMAS

Objectives

After reading this chapter, you will be able to answer the following questions:

- How do the processes of dying differ from the processes of death?
- What do most people consider to be "a good death"?
- What has been the influence of Elisabeth Kübler-Ross on people's understanding of the grieving process?
- What is social death?
- What signs might indicate that death is imminent?

A century ago, most people died from an infectious disease, often within days of contracting it. Now, most people must learn how to deal with the degenerative diseases that come with age. Dying well has become a matter of living with the knowledge that death is near for months or even years (Walker, 2003).

Dying Versus Death

The **processes of dying** involve the activities, thoughts, and feelings that a person must deal with when anticipating his or her own death. People sometimes confuse this term with the **processes of death**, which refers to what happens to bodies after death. Both involve fear.

Typically, young people fear the processes of death, such as immobility, uncertainty, isolation, and decomposition of the dead body, whereas elders usually fear the processes of dying, such as deterioration, loss of control, and dependency before they die.

When does the process of dying begin? Many people believe that dying begins at the moment of birth and continues until death. Some people believe that the process of dying begins when a physician tells someone that he or she has a terminal condition. Others may believe that dying begins when nothing more can be done to preserve life.

Many end-of-life tasks can be accomplished before death. For example, dying persons can complete unfinished business, spend time with loved ones, and resolve old hurts. The dying hope that while they are making final plans to die, they are still treated as they were when life, not death, was ahead of them.

A Good Death

A good death has been important in all cultures (Clark, 2003). Yet what is "a good death"? The answer depends on the particular society and culture (Walker, 2003). One example given by Walker is that of an elderly woman, at home, surrounded by family, who realizing that the end is near, is able to ask for Extreme Unction from a priest. To her, her family, and her neighbors, that process constitutes a good death.

Yet people do not always die where they wish or as peacefully as they desire (Smith, 2000). Too many die alone, in pain, alienated, terrified, or mentally unaware, without dignity. Even worse deaths befall people who are poor, from ethnic minorities, or socially and economically marginal.

Too often, the treatment of the dying patient is controlled by family and healthcare professionals. Patients lack autonomy over the circumstances of their dying, especially in decisions for medical treatment, including those that prolong life. The fear of death is being replaced by the fear of dying.

The process of dying should incorporate patients' views (McNamara, 2001). Patients typically want their financial, emotional, and spiritual needs to be addressed and want a chance to say goodbye (Payne, Langley-Evans, & Hillier, 1996; Steinhauser, Christakis, Clipp, McNeilly, McIntyre, & Tulsky, 2000)—things not supplied by modern medical technology.

A **good death**, whether it ends in palliative care (Chapter 4) or euthanasia (Chapter 5), is one in which the patient makes his or her personal choices about death during the final days and months. In a society that prizes individualism, a bad death is one suffered by a person who has no autonomy (Walker, 2003). The downside of individualism is that rituals and traditions are missing, the inclusion of which might help with dying. Even in religious Western societies such as the United States, individual preferences are part of a person's right to choose how to live and die, with religious or community traditions playing a lesser part. For help in charting a dying course, it is wise to yield to the experiences of hospice workers and to the stories told by those who live in the shadow of death.

Elisabeth Kübler-Ross

Possibly the most profound feeling of loss when someone is dying is the knowledge that death is imminent. A pioneer in the field of death, dying, and accompanying feelings of loss was Swiss-born Elisabeth Kübler-Ross. Her work in death, dying, and loss began after World War II when she aided survivors of concentration camps in Germany. After medical school in the 1950s, she came to the United States. Working in U.S. hospitals, her compassion and empathy for her patients became legendary.

One thing she did not understand was why, in U.S. hospitals, the dying were treated as outcasts. Once a terminal illness was diagnosed, patients frequently were left to die by themselves. No one seemed to care what they thought or how they felt. Through her work with the dying, Kübler-Ross realized that something had to be done to meet the needs of people approaching the end of life.

She initiated a project in which she interviewed a number of dying patients in the presence of medical students and nurses. On the basis of these interviews, she wrote her first and best-known book, *On Death and Dying* (1969), outlining her concept of grief about dying as progressing in stages.

The book became a great success. Innumerable seminars were held, and Kübler-Ross was invited to lecture around the world. She published close to 20 books. Hospices have been established in numerous countries where the dying are cared for according to her ideas (Byskov, 2004).

Stages of Loss for the Dying

Kübler-Ross was not the first person to propose a stage theory of dying. John Bowlby (1961, 1980) and Colin Parkes (1996) also posited stages of shock-numbness, yearning-searching, disorganization-despair, and reorganization. Bowlby's four stages are:

1. Numbing that usually lasts from a few hours to a week, which might be interrupted by outbursts of extremely intense distress and/or anger.
2. Yearning and searching for the lost person, lasting some months or sometimes years.
3. Disorganization and despair.
4. Greater or less degree of reorganization.

This four-stage model is a revision of Bowlby's earlier model (1961) which had three stages, with the initial numbing stage not included.

When discussing doctor–patient interactions leading up to death, Robert Buckman (1992) advocated a three-stage model:

1. Initial stage, when a threat is faced.
2. Chronic stage, including depression and possible resolution.
3. Final stage, in which the ability to manage the inevitable death occurs.

Kübler-Ross adapted Bowlby's and Parkes's ideas when writing about how some terminally ill patients reported their reactions to imminent death. These reports spanned from when patients found out that they had a terminal illness until they came to terms with their upcoming death.

Kübler-Ross' Five Stages of Loss

Kübler-Ross (1969) suggested that people typically pass through five psychological stages in accepting their upcoming deaths. A dying person might proceed through the stages in order, skip one or several, or go back and forth between stages. Kübler-Ross' five stages are:

1. Denial: "No, not me!"
2. Anger: "Why me?"
3. Bargaining: "Yes, me, but ..."
4. Depression: "Yes, me, and I can't change it."
5. Acceptance: "Yes, me, I'm ready."

Denial

"Not me! There must be some mistake!" In this stage, the person experiences the initial sensations of shock, disbelief, and denial upon the diagnosis of a terminal disease. These feelings also are typical when hearing that a loved one has died. One woman explained how she reacted when her physician told her that she had cancer. After he said, "I'm afraid that you have cancer," she said she looked behind her to see "who on earth is he talking to?" Of course, he was speaking with her, but she was, in effect, saying, "Not me!"

Denial is a conscious or unconscious refusal to accept reality. It is a natural defense mechanism. Some people become fixed in this stage when dealing with traumatic change, even though death is not easy to avoid or evade (Chapman, 2006).

Anger

"Why me?" Anger is a natural reaction to death—yours as well as others'. The perception of the "unfairness" or "senselessness" of the death underlies feelings of anger. A dying person might become hostile to everyone around him or her. Or, on hearing about the death of a friend, the person in grief might want to lash out at someone or something.

People who are angry might be angry with themselves or with someone else, especially someone close to them. Knowing this can help the other person to stay cool and not judge the person who is upset (Chapman, 2006).

Bargaining

"God, if you will just . . . , then I promise I will. . . ." During this stage, a person might resolve to "go to church every Sunday," in return for not dying. Or, possibly, the person might ask for a reprieve "just until after graduation," for example.

People facing death might attempt to bargain with whatever God they believe in. If they face less serious trauma, they might seek to negotiate a compromise, for example, saying "Can we still be friends?" to someone they are breaking up with. Bargaining obviously does not hold up, especially in cases of life or death (Chapman, 2006).

DEPRESSION

"It's gonna happen, and I can't do anything about it." The person generally experiences feelings of doom and tremendous loss. He or she may feel worthless or feel responsible for everyone else's emotional suffering. This stage is the point in which the person is feeling lowest.

Depression, or "preparatory grieving," is something of a dress rehearsal for the aftermath of death, although this stage can mean different things to different people. It is emotional acceptance, with sadness and regret, fear or uncertainty. It is a stage when a person has begun to accept reality (Chapman, 2006).

ACCEPTANCE

"I'm ready now." The person has not given up, but he or she is not resentful—just passive. Sometimes, this stage represents "almost no feelings," but the struggle is over, and the person is almost equal in feelings to before the eventual loss event.

Acceptance varies but generally indicates some degree of emotional detachment and objectivity. A dying person might enter this stage long before the survivors. The survivors must go through their own individual stages of dealing with grief (Chapman, 2006).

Kübler-Ross believed that, generally, women are able to move through these stages more effectively than men. Also, religious and cultural beliefs can influence how agreeable one is to progressing through the stages.

Kübler-Ross herself died in 2004, and her reaction to her impending death was different from most of the reactions reported in her book. She mainly expressed impatience and anticipation. She told people that she was trying to understand why she could not hurry up and "go on and die!" Kübler-Ross had come to believe that death was not final. Based on witnessing many deaths, especially of children, she concluded that something, the real "I," leaves the body at death, that death is merely a transition to another plane of existence (Byskov, 2004).

Over time, the principal value of Kübler-Ross' work has turned out to be that it brought greater public and professional awareness of a dying person's feelings and thoughts as well as providing useful ways to behave toward and treat that person. Knowing the Kübler-Ross stages can be helpful when dealing with a dying loved one. These stages provide knowledge of what is probably occurring psychologically to the dying person. A dying person in the second stage might be hostile toward everyone—including you, if that person is a loved one of yours. But if you know that anger can be an expected reaction, you can be supportive and allow that person to express anger and despair.

Kübler-Ross found that most people who are dying want to talk about death. If your dying loved one wants to talk, you can be a listener. Being loving and sympathetic can be especially important at that time.

Questions & Answers

Question: Do all dying people go through all of Elisabeth Kübler-Ross's stages of dying?

Answer: No. Even if they do, they might not proceed through them in the same order. Also, some people might be at the end stage of acceptance and "regress" to an earlier stage. Finally, not everyone comes to terms with (accepts) death.

Other Models of the Dying Process

Corr (1993) suggested that, in order to move beyond the limitations of stage theory, three lessons can be taken from the dying:

1. People who are dying react in their own individual ways to the challenges that confront them, and they may have unfinished needs they want to address.
2. People cannot be effective caretakers unless they listen actively to those who are coping with dying and work with them to determine their psychosocial processes and needs.
3. In order to know themselves better, people need to learn from those who are dying and coping with dying.

Zlatin (1995) focused on dying patients themselves to find out what they wanted and needed. She interviewed eight people with incurable cancer, asking them "How do terminally ill persons understand their illnesses and treatments?" She found that they gained understanding of their illness by constructing life themes based on their daily life experiences. For example, one woman characterized herself as a crusader, who told the truth and stood up against pressures. She was able to keep her life integrated despite her illness because of her sense of who she was, then as well as earlier, including what her life had meant to both herself and others. Because life themes integrate with, and give meaning to, illness, while helping explain patients' coping strategies, Zlatin recommended that healthcare providers elicit patients' life themes and use them in diagnosis and treatment. The possible benefits are better balance in doctor–patient communication and improved patient satisfaction and quality of life—not to mention helping to contain healthcare costs.

Criticisms of Kübler-Ross's Ideas

Not all workers in the field of death and dying agree with the Kübler-Ross model, and some critics believe that the stages are too rigid. Many who work with the dying found that her stages have not been very useful in practice (Klass & Hutch, 1985). Also, a major criticism is that her work was based on middle-aged cancer patients. These patients, for example, might not view death the same way young people or the elderly do.

One critic of Kübler-Ross, Charmaz (1980), suggested that existing psychiatric categories had been applied, rather than derived from, the results of the interviews, so that the results were prescriptive rather than descriptive. Also, Charmaz believed that a terminal patient's depression might be triggered by physical disability rather than emotional distress.

Kastenbaum (2004) evaluated Kübler-Ross's model and pointed out that no evidence (as of his date of publication) had been put forward to support it. Also, Kastenbaum surmised that Kübler-Ross described various patients who exhibited one of the qualities from the five different stages, but that no one patient demonstrated all five stages and of the stages completed, no patient progressed in the order presented in her model of loss.

Kaufmann (1976) noted an inconsistency between Kübler-Ross's conclusions and interviews. She held that denial is inevitable, but many of her interviewees did not admit to denial. Other criticisms are that her studies were based on subjective observation and interpretation rather than on objective scientific research procedures. In addition, some believe that the stage theory is too neat and orderly and that some stages might be experienced simultaneously. Finally, dying people might feel obligated to follow the described stages rather than spontaneously doing so.

Empirical Test of Stage Theory

From 2000 to 2003, the Kübler-Ross stages of grief were examined empirically through a survey of 233 bereaved individuals who had lost a family member—not people terminally ill themselves (Maciejewski, Zhang, Block, & Prigerson, 2007). Contrary to the Kübler-Ross stages theory as it applies to a bereaved individual, disbelief was not the initial response. Acceptance was the most frequently mentioned first response, and yearning was the chief negative response in the period from 1 to 24 months after the loss. The investigators concluded that identifying the normal stages of grief following a death from natural causes is helpful for understanding how most people process, cognitively and emotionally, the loss of a family member.

Social Death

Social death is the situation in which a person is no longer treated as a member of the group to which he or she belongs. This type of distancing is sometimes inflicted upon the dying—at the very time that a feeling of belonging is critical (Kübler-Ross, 1969). Some behaviors that contribute to social death are that the dying person:

- is referred to as if he or she were already gone, regardless of whether he or she is living at home or in an institution.
- is excluded from communications.

- is moved to a terminal hospital ward and given little care.
- overhears medical workers making negative comments about him or her.

Sometimes the living are uncomfortable being around a dying person. This uneasiness might prevent some dying people from telling family members about their terminal condition. They are attempting to preserve their family's social relationships. Eventually, whether family relationships remain positive or not, death will have its way.

Knowing It Is Time to Go

People typically do not choose how quickly or slowly they die. Some signs do indicate approaching death, though. For example, some researchers have found evidence of a **terminal drop**, or decline in mental function during the last few months before death, especially among the very old. Ferrini and Ferrini (2007) reported that it is common for the very old not only to experience a decline in abilities, but also to lose the desire to eat and drink and to become uninterested in life. These behaviors can end in death even without a terminal disease.

Terminal drop, however, is not found in all dying people. A better predictor of death might be to ask if the dying person believes he or she might soon die. Many people realize when they are about to die. Their knowledge, however, does not necessarily affect how quickly they die. Speed of death might have more to do with a person's determination to die.

Some people who do not want to live longer simply give up the struggle and die fairly quickly. Others, who are afraid of death, yet are unable to cope with the pain, go back and forth between wishing to die and hoping to live. Either way, their attitudes usually either hasten or delay death. For example, cancer patients who have a strong desire to live, many times survive longer than patients who have a weak will to live.

Fewer deaths happen before a dying person's birthday, meaning that people seem to wait until after their birthday celebration. The death rate drops 35% below normal before a big event and peaks by an equal percentage following a holiday (Phillips & Smith, 1990). Such evidence seems to support the belief that people can postpone dying.

A Day in the Life of Oscar the Cat

Oscar the Cat awakens from his nap, opening a single eye to survey his kingdom. From atop the desk in the doctor's charting area, the cat peers down the two wings of the nursing home's advanced dementia unit. All quiet on the western and eastern fronts. Slowly, he rises and extravagantly stretches his 2-year-old frame, first backward and then forward. He sits up and considers his next move.

In the distance, a resident approaches. It is Mrs. P., who has been living on the dementia unit's third floor for 3 years now. She has long forgotten her family, even though they visit her almost daily. Moderately disheveled after eating her lunch, half of which she now wears on her shirt, Mrs. P. is taking one of her many aimless strolls to nowhere. She glides toward Oscar, pushing her walker and muttering to herself with complete disregard for her surroundings. Perturbed, Oscar watches her carefully and, as she walks by, lets out a gentle hiss, a rattlesnake-like warning that says "leave me alone." She passes him without a glance and continues down the hallway. Oscar is relieved. It is not yet Mrs. P.'s time, and he wants nothing to do with her.

Oscar jumps down off the desk, relieved to be once more alone and in control of his domain. He takes a few moments to drink from his water bowl and grab a quick bite. Satisfied, he enjoys another stretch and sets out on his rounds. Oscar decides to head down the west wing first, along the way sidestepping Mr. S., who is slumped over on a couch in the hallway. With lips slightly pursed, he snores peacefully—perhaps blissfully unaware of where he is now living. Oscar continues down the hallway until he reaches its end and Room 310. The door is closed, so Oscar sits and waits. He has important business here.

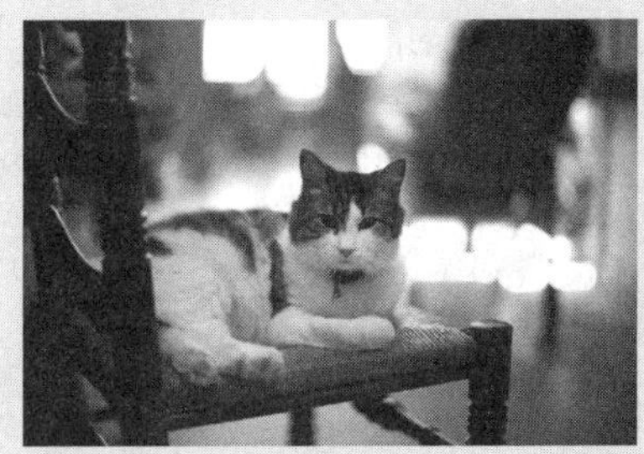

Twenty-five minutes later, the door finally opens, and out walks a nurse's aide carrying dirty linens. "Hello, Oscar," she says. "Are you going inside?" Oscar lets her pass, then makes his way into the room, where there are two people. Lying in a corner bed and facing the wall, Mrs. T. is asleep in a fetal position. Her body is thin and wasted from the breast cancer that has been eating away at her organs. She is mildly jaundiced and has not spoken in several days. Sitting next to her is her daughter, who glances up from her novel to warmly greet the visitor. "Hello, Oscar. How are you today?"

Oscar takes no notice of the woman and leaps up onto the bed. He surveys Mrs. T. She is clearly in the terminal phase of illness, and her breathing is labored. Oscar's examination is interrupted by a nurse, who walks in to ask the daughter whether Mrs. T. is uncomfortable and needs more morphine. The daughter shakes her head, and the nurse retreats. Oscar returns to his work. He sniffs the air, gives Mrs. T. one final look, then jumps off the bed and quickly leaves the room. Not today.

Making his way back up the hallway, Oscar arrives at Room 313. The door is open, and he proceeds inside. Mrs. K. is resting peacefully in her bed, her breathing steady but shallow. She is surrounded by photographs of her grandchildren and one from her wedding day. Despite these keepsakes, she is alone. Oscar jumps onto her bed and again sniffs the air. He pauses to consider the situation, and then turns around twice before curling up beside Mrs. K.

One hour passes. Oscar waits. A nurse walks into the room to check on her patient. She pauses to note Oscar's presence. Concerned, she hurriedly leaves the room and returns to her desk. She grabs Mrs. K.'s chart off the medical records rack and begins to make phone calls.

Within a half hour the family starts to arrive. Chairs are brought into the room, where the relatives begin their vigil. The priest is called to deliver last rites. And still, Oscar has not budged, instead purring and gently nuzzling Mrs. K. A young grandson asks his mother, "What is the cat doing here?" The mother, fighting back tears, tells him, "He is here to help Grandma get to heaven." Thirty minutes later, Mrs. K. takes her last earthly breath. With this, Oscar sits up, looks around, then departs the room so quietly that the grieving family barely notices.

On his way back to the charting area, Oscar passes a plaque mounted on the wall. On it is engraved a commendation from a local hospice agency: "For his compassionate hospice care, this plaque is awarded to Oscar the Cat." Oscar takes a quick drink of water and returns to his desk to curl up for a long rest. His day's work is done. There will be no more deaths today, not in Room 310 or in any other room for that matter. After all, no one dies on the third floor unless Oscar pays a visit and stays a while.

Note: Since he was adopted by staff members as a kitten, Oscar the Cat has had an uncanny ability to predict when residents are about to die. Thus far, he has presided over the deaths of more than 25 residents on the third floor of Steere House Nursing and Rehabilitation Center in Providence, Rhode Island. His mere presence at the bedside is viewed by physicians and nursing home staff as an almost absolute indicator of impending death, allowing staff members to adequately notify families. Oscar has also provided companionship to those who would otherwise have died alone. For his work, he is highly regarded by the physicians and staff at Steere House and by the families of the residents whom he serves.

Source: D. M. Dosa, A day in the life of Oscar the Cat, *New England Journal of Medicine.* July 26, Volume 357, Number 4, pp. 328–329.

A few people even seem to decide on a particular date for their death. Both John Adams and Thomas Jefferson died on July 4, 1826. Mark Twain was born the year Halley's Comet appeared in 1835, and said, "I came in with Halley's Comet, and I expect go out with it." He died in 1910, the year Halley's Comet next appeared in its 75-year cycle.

SUMMARY

- The processes of dying involve the activities, thoughts, and feelings of a person when anticipating his or her own death. End-of-life tasks that can be accomplished while living include completing unfinished business, spending time with loved ones, and resolving old hurts.
- A century ago, most people died from an infectious disease, often within days of onset. Today, how to die well is how to live for months, or even years, knowing that dying is in process.
- Swiss-born Elisabeth Kübler-Ross is considered a pioneer in the study of how people deal with impending death. On the basis of interviews with people dying of cancer, Kübler-Ross wrote her first and best-known book, *On Death and Dying* (1969), in which she outlined her concept of grief as progressing in five stages: denial, anger, bargaining, depression, and acceptance.
- The principal value of Kübler-Ross's work has been the greater public and professional awareness it has generated of a dying person's feelings and thoughts—how to behave toward and treat that person.
- Not all workers in the field agree with the Kübler-Ross model. Some critics believe that the stages are too rigid. Many who work with the dying found her stages not very useful in practice. Also, a major criticism is that her work was based on middle-aged cancer patients and that she did not follow research procedure in her interviews.
- In social death, a person is no longer treated as a member of the group to which he or she belongs. This type of distancing is sometimes inflicted on the dying—at the very time that a feeling of belonging is critical.
- People typically do not choose how quickly or slowly they die. But there is evidence of a terminal drop, or decline in mental function, during the last few months before death, especially among the very old. The death rate drops 35% below normal before a big event and peaks by an equal percentage following a holiday. Such evidence seems to support the belief that people can postpone dying.

ADDITIONAL RESOURCES

Books

Kübler-Ross, E. (1969). *On death and dying.* New York: Touchstone. This first book of Kübler-Ross's was a bestseller that is now considered a classic; after reading this book, families should better understand what's going on as the death of a loved one draws near. It is still required reading in many academic settings, including medical and nursing schools, theological seminaries, and psychology courses.

Among Elisabeth Kübler-Ross's many books, the following also stand out: *Living with Death and Dying*; *Death: The Final Stage of Growth*; *To Live Until We Say Goodbye; On Life After Death*; *On Children and Death; Death Is of Vital Importance;* and *The Wheel of Life* (her autobiography).

Miller, J. E. (1996). *How will I get through the holidays?* Ft. Wayne, IN: Willowgreen. In this book, the author draws upon his experience as a counselor and pastor to offer practical and caring suggestions for dealing with grief, including during holiday times.

Smith, H. I. (1997). *Death and grief: Healing through group support.* Minneapolis, MN: Augsburg Fortress Publishers. Found in this Bible based book is information related to fostering closeness and sharing among grief support group members.

Movie

My Life. (1993). An advertising executive (Michael Keating) learns that he is dying and consequently reexamines his life. Exemplified are the stages of loss described by Kübler-Ross.

CRITICAL THINKING

In the losses you have suffered so far, which of Kübler-Ross's stages of loss have been most prominent in your experience?

Class Activity

Watch the movie *My Life* and write a paper explaining how each of Kübler-Ross's stages are exemplified in the advertising executive's process of dying. Add to the paper a section in which you describe what you might do differently than the executive. Afterwards, share with your classmates what you might do differently and why.

References

Bowlby, J. (1961). Processes of mourning. *International Journal of Psycho-Analysis, 42*, 317–340.

Bowlby, J. (1980). *Attachment and loss, Vol. 3: Loss: Sadness and depression.* New York: Basic Books.

Buckman, R. (1992). *How to break bad news: A guide for health care professionals.* Baltimore: Johns Hopkins University Press.

Bysov, F. (2004). Death is an illusion: A logical explanation based on Martinus' worldview. St. Paul, MN: Paragon House.

Chapman, A. (2006). *Interpretation of Elisabeth Kübler-Ross's five stages of grief.* Retrieved April 30, 2008, from http://www.businessballs.com

Charmaz, K. (1980). *The social reality of death.* Reading, MA: Addison-Wesley.

Clark, J. (2003). Patient-centered death. *Student British Medical Journal, 327*, 174–175.

Corr, C. A. (1993). Coping with dying: Lessons that we should and should not learn from the work of Elisabeth Kübler-Ross. *Death Studies, 17*, 69–83.

Dosa, D. M. (2007). A day in the life of Oscar the cat. *New England Journal of Medicine, 357*(4), 328–329.

Ferrini, A. F., & Ferrini, R. L. (2007). *Health in the later years* (4th ed.). New York: McGraw-Hill.

Kastenbaum R. J. (2004). *Death, society, and human experience* (8th ed). New York: Pearson.

Kaufmann, W. (1976). *Existentialism, religion, and death.* London: New English Library.

Klass, D., & Hutch, R. A. (1985). Elizabeth Kübler-Ross as a religious leader. *Omega: Journal of Death and Dying, 16,* 89–109.

Kübler-Ross, E. (1969). *On death and dying.* New York: Touchstone.

Maciejewski, P. K., Zhang, B., Block, S. D., & Prigerson, H. G. (2007). An empirical examination of the stage theory of grief. *Journal of the American Medical Association, 297*, 716–723.

McNamara, B. (2001). A good enough death. In M. Purdy & D. Banks (Eds.), *The sociology and politics of health.* London: Routledge, 244–257.

Parkes, C. M. (1996). *Bereavement: Studies of grief in adult life* (3rd ed.). London: Routledge.

Payne, S. A., Langley-Evans, A., & Hillier, R. (1996). Perceptions of a good death: A comparative study of the views of hospice staff and patients. *Palliative Medicine, 10*, 307–312.

Phillips D. P., & Smith, D. G. (1990). Postponement of death until symbolically meaningful occasions. *Journal of the American Medical Association, 263*(14), 1947–1951.

Smith, R. (2000). A good death: An important aim for health services and for us all. *British Medical Journal, 320*, 129–130.

Steinhauser, K. E., Christakis, N. A., Clipp, E. C., McNeilly, M., McIntyre, L. M., & Tulsky, J. A. (2000). Factors considered important at the end of life by patients, family, physicians, and other care providers. *Journal of the American Medical Association, 284*, 2476–2482.

Walker, T. (2003). Historical and cultural variants on the good death. *British Medical Journal, 327*, 218–220.

Zlatin, D. M. (1995). Life themes: A method to understand terminal illness. *Omega, 31*, 189–206.

Chapter 8

End-of-Life Issues

Dying is an art, like everything else.
—Sylvia Plath

Objectives

After reading this chapter, you will be able to answer the following questions:

- How are caregivers affected by long-term caregiving?
- What is an advance care directive, and how is one created?
- What various medical procedures can be used to prolong life?
- What is a Do Not Resuscitate (DNR) order, and how is one created?
- What cultural issues affect decision making at the end of life?
- What do most elderly people want at the end of life?
- What spiritual issues come into play at the end of life?
- What is meant by the phrase "ambiguous death"?

As people approach the end of their lives, they and their families commonly face many decisions and tasks (APA Working Group, 2007), including:

- what kind of care they want or need;
- whether they want care at home or in an institutional setting;
- the degree of family involvement in decision making and care; and
- legal decisions about wills, advance directives, and durable powers of attorney.

Who Gives Care?

Most caregiving is provided by family members in the home. Half of elders with no family are in institutions, but only 7% of elders with a family caregiver are in institutions (Ferrini & Ferrini, 1999).

From 59% to as many as 75% of caregivers are women (Arno, 2002). Another might be the fact that many men, at least of past generations, viewed caregiving as "woman's work." Yet, after caring for children, aging parents, and an aging husband, a woman often is left alone, with no family to care for her.

Adults who take care of elderly parents report a wide range of emotions (see Table 8.1). Most of

Table 8.1 EMOTIONAL RESPONSES OF ADULTS CARING FOR ELDERLY PARENTS

Emotion	Percent (%)
Loving	96
Appreciated	90
Proud	85
Hopeful	78
Worried	53
Frustrated	37
Sad/Depressed	28
Overwhelmed	22

Source: Modified from Kaiser Family Foundation, National survey on health care and other elder care issues, 2000. Available at www.kff.org/mediapartnerships/loader.cfm?url=/commonspot/security/getfile.cfm&PageID=13426

these emotions are positive, but sometimes caretakers can feel good and bad at the same time.

Caregiving Stress

Whether the caregiver is male or female, the emotional stress and physical strain of caregiving can take its toll. In a survey by the National Institute on Aging (2000), more than twice as many women as men caretakers reported physical strains, and 30% of women caretakers reported being emotionally stressed, compared to 13% of men. These stressors also were reported as causes of mental health problems for caretakers by 17% of women and 9% of men.

Women live longer, so caring for them lasts longer. Caregivers, especially of women, therefore might become very fatigued. If caregivers begin feeling "forced" to do routine tasks and wish to be someplace else, they are probably experiencing caregiver burnout. If so, finding someone who can help the caregiver discuss her feelings can be helpful. Joining a caregiver support group is ideal.

Both those receiving care and their caregivers may experience mental health problems such as depression. More than half of caregivers are clinically depressed, and caregivers who experience mental or emotional strain associated with depression have a higher risk of dying than do noncaregivers (Family Caregiver Alliance, 2003). In general, depression among men is believed to have more negative effects, including death, than for women. Elderly women may have more depression, but it is not associated with death as strongly as it is for men.

Many caretakers lose friends, become ill, experience exhaustion, become anxious, or are physically or verbally abused by the elder person for whom they are caretaking. Even with enough money to secure outside-the-home caretakers and hospitalization, surviving the caretaking experience can be psychologically draining, especially if the elder is a manipulating, enraged person.

Caregiving Expense

Financial strains present problems for many unpaid family caretakers. Obvious expenses include food and medicine. Other expenses not paid by insurance might include grab bars or shower seats, wheelchairs, railings, call device systems, and outside ramps. Another expense can be hiring a cook, which is most often done by male caretakers. In addition to caregiving, men of earlier generations considered cooking, along with shopping and housework, to be "woman's work." Younger men are less concerned about chores divided by gender.

Men Needing Care

In old age, many men, who once believed they were "in charge," find themselves needing help. An older man might have the attitude, "I don't need help from anyone. If I have a problem, I'll take care of it." Upon needing help in old age, the same man might say, "For the first time in my life I don't know how or where to go to fix the problem I have." Older men's reluctance or bafflement might be the first issues with which caregivers must deal.

Elderly men in need of caretakers are likely to have one or more disabling conditions: arthritis (17.1%), heart trouble (11.1%), high blood pressure (5.2%), diabetes (3.9%), blindness and other visual problems (3.6%), and deafness or hearing troubles (2.6%). These conditions can occur along with heart disease, cancer, and stroke (U.S. Department of Health and Human Services, 2000).

Jacqueline Marcell's Experience

Jacqueline Marcell (2000) was a busy television executive who attempted to hire caregivers to help her take care of her aging parents. Marcell said that she could not get caregivers to stay because her 85-year-old, 185-pound father, who suffered from dementia and rage, would physically throw them out of the house.

Eventually, Marcell's father even choked her! He was taken to a psychiatric hospital four times for violent behavior. He was released each time because he would "act normal" in front of the doctors. As Marcell said, "Demented does not mean stupid."

Unlike elderly women, elderly men's perceptions of their health turn out to be good predictors of their risk of death. For example, elderly men who rated their health as fair or poor were nearly five times more likely to die than men who rated their health very good or excellent. This research result indicates that men have an accurate "feel" for any potentially life-threatening conditions (Benjamin, Leventhal, & Leventhal, 2000).

End-of-Life Decisions and Tasks

As life comes to an end, some people reflect on the meaning of life; conduct a life review or deal with unfinished business; and/or plan rituals for before or after death (APA Working Group, 2007). In some religious traditions, end-of-life activities include confession of sins, preparation to "meet one's maker," or asking forgiveness from others. Medical decision making often is the most challenging end-of-life task. For example, in Western medicine, individual autonomy and informed consent are primary. By contrast, in many cultures interactive family or community decision making is the ideal. In some cultural traditions, planning or even discussing death is viewed as inviting it (Carrese & Rhodes, 2000).

Discontinuing life-extending treatment for a critically ill person might seem to be a simple decision, particularly if it is based on the medical conclusion that further intervention will not

Two Responses to Needing Care

Kathleen Lavanchy, director of counseling for caregivers in a small Pennsylvania town, recalled a situation in which a nephew promised his aunt that she would not have to go to a nursing home. The aunt's care fell to the nephew's wife. The wife was taking care of a belligerent old woman who kept saying, "I don't like what you feed me. I'm too cold. I'm too hot." One day, the wife snapped and slapped the aunt. That action was not typical for the wife; she just acted out of frustration and tiredness before she had a chance to think rationally.

For his book, *Tuesdays with Morrie*, Mitch Albom (1997) interviewed his former college professor, Morrie Schwartz, who was dying. Schwartz had reached the stage of his disease where, except for breathing and swallowing, he was dependent on others. At first, he said that he was ashamed, because American culture says that "people should be ashamed if they cannot wipe our own behinds." Then, he said that he decided to enjoy his dependency. When caretakers turned him on his side to rub cream on him, or when they wiped his brow or massaged his legs, he said, "It seems very familiar to me. It's like going back to being a child again. We all know how to be a child. It's inside all of us. For me, it's just remembering how to enjoy it." At age 78, Morrie Schwartz had made the best out of what life he had left.

improve quality of life and only prolong dying. That decision, however, might be influenced by the emotional state of family members and the dying person. Family members might oppose a physician's recommendation to discontinue life support, or they might disagree among themselves about what future treatment should be used.

Other factors that complicate a decision about continuing life support include legal or ethical issues, and issues of resource allocation. Some regard discontinuance of life support as a social good, as well as good for individuals and family. Others warn of using cost as a motive, which discriminates against those among the dying whose resources are limited.

Advance Care Directives

Do you want to make sure your wishes for your last days are honored? One way is to create an **advance care directive** (APA Working Group, 2007). After you no longer can decide on your care, the directive tells family and healthcare providers what you want. An advance care directive should contain the following:

- Descriptions of when you want, and do not want, treatment
- What extraordinary measures (if any) you want taken to preserve life
- What kind of pain management you want at the end
- Instructions regarding organ donation and permission to perform an autopsy

Advance directives, however, are not a cure-all; they also present problems. For instance, many people do not prepare advance directives because they do not want to think about death. Or, the directions specified by an individual might not be followed by his or her family members. Moreover, advance directives might go against the values of many cultural and religious communities or against the duties that dying persons and their families perceive they have.

Other unexpected wrinkles in the application of advance directives include:

- What a person wants in the way of life-sustaining medical treatments can change over time.
- People might be unable to predict what their preferences will be after their health becomes impaired.
- Terminally ill people in hospice care sometimes want to live and sometimes not.
- Depression and presence or absence of family support can affect the refusal of life-sustaining treatment.

Given these possible complications, healthcare providers, in dealing with patients who have advance directives, must be sensitive to the:

- limitations of an advance directive for a particular individual over time.
- need for continuing attention to the desires and needs of dying people and their loved ones.
- possibility that a directive might conflict with a person's values and traditions.

Advance directives include two legal documents. They include the Directive to Physician and Family or Surrogates (living will) and the Medical Power of Attorney (or healthcare proxy; Caring Connections, 2007).

In a **living will** (also referred to, in general, as an *advance care directive*), medical personnel (at a time when the individual might be incapacitated) are instructed to withdraw or withhold life-prolonging treatments. In a **durable power of attorney**, or *healthcare proxy*, another person is designated to make such decisions. To be honored, these documents need to be in writing. A notary or a lawyer is not required to draft the documents. All that is needed is two witnesses to the signature. The requirements for these witnesses are fully explained in the instructions for completing the documents.

These documents were devised to help resolve the basic conflict between medical and health professionals who feel an obligation to prolong the lives of others and those who believe that an individual has a right to choose his or her destiny (Cicirelli, 1998). At least one form of advance directive is now available in all 50 states (Choice in Dying, 1993).

Through such instruments and the force of the 1991 Patient Self Determination Act (Kastenbaum, 2004), society has acknowledged patients' rights to withdraw or withhold treatments. Many people in society still frown on suicide, although the suicide rate has been increasing among the elderly (Kastenbaum & Kastenbaum, 1993; "Suicide rate among the elderly climbs by 9% over 12 years," 1996).

Living Will

A living will (see Figure 8.1) is used to inform loved ones and healthcare team members of the patient's wishes about medical treatment when that patient is no longer able to speak for him- or herself. (In this situation, the medical power of attorney is used to appoint a person who will speak for the patient.) Before a living will can take effect, two physicians must certify that the patient is unable to make medical decisions and is in the medical condition specified in the state's living will law (such as "terminal illness" or "permanent unconsciousness"). Other requirements might also apply, depending on the state.

Medical Power of Attorney

A **medical power of attorney**, or *healthcare proxy*, is used to appoint a person to act as the patient's healthcare agent (or surrogate decision maker). This person is then authorized to make medical decisions on the patient's behalf. An individual is allowed to write his or her own healthcare proxy (see Figure 8.2 for an example). Before a medical power of attorney goes into effect, a physician must conclude that the patient is unable to make medical decisions. In addition, if the patient

Figure 8.1 EXAMPLE OF A LIVING WILL.

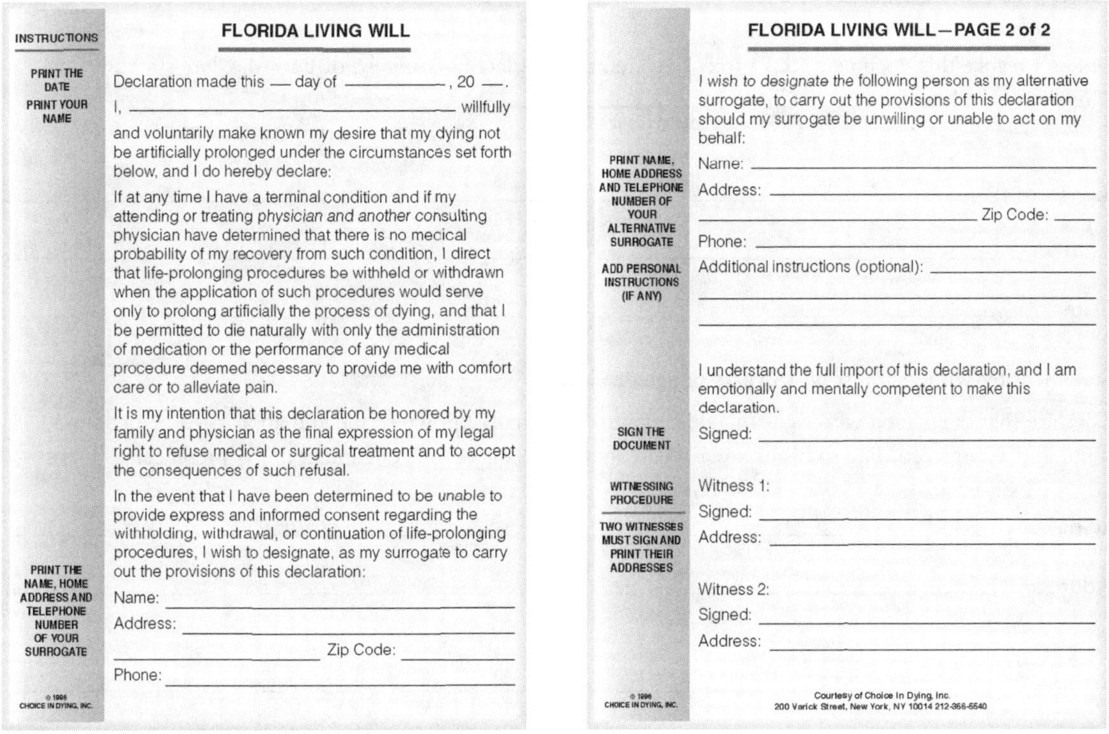

INSTRUCTIONS

FLORIDA LIVING WILL

PRINT THE DATE

PRINT YOUR NAME

Declaration made this ___ day of __________, 20 ___.

I, ______________________________ willfully and voluntarily make known my desire that my dying not be artificially prolonged under the circumstances set forth below, and I do hereby declare:

If at any time I have a terminal condition and if my attending or treating *physician and another* consulting physician have determined that there is no mecical probability of my recovery from such condition, I direct that life-prolonging procedures be withheld or withdrawn when the application of such procedures would serve only to prolong artificially the process of dying, and that I be permitted to die naturally with only the administration of medication or the performance of any medical procedure deemed necessary to provide me with comfort care or to alleviate pain.

It is my intention that this declaration be honored by my family and physician as the final expression of my legal right to refuse medical or surgical treatment and to accept the consequences of such refusal.

In the event that I have been determined to be *unable* to provide express and informed consent regarding the withholding, withdrawal, or continuation of life-prolonging procedures, I wish to designate, as my surrogate to carry out the provisions of this declaration:

PRINT THE NAME, HOME ADDRESS AND TELEPHONE NUMBER OF YOUR SURROGATE

Name: ______________________________

Address: ______________________________

______________________________ Zip Code: __________

Phone: ______________________________

© 1996 CHOICE IN DYING, INC.

FLORIDA LIVING WILL—PAGE 2 of 2

I wish to designate the following person as my alternative surrogate, to carry out the provisions of this declaration should my surrogate be unwilling or unable to act on my behalf:

PRINT NAME, HOME ADDRESS AND TELEPHONE NUMBER OF YOUR ALTERNATIVE SURROGATE

Name: ______________________________

Address: ______________________________

______________________________ Zip Code: ______

Phone: ______________________________

ADD PERSONAL INSTRUCTIONS (IF ANY)

Additional instructions (optional): ______________________________

____

____

I understand the full import of this declaration, and I am emotionally and mentally competent to make this declaration.

SIGN THE DOCUMENT

Signed: ______________________________

WITNESSING PROCEDURE

TWO WITNESSES MUST SIGN AND PRINT THEIR ADDRESSES

Witness 1:

Signed: ______________________________

Address: ______________________________

Witness 2:

Signed: ______________________________

Address: ______________________________

© 1996 CHOICE IN DYING, INC.

Courtesy of Choice In Dying, Inc.
200 Varick Street, New York, NY 10014 212-366-5540

Figure 8.2 EXAMPLE OF A HEALTHCARE PROXY FORM.

I, ________________________________, hereby appoint ________________________________
(name, home address, and phone number)
as the healthcare agent who will make any and all healthcare decisions for me. This proxy takes effect if/when I become unable to make my own healthcare decisions.

Optional instructions: I direct this agent to make healthcare decisions only in accord with my wishes and limitations as stated below.

____

____

____

(If your agent does not know your wishes about artificial nutrition and feeding tubes, he or she will not be allowed to make those decisions.)

Name of substitute person if person I appoint (name above) is unable, unwilling, or unavailable to act as my healthcare agent.

____
(name, home address, and phone number)

Unless I revoke this document, this proxy shall remain in effect indefinitely, or until the date stated below. This proxy shall expire ________________________________.
(specific date if desired)

Signature ____

Address ____

Date ____

Statement by Witness (must be 18 years of age or older)

I declare that the person who signs this document is personally known to me and appears to be of sound mind and acting according to his/her own free will. He/she signed this document in my presence.

Witness 1 ____

Address ____

Witness 2 ____

Address ____

EMTs and Advance Directives

EMTs (emergency medical technicians) are not allowed to abide by advance directives. They must do what is necessary to stabilize a person on the way to a hospital. Only after a physician evaluates the patient's condition and determines underlying conditions can an advance directive be followed.

regains the ability to make decisions, the agent cannot continue to act on his or her behalf.

Many states have additional requirements that apply only to decisions about life-sustaining medical treatments. For example, before an agent can refuse a life-sustaining treatment on a patient's behalf, a second physician might have to confirm the first doctor's assessment that the patient is incapable of making treatment decisions.

Who Should Have an Advance Care Directive?

Advance directives are not just for the elderly. (See the case of Terri Schiavo, described in Chapter 5.) You could be involved in a car accident that leaves you in a coma. Would anyone know your wishes? Maybe you would want everything tried, even if you are unlikely to live.

Maybe your ethnic/cultural background dictates the outcome. For example, in the African American population, people generally want aggressive treatment, even if it means feeding tubes, pain, or financial drain, because doing everything is a sign of respect (Cloud, 2000).

Maybe you would refuse life-extending measures for fear of prolonged suffering or financially draining your family. If, in the end, there is nothing left to do, you might want at least to be made comfortable. Whatever your wish, be sure to make it known.

When Do Advance Care Directives Apply?

Advance directives are legally valid in every state (Caring Connections, 2007). An advance directive becomes valid as soon as it is signed in front of the required witnesses. The laws governing advance directives vary from state to state (as do the titles in some cases), so it is important to complete one that complies with the law in your state.

An advance directive created in one state might not be recognized and followed in another state. Some states do honor advance directives from other states; others will honor out-of-state advance directives as long as they are similar to the state's own law; and some states do not have a policy in place. If you spend a significant amount of time in more than one state, it is advisable to complete the forms for each state. State-specific advance directives are available at www.caringinfo.org.

Advance directives do not expire; they remain in effect until changed. Nevertheless, it is a good idea to review your advance directive periodically to make sure it still matches what you want. To make any changes, you should complete a new directive.

Preparing an Advance Care Directive

Before you prepare a directive:

- Find out what types of life-sustaining treatments are available.
- Decide what types of treatment you want or do not want.
- Share your wishes and preferences with others involved.

Read all of the instructions carefully to make sure you have included all of the necessary information and that your documents are properly witnessed. In most states, you can include special requests, such as organ donation, cremation, or burial. Inform your physician and loved ones of your specific requests so that appropriate arrangements can be made. When you are finished completing the documents, ask someone to look them over to make sure that you have filled them out correctly.

After your advance directive is completed and signed, make several photocopies. Give copies to your agent and alternate agent. Note on the photocopies the location where the originals are kept. Keep the original documents in a safe but easily accessible place, and tell others where they are placed. Do not keep advance directives in a safe-deposit box. Other people might need access to them.

Be sure your doctor(s) has/have copies of your advance directives, and give copies to everyone who might be involved with your health care, such as your family, clergy, or friends. Your local hospital also may be willing to file your advance directives in case you are admitted in the future.

It is important that anyone who might be involved in your care at end of life be aware of your wishes. Many people who have been nominated to help or take charge did not know they were picked (Cloud, 2000).

Notify family members, loved ones, and your healthcare providers. You want them to know how you want to be treated at the end of life.

Life-Sustaining Treatments

The most common end-of-life medical decisions made are those involving medical procedures to keep a person alive, such as cardiopulmonary resuscitation (CPR), intubation, and artificial nutrition and hydration (Caring Connections, 2007).

As explained in Chapter 2, cardiopulmonary resuscitation (CPR) is a group of procedures used on a person when the heart stops (cardiac arrest) or breathing stops (respiratory arrest). For **cardiac arrest**, the treatment might be chest compressions, electrical stimulation, or use of medication. For **respiratory arrest**, treatment might include **intubation**, insertion of a tube connected to a mechanical ventilator through the mouth or nose into the trachea (windpipe that connects the throat to the lungs).

Performing CPR can be risky. The success rate is extremely low in very ill persons. Even successful CPR usually produces additional problems such as broken bones (from chest compression), brain damage, or dependency on a ventilator. Therefore, it is very important to think about these possible complications in advance.

Artificial nutrition and **hydration** are processes whereby a person is given nutrition (food) and hydration (fluid) when they can no longer be taken by mouth. The most common forms are:

- **Intravenous (IV) fluids:** A chemically balanced mix of nutrients and fluids given to a person using an intravenous catheter (a tube and needle placed into a vein).
- **Nasogastric tube:** Flexible plastic tube placed directly through the nose into the stomach by way of the esophagus.
- **Gastrostomy:** Making a small incision through the abdomen and placing a flexible plastic tube into the stomach.

Common side effects of artificial nutrition include:

- Damage to the inside of the nose, esophagus, stomach, or intestine
- Infections of the skin or in the stomach or intestines
- Imbalances of electrolytes (important chemicals in the bloodstream) in the body due to fluid overload
- Nausea and diarrhea
- Bloating, cramping, or vomiting
- Cough or pneumonia

Do Not Resuscitate Orders

A **DNR (Do Not Resuscitate)** order is a written physician's order not to initiate CPR. The physician writes and signs a DNR at the patient's request or at the request of the family or appointed healthcare agent, if expressed in a patient's living will. If a person requests a DNR order, the physician might ask if a "do-not-intubate" order is also desired. Refusal of intubation does not mean refusal of other techniques of resuscitation. DNR orders can be canceled at any time by letting the doctor who signed the DNR know that the patient has changed his or her mind.

DNRs remain in effect after transfer from one healthcare facility to another, depending on the arrival facility's policy. The DNR might not be honored, however, if the patient is discharged from the facility to home, if the state does not have an out-of-hospital DNR policy. DNRs should be posted in the home if that is where a person is receiving care. DNRs might not be followed during surgery, so that should be discussed with the surgeon and anesthesiologist before surgery.

Cultural Issues at the End of Life

Cross-cultural communication becomes especially important when dealing with end-of-life issues. For example, decision making might be very difficult for a patient who believes that someone else should make decisions about issues such as withholding resuscitation efforts. In many cultures, decision-making power for family members is given to the member of highest status, which may be the eldest male.

Kagawa-Singer and Blackhall (2001) identified issues related to end-of-life care that may be influenced by cultural beliefs and should be taken into account by healthcare professionals:

- Religion and spirituality should be acknowledged and respected.
- An increased desire for futile care at the end of life may exist, and possibly a lack of interest in hospice services, because of an underlying concern that not all the best options are being offered.
- People in many cultures believe that informing the patient of a terminal diagnosis may hasten death. Thus, an agreement needs to be reached between the physician and the patient and patient's family on withholding a terminal diagnosis. Questions to ask a patient include: "How much do you want to know about your illness?" or "Do you prefer that I discuss (or not discuss) your diagnosis with you or with your family?"

Different forms of grief expression also need to be understood. For example, loud wailing at the death of a loved one is common in some Middle Eastern cultures (Galanti, 1997). Beliefs regarding postmortem testing also are shaped by cultural norms. For example, both Orthodox Jewish and Muslim family members might not be willing to consent to an autopsy.

What Do Elderly People Want at End of Life?

As life expectancy increases, many older people suffer physical pain, mental suffering, immobility, and significant dependency. Some consider these conditions so repugnant that death is seen as a welcome alternative (Corr, Nabe, & Corr, 1997). Given this consideration, systematically determining older people's preferences for various end-of-life choices can offer a basis for helping them make better actual end-of-life decisions (Cicirelli, 1998).

Despite all the media attention on assisted suicide and euthanasia, slightly over half of older people questioned wanted to continue living for as long as possible, regardless of a poor quality of life or a terminal condition. This preference seems not to be related to a religious affiliation (Cicirelli, 1998).

Nearly a third of elders would give the decision to continue or end their lives to someone else. These elders are willing to place one of their most important decisions in the hands of others whom they trust (family, friends, or physicians), reflecting a strong need to depend on others to make complex decisions (High, 1993). A significant minority of elders reported that they would prefer to take active steps to end their lives rather than continue living with a quality of life unbearably low. Apparently a life without quality or dignity was seen by these elders as not worth living (Cicirelli, 1998). (See Table 8.2.)

The lesson here is that healthcare counselors who work with older adults should explore all the available end-of-life choices with a patient and significant others or family members—and do so while the patient feels reasonably well. More than one-third of

Table 8.2 ELDER END-OF-LIFE CHOICES

Choice	Percent in Favor
Try to continue living	52
Refuse or withdraw treatment	47
Let someone close decide what is best	36
Let a physician or someone else make the decision to end their life	19
Ask someone else to help them take their own life	12
Ask someone else to end their life	12
It is ok to take their own life	7

Note: Percentages total more than 100% because participants tended to find more than one option acceptable.

Source: Cicirelli (1998).

elders who made "do not resuscitate" decisions on entering a hospital rescinded them after they get better (Potter, Stewart, & Duncan, 1994). This decision reversal suggests that counselors should record preferences before the patient becomes very ill and depressed or otherwise highly emotional.

Why is it important for counselors to spend time with people at the end of life? One reason is that when doctors spend 10 minutes more than they normally do listening to the families of people dying in an ICU and provide them with a brochure on bereavement, those family members were less likely to suffer from stress, anxiety, or depression after the death of the loved one (Lautrette et al., 2007).

If you have a family member in crisis, and the doctor or healthcare team does not approach you, be proactive by asking for a meeting with the doctors and nurses involved and have all important family members present. Also, come prepared to talk about what the goals of care should be and talk about the loved one's values, including what kind of functional outcome he or she would want. Good communication helps everyone understand the available options and what to expect (Lilly & Daly, 2007).

Spiritual Issues at the End of Life

Among the common fears and concerns of people nearing the end of life is reconciling their spiritual selves. These concerns are shared by family and caregivers (GP Clinical, 2004). For many patients and family members, spiritual (not necessarily religious) issues become important as the end nears. The more open family, caregivers, and medical staff are regarding discussing spiritual issues, the more willing patients are to talk about them. The medical team especially should be aware of these issues, as they bear on each patient, so as to integrate spiritual care with health care. It might be helpful for a chaplain or spiritual counselor to call on the patient, especially toward the end, if the patient asks for it. A chaplain also can help a patient make treatment decisions, for example, about how long he or she wants medical intervention.

Ambiguous Dying

Up until the twentieth century, little could be done medically to affect the process of dying (Bern-Klug, Gessert, & Forbes, 2001). Within a week of serious injury or the onset of serious illness, a person either died or recovered (Tilden, Tone, Nelson, Thompson, & Eggman, 1999). The move from home to hospital for end-of-life care and treatment has led to the development of hospice and palliative care to make dying easier and more dignified.

This shift has made it more difficult, however, to determine when the end of life begins and, thus, who would benefit from end-of-life care (Bern-Klug, 2004). People who die in advanced old age often have multiple chronic conditions, all of which can affect the nature and timing of dying. They are more likely to have lived months or years in a state of vulnerable frailty.

Many people assume their doctor will tell them when they are at the end of life, but this does not always happen. Not only that, most people avoid admitting they are dying until death is upon them, and thus, they do not complete important tasks, make plans for dispersing resources, seek for spiritual meaning, or complete important relationships, and forfeit the help and palliative care otherwise available to the dying.

Even living wills do not always work as designed. Because many people will never be declared terminal, their living will might never be invoked or it might be invoked just hours or days before they die. Advance directives, in general, are not consulted until patients are seen as "absolutely hopelessly ill" or "actively dying" (Teno, Stevens, Spernak, & Lynn, 1998, p. 442). Teno and colleagues thus recommended advance care planning (a series of discussions over time with the patient, family, and doctors and other healthcare professionals), based on understanding that it might not be clear how close the person is to death. Discussions about peace of mind can be important. A person's sense of being sick or being terminally ill also can affect how care is planned.

What else can help dying patients and their families? Give clients and families the opportunity to express the feelings of frustration, anxiety, bewilderment, despair, uncertainty, and grief often associated with an ambiguous prognosis or advisability of medical interventions as the end of life draws near. Some families might find that speaking with a member of the clergy, a counselor, or a good friend will help them and the patient make the transition to dying (Welk, 1996).

Summary

- As people approach the end of their lives, they, as well as their family members, commonly face many decisions and tasks. One decision to be made is what kind of care they want or need, including whether they want care at home or in an institutional setting.
- From 59% to as many as 75% of caregivers are women. The emotional stress and physical strain of caregiving can take a toll on caregivers, especially women caregivers. Financial strains also can present problems for unpaid family caretakers.
- In some religious traditions, end-of-life activities include confession of sins, preparation to "meet one's maker," or asking forgiveness from others. Medical decisions often are the most challenging. For example, in Western medicine individual autonomy and informed consent are primary. By contrast, in many cultures interactive, family or community decision making is the ideal. In some cultural traditions, planning or even discussing death is viewed as inviting it.
- In an advance care directive, family and healthcare providers are informed about what a patient wants once he or she is no longer able to direct his or her health care. In an advance care directive, when treatment should be provided or withheld is presented, as are what extraordinary measures (if any) should be taken to preserve a person's life; what kind of pain management is desired; instructions as to organ donation; and permission to perform an autopsy.
- A DNR (Do Not Resuscitate) order is a written physician's order not to initiate CPR. DNR is implemented at the patient's direct request or from instructions contained in his/her living will. A DNR order can be canceled at any time. They remain in effect after transfer from one healthcare facility to another, depending on the arrival facility's policy. They may not be honored on discharge to home, however, if the state does not have an out-of-hospital DNR policy. In addition, a DNR might not be followed during surgery. Also, DNR orders do not automatically include a "do-not-intubate" order.
- Cross-cultural communication is important when dealing with end-of-life issues. For many patients and family members, spiritual (not necessarily religious) issues become important as the end nears.

Additional Resources

Books

Preston, T. (2000). *Final victory: Taking charge of your life when you know the end is near.* Rocklin, CA: Prima Publishing. In clear language aimed at patients, family members, and their friends, Preston explains how to create a peaceful end through a living will, designation of durable power of attorney, and candid conversations with one's family and doctor, as well as how to plan for the death of a terminally ill child.

Wanzer, S. H. (2007). *To die well: Your right to comfort, calm, and choice in the last days of life.* NY: Da Capo. In this book, the rights of patients are outlined, including advice about how to appoint a healthcare proxy and how to refuse unwanted treatments. Wanzer supports hospice care and focuses on minimizing pain and making patients comfortable. Also emphasized in this book is the need to differentiate between a rational decision to end life and suicidal depression.

Movie

The Bucket List. (2007). In this movie, the tale is humorously told of two terminally ill men, who escape from a cancer ward and head off on a road trip with a wish list of to-dos before they die.

CRITICAL THINKING

1. Provide three reasons why you would (or would not) want a doctor to tell a loved one that he or she has a terminal illness with only a short time to live.
2. Give three reasons why you would (or would not) want a doctor to tell *you* that you have a terminal illness and how long you are expected to live.

CLASS ACTIVITIES

1. Discuss how each class member feels about preparing a living will.
2. Invite to class, and interview, an EMT or emergency room worker about his or her experience with resuscitations. Ask if he or she recommends or does not recommend DNRs.

REFERENCES

Albom, M. (1997). *Tuesdays with Morrie.* New York: Doubleday.

APA Working Group. (2007). *Assisted suicide and end-of-life decisions.* Washington: DC: American Psychological Association.

Arno, P. S. (2002, February). *The economic value of informal caregiving, U.S., 2000.* Paper presented at the annual meeting of the American Association for Geriatric Psychiatry, Florida.

Benjamin, Y., Leventhal, E. A., & Leventhal, H. (2000). Gender differences in processing information for making self-assessments of health. *Psychosomatic Medicine, 62*, 354–364.

Bern-Klug, M. (2004). The ambiguous dying syndrome. *Health and Social Work, 29*(1), 55–65.

Bern-Klug, M., Gessert, C., & Forbes, S. (2001). The need to revise assumptions about the end of life at the beginning of the 21st century: Implications for social work practice. *Health & Social Work, 26*(1), 38–48.

Caring Connections. (2007). *National Hospice and Palliative Care Organization, 2007.* Alexandria, VA: NHPCO. Retrieved May 1, 2008, from www.caringinfo.org

Carrese, J. A., & Rhodes, L. A. (2000). Bridging cultural differences in medical practice. The case of discussing negative information with Navajo patients. *Journal of General Internal Medicine, 15*(2), 92–96.

Choice in Dying. (1993). *State statutes governing living wills and appointment of health care agents.* New York: Choice in Dying, Inc.

Cicirelli, V. G. (1998). Views of elderly people concerning end-of-life decisions (Abstract). *Journal of Applied Gerontology, 17*(2), 186–197.

Cloud, J. (2000, September 10). A kinder, gentler death. *Time.* Retrieved May 1, 2008, from http://www.time.com/time/magazine/article/0,9171,997968,00.html

Corr, C. A., Nabe, C. M., & Corr, D. M. (1997). *Dead and dying, life and living* (2nd ed.). Pacific Grove, CA: Brooks/Cole.

Family Caregiver Alliance. (2003). *Women and caregiving: Facts and figures.* Retrieved May 1, 2008, from www.caregiver.org/caregiver/jsp/content_node.jsp?nodeid=892

Ferrini, A. F., & Ferrini, R. L. (2000). *Health in the later years* (3rd ed). New York: McGraw-Hill.

Galanti, G. (1997). *Caring for patients from different cultures.* Philadelphia: University of Pennsylvania Press.

GP Clinical. (2004, October 22). Palliative care in motor neuron disease. *GP Magazine,* 61.

High, D. M. (1993). Why are elderly people not using advance directives? *Journal of Aging and Health, 5*(4), 497–515.

Kagawa-Singer, M., & Blackhall, L. J. (2001). Negotiating cross-cultural issues at the end of life: "You got to go where he lives." *Journal of the American Medical Association, 286*, 2993–3001.

Kaiser Family Foundation. (2000). *National survey on health care and other elder care issues.* Retrieved May 1, 2008, from www.kff.org/mediapartnerships/loader.cfm?url=/commonspot/security/getfile.cfm&PageID=13426

Kastenbaum, R., & Kastenbaum, B. (1993). *Encyclopedia of death.* New York: Avon.

Kastenbaum, R. J. (2004). *Death, society, and human experience* (8th ed.). New York: Pearson.

Lautrette, A., Darmon, M., Megarbane, B., Joly, L. M., Chevret, S., Adrie, C., et al. (2007). A communication strategy and brochure for relatives of patients dying in the ICU. *New England Journal of Medicine, 356*(5), 469–478.

Lilly, C. M., & Daly, B. J. (2007). Editorial: "The healing power of listening in the ICU." *New England Journal of Medicine, 356*(5), 513–515.

Marcell, J. (2000). *Elder rage, or take my father . . . please! How to survive caregiving aging parents.* Irvine, CA: Impressive Press.

National Institute on Aging. (2000). Caregiving: Helping the elderly with activity limitations. *National Academy on an Aging Society,* 7(5), 1–6.

Potter, J. M., Stewart, D., & Duncan, G. (1994). Living wills: Would sick people change their minds? *Postgraduate Medical Journal, 70*, 818–820.

Suicide rate among elderly climbs by 9% over 12 years. (1996, January 12). *New York Times*, p. A11.

Teno, J. M., Stevens, M., Spernak, S., & Lynn, J. (1998). Role of written advanced directives in decision making: Insights from qualitative and quantitative data. *Journal of General Internal Medicine, 13*(7), 439–446.

Tilden, V. P., Tone, S. W., Nelson, C. A., Thompson, M., & Eggman, S. C. (1999). Family decision making in foregoing life-extending treatments. *Journal of Family Nursing,* 5(4), 426–442.

U.S. Department of Health and Human Services. (2000). *Healthy people 2010*. Washington, DC: Government Printing Office.

Welk, T. (1996, January–February). Ministering to those in the dying role. *Healing Ministry,* 6–8.

Chapter 9

Death of a Loved One

Even the death of friends will inspire us as much as their lives . . .
Their memories will be encrusted over with sublime and pleasing thoughts,
as monuments of other men are overgrown with moss;
for our friends have no place in the graveyard.
—Henry David Thoreau

Objectives

After reading this chapter, you will be able to answer the following questions:

- How are people typically affected by the death of a parent?
- How are people typically affected by a death of a spouse/partner?
- How are people typically affected by the death of a child?
- How are people typically affected by the death of friend?
- How are people typically affected by the death of a pet?

Throughout history, people have had a hard time imagining that a family member could die. But each year approximately 8 million people in the United States experience the death of a parent, child, sibling, or grandparent ("Divorce and Death," 2008). Many others lose a friend to death. Finally, the death of a pet, which might seem inconsequential to some people, is typically a cause for real grief on the part of the person who lost the pet.

Death of a Parent

Almost everyone must deal with the death of a parent sooner or later, but most typically hope that it comes later. Yet, by the age of 18, approximately 2 million young people in the United States have had a parent die (Christ, 2001).

Worldwide, 13.4 million children have lost one or both parents to AIDS. This phenomenon has hit particularly hard in Africa, home to 95% of those

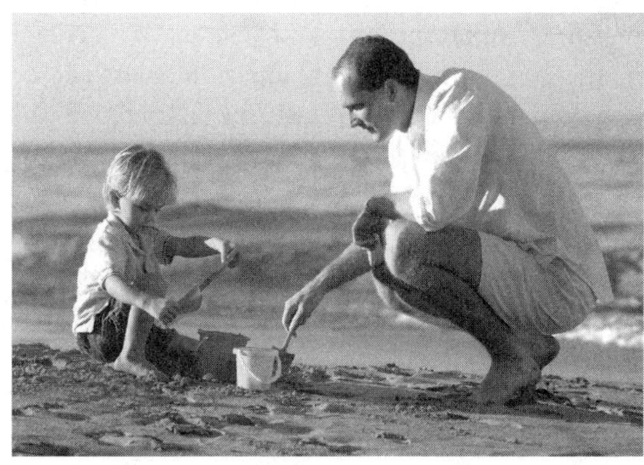

dying from AIDS, even though it has only 10% of the world's population (Glasser, 2004).

Impact of Parental Death

The death of a parent is considered to be the worst thing that can happen in a child's life. Particularly, the death of a parent seems to hit very young children (under 5) and adolescents the hardest (Fristad, Jedel, Weller, & Weller, 1993). Children who lose a parent to death can develop an internal sense of the parent's presence. They might silently talk to that image at times of stress or joy (Jellinek, 2003).

Most children who lose a parent to death experience sadness, grief, and despair. Some children exhibit stronger symptoms, such as anxiety, depression, angry outbursts, and developmental regression. The latter is worst for children who are already emotionally disturbed, whose parent died from trauma or suicide, and whose surviving parent is having difficulty dealing with the death of a spouse (Cerel, Fristad, Verducci, Weller, & Weller, 2006; Dowdney, 2000; Pfeffer, Karus, Siegel, & Hang, 2000).

The less depressed a surviving parent is, the better is the child's recovery from losing a parent. Socioeconomic status also is a factor in a child's recovery, perhaps because intensifying financial struggles after parental death cause additional stress on survivors. Anticipation of death seems not to be a factor for children's recovery. A sudden death is shocking, but living with a dying parent is equally stressful (Cerel et al., 2006).

Even if a child seems to adjust to a parent's death, trouble can emerge later. As the child matures, important family life events (remarriage of the surviving parent, graduation, marriage of the grown child, and so on) can trigger delayed grief and renewed difficulties in adjusting (Raveis, Siegel, & Karus, 1999).

The process of mourning the death of a parent for children aged 9 to 14 is more complex than it is for younger children. Many of these children feel overwhelmed by emotional pain. To deal with it, they sometimes bury their feelings, are unwilling to talk about the death, and escape by doing familiar things and being with friends.

The avoidance and self-centeredness of adolescents 12 to 14 years of age is sometimes the hardest thing with which surviving parents must cope. For example, a 13-year-old, when told her father was dying, went to a party. "What was I supposed to do?" she asked her mother, "stay home and cry?" (Christ, 2000). Most adolescents do not want to know the nature of a fatal illness or talk about a parent's death. They miss the parent but hate the idea of showing emotion.

Adolescents 15 to 17 years of age mourn like adults, but not for as long. They can be supportive of the surviving parent. "I'm trying to deal with two things at once—help my mom and help myself. It's hard, but I'm toughing it out," said one boy, age 16 (Christ, 2000).

For children of college age who have lost a parent, differences arise on some counts, but not others. When it comes to psychological distress, young women and men essentially suffer in the same ways. But many females engage in avoidance behavior because they are depressed, which is not usually the case for males. The other difference among those in this age group is the reaction to which parent has died. The ones who lost a mother are more likely to be depressed, feel hopeless, and think about suicide than those who lost a father (Lawrence, Jeglic, Matthews, & Pepper, 2006).

Adults whose parent(s) died when they were children are closer to their siblings than are those who grew up in intact families. Adults who lost a mother as children, however, have less contact with siblings in adulthood than do those who lost a father (Mack, 2004).

Importance of Involvement and Communication

Is a child prepared for the funeral experience? Should a child be involved in the wake or funeral? Should a child be permitted to view his or her parent's body? The answers to these questions have a strong impact on a child's postdeath adjustment (Worden, 2002).

Tips for parents who want to help their children understand death (Wolfelt, 1999) include the following:

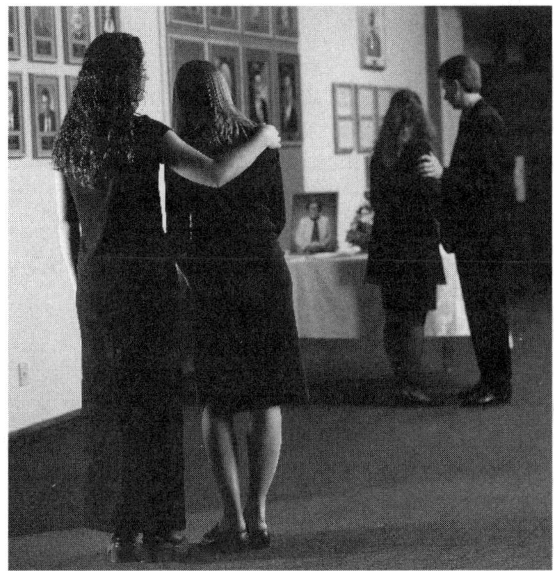

- Allow children to attend the funeral of a person they loved. Prepare them for the experience, and recognize that sometimes a child who is innocent about life might actually be wiser and better able to heal than someone with more life experiences.
- Do not lie or tell half-truths. People, in general, and children, specifically, can usually cope with what they know; it is trying to handle what they do not know can be a problem.
- Many people think that children should reach a particular age before being told anything about death. Actually, no such age exists. Children are never too young to experience loss, be it the loss of a friend who moves away or the death of a pet.
- Children typically would rather have adults they trust talk about the experience with them than go through it all alone.

Children are curious about death and should be encouraged to ask questions about it.

A child's healthy adaptation to the loss of a parent is also more likely if the family shares information and openly expresses feelings about the dead person. If the family remains silent or says little about the death, however, the child is more likely to suffer, to deny, to act out, or to feel guilty about causing the death (Raveis et al., 1999). After a period of mourning, most children (84% of 157 young people ages 3 to 17 in a study group of 88 families) get back to normal (Christ, 2000).

The loss of a parent represents not only the loss of that person from a life, but all the future events that would have included them. Moreover, the survivor's feelings along the way, primarily sadness, would be very different if the parent were there. By expressing these feelings, most people adjust over time.

After the Death of a Parent

There is an expression, "Death ends a life, but not a relationship." Most people spend the rest of their lives missing a dead parent. For example, Sadie Delaney (Hearth, 1993) found her younger sister Bessie, who was in her 90s, crying, and asked her, "What are you crying about?" Bessie replied, "I miss Mama."

Besides missing the dead parent, the surviving child can have feelings of anger, guilt, and loneliness—and sometimes relief, if the parent was in intense

Loss of a Father

Terri Ouellette, whose father died of a heart attack at age 54, reported that she had good memories of her dad telling her how he would protect her. After he died, that was one of the things she missed most. One day, when she and her best friend were "oogling some guy," her friend's dad said to her friend, "If I ever see you with him, I will kick your butt." Then he looked at her [Terri] and said, "That goes for you, too." Terri said that meant a lot to her because she then felt supported by a father figure. She said, "Fathers always talk about having to chase the boys away" (Kelly, 2000, p. 88).

MY STORY

It seemed like an ordinary day that evoked a "just-another-day" feeling. If anything, the day started on the more positive side of ordinary. After all, the predicted warmer temperature would rid the university of most of its ice patches that had been plaguing its students. The weather difficulties compounded the existing difficulties of an almost-50-year-old entering a doctoral program. One major apprehension was the concern of being too old to pursue a lifelong desire to teach. Was teaching really important enough to give up the comforts of home? Interestingly, the day progressed to a point that the answer came without any reservation.

To explain, as a teaching assistant, I was waiting for the last student in a Health Education 101 class to complete a required pretest. I walked to an open window, and my ear became attuned to a somewhat familiar repeating sound. Squeak, squeak—pause—squeak, squeak. Moreover, a lone-ago-remembered chatter permeated the squeaks. As I glanced down, I saw a small playground. Oh, how warm I felt! Those were the sights and sounds that always felt best. It was recess. People had been learning! Yes, I was supposed to be a teacher! However, no one shouted, "Yes, you are finally where you should be!" No car horns honked. No congratulatory speeches were given. It was just another day.

Later that day, I received a call from my sister, who told me that my mother had just been found dead. How could my mother be dead? I had just determined my reason for existence. How could I tell her? She wouldn't see me graduate. She had said she would be there. She was the one who would have been most proud of me.

As I prepared to go home for the funeral, I had many flashbacks of the life with my mother. I had learned many lessons from her that I would make sure lived on. I would share them with my students. "You know that everything happens for a reason," she had said. Yes, she would be proud of me.

No horns honked. Everyone laughed and joked. It was just another day.

pain for a long time. Many people report having dreams in which they spoke with their dead parent(s). This process can provide a feeling of ongoing connection.

Recovering from the death of a parent is more likely if the survivor talks with friends and receives support from adults. Essential, however, is that anyone who is suffering serious or long-lasting depression over the loss of a parent see a therapist.

Death of Partners/Spouses

Losing a spouse is one of the most stressful experiences a person can have. (A woman whose spouse has died is termed a **widow**; a man in similar circumstance is called a **widower**.) Approximately 45% of married women and 14% of married men eventually are widowed—percentages that would be even higher were not for the number of divorces (Kastenbaum, 2004).

The older people get, the more widows and widowers there are, with the number of widowed persons increasing rapidly after age 55. The U.S. Census Bureau (2002) reported that among people 65 or older, approximately 8.5 million are widows and about 2 million are widowers. By age 85 and older, 80% of women are widows and 43% of men are widowers. Widows outnumber widowers in all population groups (Caucasian, African American, Hispanic).

Men and women often have very different types of personal relationships. Women might have friends to turn to for support during the process of becoming widowed. Men tend to withdraw from others and seek closeness only from their dying wives (Carr, House, Wortman, Nesse, & Kessler, 2001).

Rapin (as quoted in Brunk, 2006) offers the following tips on getting through the death of a spouse:

- Maintain social ties. Typically, a man alone is uncomfortable without his spouse. Women network socially, and the network is very supportive. Men who lose wives should go out when invited to maintain the social connections the couple once had together.
- Take some time off from work, at least a 2-week break, just to get things settled.
- Don't make drastic changes right away. Take at least a year before selling the house, moving elsewhere, or getting remarried. Within a year, the survivor is emotionally more stable and better able to make those decisions.
- Get professional help if needed. Signs suggesting that help is needed include irritability, insomnia, feelings of guilt, significant changes in eating patterns, and seeming to walk around in a daze.

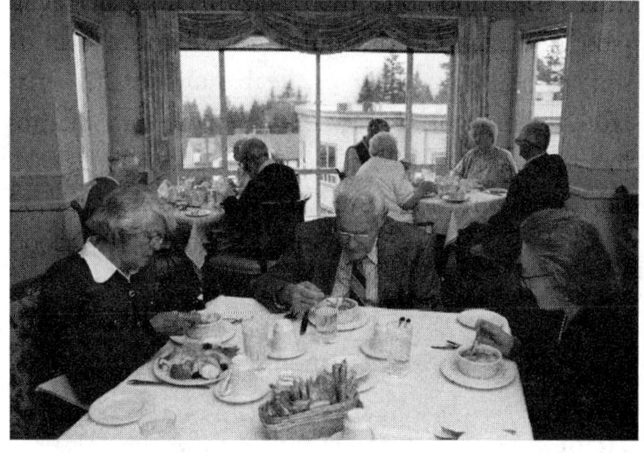

Losing a Spouse When Older

Most older adults recover better than younger adults do from the loss of a spouse, returning to earlier levels of physical and psychological health within a year and a half. A common belief exists that a survivor suffers more when a spouse dies suddenly than after a long illness. This occurrence is not always true, especially for older men. They handle the sudden death of a spouse more easily than a delayed death. The reverse is generally true for widows; women do not take a lingering death as hard as a sudden one, perhaps because they are more willing caretakers. Widows who depended on their husbands for such tasks such as financial management and home repairs are likely to suffer high levels of anxiety (Carr et al., 2001).

Someone who is intelligent, well-educated, financially well off, and who has had a stable, harmonious marriage can easily handle the loss of a spouse, right? Wrong. They are at risk for more severe and longer term depression than people who are less successful, have stormier marriages, and do not feel as good about themselves. Most older women and men can, and do, recover from the death of a spouse, however stressful it is (Carr et al., 2001).

Death of a Partner

Marriage partners are usually closer to each other than to anyone else in the world. Sometimes the dying one or the survivor has one last chance to express intense love. For example, a nurse described parting words she overheard an older woman say to her dying husband. The dying man had stopped breathing, but his heart was still beating. When the nurse tried to rush the wife out of the room, the elderly woman asked if she could speak to her husband to give him a final goodbye. She took his hand and said, "Thank you for being the best husband I could have ever had and for being such a wonderful father to our kids." She then said, "Goodbye; I'll miss you and I'll always love you." She kissed his forehead and tearfully left the room.

Widowhood

Women are living longer, healthier lives, with a current life expectancy of almost 80 years for those in the United States. The bad news is that they typically outlive their spouses. Men's life expectancy is a bit less than 75 years. So, once women enter their 70s, chances are that they will become first a caretaker and then a widow, facing their last years alone. Almost half of women over 65 are widows, and once they pass age 65, only 2% of widows remarry (Schneider, 2003).

Older widows frequently become so depressed that they no longer enjoy life. Yet there are ways for the elderly to combat the loneliness, fear, and sadness of widowhood—through activity. Physicians still put such patients on antidepressants or sleeping pills, but they also are more often prescribing social activity and fitness.

Exercise, in particular, not only has shown positive physical effects, but it also can provide older, lonely women a badly needed social outlet. One widow reported that, although she did not enjoy working out at a health club, she realized that it had definite benefits: she sleeps better at night; she doesn't feel so sad, which occurred especially at suppertime; and she finds the social contacts at the club beneficial. On the one-year anniversary of her husband's death, she felt she had turned a corner when she finally felt that she was going to "make it" (Schneider, 2003).

Losing a Spouse to Cancer

The onset of cancer changes the household dynamic. If a husband has cancer, his wife often finds that he will not talk about it, and she withdraws. If a wife has cancer, it might be hard to get her husband to listen so she can talk about it. These difficulties create a distance between the two. Moreover, cancer can play havoc with all other aspects of a relationship (Lalley, 2007), including the:

- financial strain of paying for treatment.
- household upheaval caused by changes in traditional roles.
- possibly negative effect on sexual intimacy.
- immediate fear that the partner may die.

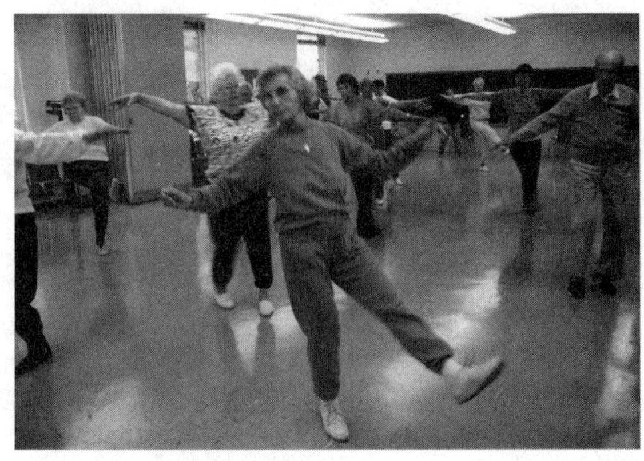

The biggest issue of all in the onset of cancer is death. For some couples, it is a subject neither wants to address. The sick partner might not want to frighten the other partner by talking about it. The well partner might not want the sick partner to think he or she has given up hope. But silence is worse than talking. Support groups can help, even though many couples avoid them. They should not, though. The purpose of a support group is simply to coach people about how to work through the practical daily life issues of sex, money, children, and chores.

The experience of going through treatment for cancer, in time, can bring a couple closer together. Many husbands, who at first hold back out of fear, become supportive and participative. Many couples develop a deeper and closer relationship than they thought possible, making it easier for the survivor to recover.

Death of a Child

In the 1900s, children accounted for 53% of total deaths in the United States. Today, children account for only 3% of total deaths. Although the percentage is much lower now, about 43,000 infants and children aged 0 to 14 die in the United States each year (Fletcher, 2002). Each week, approximately 1900 American families are faced with the death of a child (Rosof, 1995). According to parents who have had a child die, the grief is unlike any other. The death of a child typically "robs parents of whom they loved most, isolates parents from one another, and deafens them to the cries of their other children" (Rosof, 1995).

So, how do parents deal with the death of a child? They need to know that grief, an emotion, is permanent. It will not go away. Grieving, however, does not have to be permanent. Basically, grieving is a slow coping process that parents can move through. In fact, they must move through it if they expect to become normal again.

Hard emotional work is required to remake the world, find a way to say goodbye, put the dead child's life in an acceptable context, and learn to live again. While learning to live again, though, a parent does not forget.

Also, the age of the child, born or unborn, has nothing to do with the intensity of the grief or the length of the grieving process. One woman explained that she would never forget how her 96-year-old grandmother, on her deathbed, spoke of a stillborn daughter.

Family Bereavement

The death of a child affects a family profoundly. More than the loss of a person, it is the loss of hopes, dreams, identities, relationships, and family cohesion. The individuals who are left must re-create the family anew (Fletcher, 2002).

Each family member grieves alone. Grief can pull parents together or push them apart. Parents might become overprotective of surviving children, emotionally abandon them, or try to use a surviving child or later children as a replacement.

Why does the death of a child severely dislocate a family?

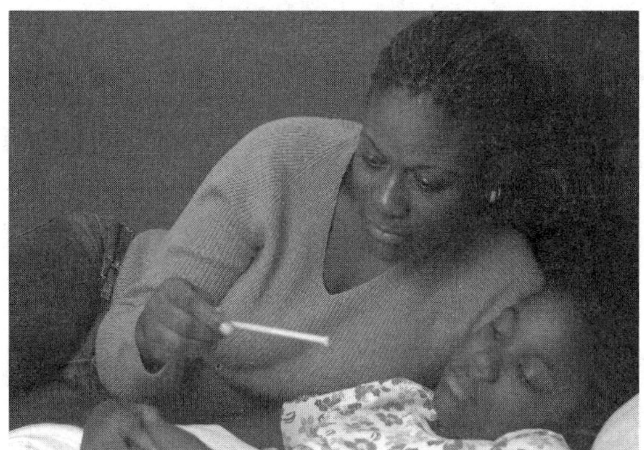

- The death of a child is unnatural.
- Parents might feel like failures as protectors.
- Family boundaries must be reorganized and roles reassigned.
- Family communication breaks down. Families with open communication seem to cope with the loss better than families with closed or no communication.

Families, in addition to existing as a whole, exist as subparts. In a family of four, for instance, a father and the two children are a family triad, which often acts as a group, shopping (say) for a gift for mother's day. If one of the children dies, the other family members grieve individually, and the father and the surviving child grieve the loss of their triad and the activities it had.

Consider the family impact of a child's death quantitatively (Detmer & Lamberti, 1991). A family of four has six dyads:

- The two parents
- The two children
- Mother and one child
- Father and one child
- Mother and the other child
- Father and the other child

and four triads:

- Mother and two children
- Father and two children
- Parents and one child
- Parents and the other child

The loss of one family member reduces the number of dyads to three:

- The two parents
- Mother and surviving child
- Father and surviving child

and the triads to one: mother, father, surviving child. The end result of the turmoil is reconfiguration of the family, with an alternate plan for each of its members (Fletcher, 2002).

How a Therapist Can Help

The role of a therapist in treating families includes:

- facilitating resolution of the family's identity crisis;

- ensuring that communication occurs; and
- promoting family reunification.

Because mothers experience grief differently than do fathers, therapists should not overlook the father as an individual, and the couple as a whole, when counseling bereaved parents (Fletcher, 2002).

Effect on Doctors and Nurses

Most physicians and nurses can rationalize the death of an adult, but the death of a child is viewed as unfair and cruel and a very painful experience (McKelvey, 2006). Nurses usually give emotional support to one another, though. They also get it from other health professionals. This process enables nurses, in turn, to support surviving children and families. But some nurses believe their code of conduct dictates that emotions should be tamped down, or at least not shown (Davies et al., 1996).

Some nurses begin withdrawing from the child and family when death becomes inevitable. This separation enables them to carry out tasks that need to be accomplished. If this strategy is the only one for dealing with distress, however, withdrawal comes to lose its usefulness.

After recognizing that a child's death is inevitable, nurses often face the dilemma of their obligation to follow physicians' orders and their belief that children should be allowed to die peacefully, without unnecessary pain. Some nurses deal with this dilemma by spending time with the child through sitting, listening, providing company, and accompanying them during vulnerable moments, such as during painful procedures or when talking about death. Some nurses follow through even further by staying with the child until death occurs. After the child's death, some nurses make a special effort to talk with the parents and even attend the child's funeral.

What prevents many (typically male) physicians from sharing their response to a child's death is their concern that expressing their feelings will lead to criticism from peers and attending physicians. Attending physicians rarely speak with anyone about a child's death. But they are still vulnerable to the emotional impact (McKelvey, 2006).

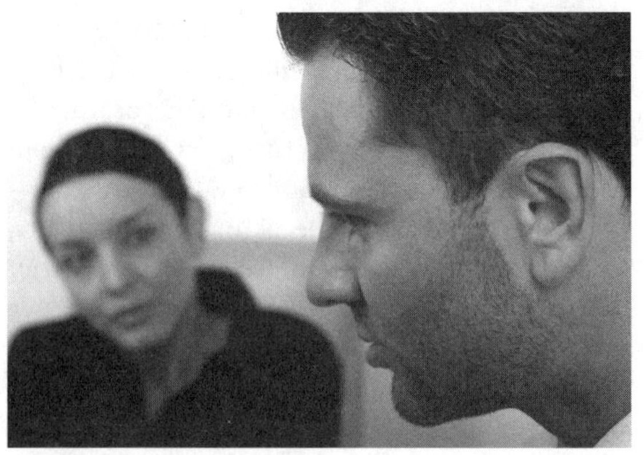

What can be done to help nurses and physicians deal with the deaths of children? Some fear that talking about how they feel might make them appear unprofessional or that discussing a sensitive case might compromise them if it comes to a malpractice lawsuit. But counseling services are a must. Without them, nurses and physicians likely will go to less demanding settings or leave medicine altogether. As a nurse may say, "There is a black hole within me that keeps growing and growing. Eventually, I'll have to do something else."

Death of a Friend

The death of a friend causes sadness. If the person was a close friend, the grieving is intense. The death of a friend hits children and young people especially hard, because it is unnatural. Death is something either not understood (for children) or far away (for young people) and not something they normally think about—until it happens. Adults grieve for the death of a friend, but greater life experience usually helps them deal with it, especially in later years when death is not as unexpected.

Children

Children respond to death differently at different ages. Preschoolers do not yet recognize the finality of death; therefore, they generally continue to bring it up. Later, they usually are more developmentally able to work through the experience with a more mature understanding (Essa, Murray, & Everts, 1995).

The ages between 5 and 7 are key to developing an understanding of death (Speece & Brent, 1984; Stambrook & Parker, 1987). During this stage, children begin to realize that death is not temporary, that one cannot come back to life under any circumstances. Also, they typically realize that death happens to everyone (Essa & Murray, 1994).

Although children's concrete responses to illness and death can seem ghoulish to adults, they reflect children's curiosity and need to know. Children almost always ask numerous questions about illness and death, and parents can expect recurring conversations and questions. Allowing children to process their questions helps them deal with their fears, anger, and/or confusion (Essa et al., 1995).

The following tips can help children in dealing with a death:

- Create an accepting atmosphere that allows children the opportunity to discuss someone's death. Do not try to protect them from the facts. Having a friend disappear without knowing what has happened can be more distressing than learning of a death (Fox, 1985; Wolfelt, 1983).
- Make it clear that it is all right to be sad, grieve, and/or feel uncertainty. Also, make sure that children know that someone would care if they became seriously ill or died.
- Be aware that children's behavior can change because of fear, anger, distress, and/or feelings of loss (Fox, 1985).
- Keep explanations simple and honest. Present the basic facts and then allow children to ask questions. Children's questions usually are concrete and reflect concern about themselves (e.g., Could they also become sick?; Fox, 1985; Grollman, 1967; Wass & Corr, 1984).
- Know that children do not all react in the same way to death; some might not react visibly at all (Wolfelt, 1983). Some may seem callous. Some are eager to play with a sick friend; others remain aloof.

Death of a Classmate

A boy in school became very sick (and eventually died). His classmates reacted in typical ways. They asked lots of questions. Why did he get the illness? Would they catch it? Would he return to class? Is he going to die? Some students talked about him every day; others never mentioned him.

After he came home from the hospital, he was invited to visit the class. The teachers discussed the visit beforehand, saying that he might look a little different, but that he was the same person they knew. At first, he was hesitant to talk about his illness, as were some of his classmates. But their natural curiosity about what had happened to him helped break the ice. They did react in different ways: one wanted to play with him, another did not want to be around him at all.

When he died later that year, many of his classmates attended the funeral service. Some of the children wandered to the edge of the group and played. Some looked at a scrapbook full of pictures and other mementos.

His friends brought up his death at school and home and continue to do so five years later. One girl, who was four when he died, at first asked, "He is dead, right? He won't ever come back, right?" Now she remembers that he is dead and mentions that he is under the ground. Sometimes she wonders if he is up in the air and if he still has bones.

His picture is posted on the bulletin board in his former classroom. When a child asks a question like, "Who is that?" the teacher names him, and says that the picture reminds students that he was in their class and that they like to remember him (Essa et al., 1995).

- Help children work through feelings indirectly via play (e.g., hospital props in play areas; Tait & Depta, 1993).
- Have children read books about illness and death, but be careful in book selections. Screen the books for age appropriateness, situation appropriateness, and religious overtones. Only a few books are appropriate for young preschoolers (Ordal, 1983). The message from some books can be more confusing than helpful or too removed from the reality of losing a friend. Instead of feeling better, children might fear losing a person important to them.

Adolescents and Young Adults

Regardless of whether a friend died in a car accident or from a shooting, a drowning, cancer, AIDS, or one of many other possible causes, the death of a young adult friend never comes at a good time. The grief young people experience might overwhelm them and their world might seem to be shattered, but one thing is for sure—their feelings about the friend's death become part of their lives forever.

Sometimes the unreality and pain surrounding a friend's death can cause young people to experience serious depression. Feelings of sadness are normal when a friend dies, but a young person might want to see a family doctor or speak with a counselor if any of the following symptoms of depression are severe or last too long:

- Sleeping difficulties
- Low self-esteem
- Failing grades in school
- Relationship problems with family and friends
- Drug or alcohol abuse
- Tendency to get into fights

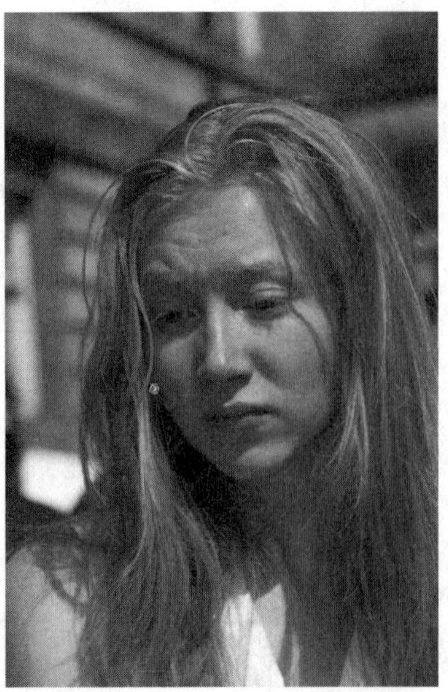

One of the best ways for a young person to recover after the death of a friend is to attend peer support groups. Group members with similar needs meet periodically and encourage each other to tell their stories as often as they like. It is a place to openly express feelings. Group support helps each person, because as members share their grief stories, the intensity of grief often is lessened. If a local support group for young people who have experienced a friend's dying is not available, perhaps a group of young people can start one.

Death of a Pet

The death of a pet might seem unimportant—until it happens to you. The grief is very real, and reactions to the death of a pet can be extreme, with some people even committing suicide following their pet's death. Some say that they would rather lose a husband or wife than a pet (Carmack, 1985).

To understand the impact of the death of a pet, it is important to first understand the nature and extent of human–animal attachments (Sharkin & Knox, 2003). Since the beginning of civilization, humans have had loving relationships with pets. For example, a 14,000-year-old human skeleton was discovered by archeologists with its hands wrapped around a dog skeleton (Arkow, 1987).

Pets typically have a shorter life span than humans. Dogs, for example, usually live 12 to 15 years, and cats 18 to 20 years. It is no wonder, then, that the loss of a pet is, for many people, their first experience of the death of a loved one.

A pet death, if it is the first death a person has experienced, can help prepare the person for other losses. The rituals of saying goodbye to a pet can be similar to those used in saying goodbye to other loved ones. Ways of saying goodbye to pets and people include touching them, sitting with them after death, preparing a final place of rest, and placing keepsakes, all of which help people accept the finality of a death (McElroy, 1998).

The pattern of grief following the death of a pet parallels the pattern of bereavement for the death of a person (Archer & Winchester, 1994), although it is generally less pronounced. Grief patterns include:

- initial numbness or disbelief;
- preoccupation with the loss;
- a loss of part of themselves;
- being drawn toward reminders of the pet;
- an urge to search for the missing pet;
- avoidance or mitigation strategies; and
- anger, anxiety, and depression.

The intensity of grief is greater the stronger the attachment to the pet, the suddenness of the death, and if the owner lives alone, thus lacking social support.

An additional aspect of grief over the death of a pet is that it is often **disenfranchised grief** (Doka, 1989). That is, the grief is not recognized by others as important, so the social support is not there—except in the case of a family loss of a pet, when everyone in the family grieves the loss.

As the concept of a traditional family becomes more varied, it seems natural to assume that pets will play a larger role now than ever before in the dynamics of family systems. Today, adolescents, many of whom have both parents working outside of the home, are spending more time alone than youth in past generations. The family pet, therefore, might take on the role of daily companion in the home. Many children say that their pet is their best friend.

The relationship with a pet is seen as pure, meaning that the bond is based on a genuine and consistent sense of unconditional, nonjudgmental love and acceptance—something that may be difficult to obtain or sustain in relationships with people (Allen, Blascovich, & Mendes, 2002).

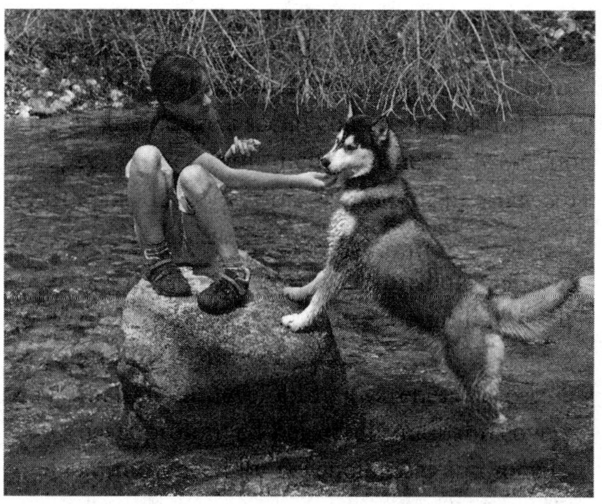

Many pet owners celebrate their pets' birthdays, carry pictures of them, and confide to them. In fact, animal companionship can have very positive effects on people's emotional, social, psychological, and physical well-being (Sharkin & Knox, 2003). For example, pets can provide a sense of being needed, lessen the effects of loneliness, and boost self-esteem.

Euthanasia of a Pet

In veterinary practice, euthanasia is accomplished by intravenous injection of a concentrated dose of pain medication. The animal might feel slight discomfort when the needle pierces the skin, but this sensation is no greater than for any other injection. The euthanasia solution takes only seconds to induce a total loss of consciousness, which is soon followed by a stopped heart.

Doctors of veterinary medicine do not take lightly the difficult decision an owner makes to have a pet euthanized. A veterinarian's medical training is dedicated to treatment for animals, and he or she is very much aware of the balance between extending an animal's life and its suffering. Euthanasia is used as a last resort to mercifully end a pet's suffering. Although this act to prevent a terminally ill pet from further suffering is an act of kindness, people sometimes feel guilty for having a pet euthanized.

SUMMARY

- Each year, approximately 8 million people in the United States experience the death of a parent, child, sibling, grandparent, or a pet.
- Death of a parent typically hits very young children (under 5) and adolescents very hard. Children losing a parent recover better if the surviving parent is not depressed. Mourning the death of a parent for children aged 9 to 14 is more complex than for younger children. These children typically bury their feelings, are unwilling to talk about the death, and escape by doing familiar things and being with friends.
- Adolescents 15 to 17 mourn like adults, but generally not for as long.
- College-age females who have lost a parent are more likely to engage in avoidance behavior, because they are depressed, which is not usually the case for males. Those who lost a mother are more likely to be depressed, feel hopeless, and think about suicide than those who lost a father.
- Tips for helping children understand death include, in part, allowing them to attend the funeral and being truthful about death.
- Someone who is suffering serious or long-lasting depression over the loss of a parent should see a therapist.
- A woman losing a spouse to death is a *widow*; a man is a *widower*. Approximately 45% of married women and 14% of married men eventually are widowed. Widows outnumber widowers in all population groups. Women may have friends to turn to for support during the process of becoming widowed. Men tend to withdraw from others.
- Most older adults recover better than young adults from the loss of a spouse. Older men handle the sudden death of a spouse more easily than a delayed death. The reverse is generally true for widows.
- Women have a current U.S. life expectancy of almost 80 years. Men's life expectancy is a bit less than 75 years. Almost half of women over 65 are widows, and once they pass age 65, only 2% of widows remarry.
- In the 1900s, children accounted for 53% of all deaths in the United States. Today, children account for only 3% of deaths. About 43,000 infants and children aged 0 to 14 die in the United States each year. Each week, approximately 1,900 American families are faced with the death of a child.
- According to parents who have a child die, the grief is profound and unlike any other. Grief can pull parents together or push them apart. Parents might become overprotective of surviving children, emotionally abandon them, or try to use a surviving child or later children as a replacement.
- Counseling services are available to help nurses and physicians deal with the deaths of children.
- Children respond to the death of a friend differently at different ages. Preschoolers do not yet recognize the finality of death. The ages between 5 and 7 are key for developing an understanding that death is permanent and universal.
- For young adults, the death of a friend is untimely. It can cause serious depression. See the family doctor or speak with a counselor in the school or community if the following symptoms of depression are severe or last too long: sleeping difficulties, low self-esteem, failing grades in school, relationship problems with family and friends, drug or alcohol abuse, or tendency to get into fights. Peer support groups can be helpful as a place to express feelings openly.
- The grief on the death of a pet is very real, and reactions to the death of a pet can be extreme. Dogs usually live 12 to 15 years, and cats 18 to 20 years. Thus, for many people, a pet's death is their first experience

of a meaningful death and, as such, can serve as a model for other losses. The pattern of grief following the death of a pet parallels the pattern of bereavement for the death of a person.

- Euthanasia of a pet is done by intravenous injection of a concentrated dose of pain medication. Doctors of veterinary medicine do not take lightly the difficult decision an owner makes to have a pet euthanized. Euthanasia is used as a last resort to mercifully end a pet's suffering.

Additional Resources

Books

Bartocci, B. (2000). *Nobody's child anymore: Grieving, caring, and comforting when parents die.* Notre Dame, IN: Sorin Books. The author shares her thoughts on illness, death, and coping and offers advice at the end of each chapter, which ranges from healthy ways to express anger to comforting methods to keep the memory of one's parents and their traditions alive after they're gone.

Carmack, B. J. (2003). *Grieving the death of a pet.* Minneapolis, MN: Augsburg Fortress Publishers. The death of a pet is like no other loss. This book reveals the author's own experience and interviews with dozens of pet lovers to guide the reader through the experience of losing a pet.

Cochran, B. (2007). *The forever dog.* New York: HarperCollins. Losing a pet can be heartbreaking to anyone who has experienced it. The reader of this book becomes familiar with Mike, who loses his dog, Corky, "one of those dogs that seemed to be built from other dogs' spare parts." His mother tells Mike that "Corky's a part of you now. He lives in your heart."

Dower, L., & Lister, E. (2001). *I will remember you: What to do when someone you love dies, a guidebook through grief for teens.* New York: Scholastic. Using stirring words by well-known personalities, as well as from fellow teens who have lost a loved one, this book is used to encourage teens to explore the grieving process and to keep going in the face of terrible loss and sadness.

Rosof, B. D. (1994). *The worst loss: How families heal from the death of a child.* New York: Henry Holt & Co. After describing the many ways children die, the author uses anecdotes from her practice to explain why grieving is crucial to recovery, how the parental relationship may be affected, and the ways surviving siblings grieve. Throughout, the author stresses that parents will never be the same as they were before. Included in the book is a list of national organizations that support bereaved parents.

Movies

Ghost. (1990). Issues of living, dying, and grieving are portrayed in this movie. In addition, the movie is a love story, mystery, comedy, and supernatural tale!

P.S. I Love You. (2007). This story involves accounts of the struggles of a grief stricken young wife who has lost her husband to death and is trying to move on with her life.

Critical Thinking

1. What are the implications of a fictional account, as in *Ghost,* in which a dead person comes back to interact with a living one?
2. What are the pros and cons of believing that the dead can interact with the living?
3. Could there be anything "good" for you if a loved one dies?
4. What would you say to an 8-year-old whose puppy just died?

Class Activity

1. Write a letter addressed to someone (dead or alive) to resolve an issue that is troubling for you—but keep it. Then, write a paper describing how you felt about writing the letter; discuss this paper with your classmates.
2. Engage in a class discussion about the movie *P.S. I Love You.*

References

Allen, K., Blascovich, K., & Mendes, U. B. (2002). Cardiovascular reactivity and the presence of pets, friends, and spouses: The truth about cats and dogs. *Psychosocial Medicine, 64*(5), 727–739.

Archer, J., & Winchester, G. (1994). Bereavement following death of a pet. *British Journal of Psychology, 85*(2), 259.

Arkow, P. (1987). *The loving bond: Companion animals in the helping professions.* Saratoga, CA: R&E Publishers.

Brunk, D. (2006). Coping with the loss of a spouse. *OB/GYN News, 41*(13), 38.

Carmack, J. (1985). The effects on family members and functioning after death of a pet. *Marriage and Family Reviews, 8*(3/4), 149–161.

Carr, D., House, J. S., Wortman, C. B., Nesse, R. M., & Kessler, R. C. (2001). Psychological adjustment to sudden and anticipated spousal death among the older widowed persons. *Journal of Gerontology: Social Sciences, 56B*(4), S237–S248.

Cerel, J., Fristad, M. A., Verducci, J., Weller, R. A., & Weller, E. B. (2006). Childhood bereavement: Psychopathology in the two years postparental death. *Journal of the American Academy of Child and Adolescent Psychiatry, 45*(6), 681–690.

Christ, G. H. (2000). *Healing children's grief: Surviving a parent's death from cancer*. New York: Oxford University Press.

Christ, G. H. (2001). Facilitating mourning following parental death. *Psychiatric Times, 18*(9), 1–9.

Davies, B., Cook, K., O'Loane, M., Clarke, D., MacKenzie, B., Stutzer, C., et al. (1996). Caring for dying children: Nurses' experiences. *Pediatric Nursing, 22*(6), 500.

Detmer, C., & Lamberti, J. (1991). Family grief. *Death Studies 15*, 363–374.

Divorce and death: Their social and social-psychological impacts. (2008). Retrieved May 2, 2008, from http://www.trinity.edu/~mkeal/fam-div.html

Doka, K. J. (Ed.). (1989). *Disenfranchised grief: Recognizing hidden sorrow.* Lexington, MA: Lexington Books.

Dowdney, L. (2000). Childhood bereavement following parental death. *Journal of Child Psychology and Psychiatry, 41*(7), 819–830.

Essa, E. L., & Murray, C. I. (1994). Young children's understanding and experience with death. *Young Children, 49*(4), 74–81.

Essa, E. L., Murray, C. I., & Everts, J. (1995). Death of a friend. *Childhood Education, 71*(3), 130.

Fletcher, P. N. (2002). Experiences in family bereavement. *Family and Community Health, 25*(1), 57.

Fox, S. S. (1985). *Good grief: Helping groups of children when a friend dies.* Boston: The New England Association for the Education of Young Children.

Fristad, M. A., Jedel, R., Weller, R. A., & Weller, E. B. (1993). Psychosocial functioning in children after the death of a parent. *American Journal of Psychiatry, 150*, 511–513.

Glasser, J. (2004). *Address.* American Public Health Association (APHA), San Francisco.

Grollman, E. A. (Ed.). (1967). *Explaining death to children.* Boston: Beacon Press.

Hearth, A. H. (1993). *Having our say: The Delaney sisters' first 100 years*. New York: Kodansha America, Inc.

Jellinek, M. S. (2003). The varying faces of grief. *Pediatric News, 37*(4), 21.

Kastenbaum, R. J. (2004). *Death, society, and human experience* (8th ed.). New York: Pearson.

Kelly, L. (2000). *Don't ask for the dead man's golf clubs*. New York: Workman.

Lalley, H. (2007, April 10). Coping with cancer. *Spokane (WA) Spokesman-Review.*

Lawrence, E., Jeglic, E. L., Matthews, L. T., & Pepper, C. M. (2006). Gender differences in grief reactions following the death of a parent. *Omega: The Journal of Death and Dying, 52*(4), 323.

Mack, K. Y. (2004). The effects of early parental death on sibling relationships in later life. *Omega: The Journal of Death and Dying, 49*(2), 131.

McElroy, S. C. (1998, October). The gift of grief. *Vegetarian Times, 254,* 128.

McKelvey, R. S. (2006). Coping with the death of young patients. *Clinical Psychiatry News, 34*(2), 18.

Ordal, C. C. (1983). Death as seen in books suitable for young children. *Omega: The Journal of Death and Dying, 14*(3), 249–277.

Pfeffer, C. R., Karus, D., Siegel, K., & Hang, H. (2000). Child survivors of parental death from cancer or suicide: Depressive and behavioral outcomes. *Psycho-oncology, 9*(1), 1–10.

Raveis, V. H., Siegel, K., & Karus, D. (1999). Children's psychological distress following the death of a parent. *Journal of Youth and Adolescence, 28*(2), 165.

Rosof, B. D. (1995). *The worst loss: How families heal from the death of a child.* New York: Owl Books.

Schneider, J. M. (2003, June 2). Coping with a spouse's death. *U.S. News & World Report,* 54.

Sharkin, B. S., & Knox, D. (2003). Pet loss: Issues and implications for the psychologist. *Research & Practice, 34*(4), 414–421.

Speece, M. W., & Brent, S. B. (1984). Children's understanding of death: A review of three components of a death concept. *Child Development, 55*, 1671–1686.

Stambrook, M., & Parker, K. C. (1987). The development of the concept of death in children: A review of the literature. *Merrill-Palmer Quarterly, 33*, 133–157.

Tait, D. C., & Depta, J. (1993). Play therapy group for bereaved children. In N. B. Webb (Ed.), *Helping bereaved children: A handbook for practitioners.* (pp. 169–185). New York: Guilford Press.

U.S. Census Bureau. (2002). *Historical statistics of the United States, colonial times to 1970, 1975.* Statistical Abstract of the United States.

Wass, H., & Corr, C. A. (1984). *Helping children cope with death: Guidelines and resources* (2nd ed.). New York: Hemisphere Publishing.

Wolfelt, A. (1983). *Helping children cope with grief.* Muncie, IN: Accelerated Development, Inc.

Wolfelt, A. (1999). Coping with death. *Alberta Report, 26*(6), 38.

Worden, J. W. (2002). *Grief counseling and grief therapy: A handbook for the mental health practitioner* (3rd ed.). New York: Springer.

Chapter 10

Grief and the Process of Grieving

Well, everyone can master a grief but he that has it.
—Shakespeare, in *Much Ado About Nothing*

Objectives

After reading this chapter, you will be able to answer the following questions:

- What is grief, and how does it differ from grieving and bereavement?
- What are some common patterns of grief?
- What is acute grief, and what are some of its symptoms?
- How can a person transform his or her grief?
- How can storytelling and spirituality aid in grieving?
- What is anticipatory grief, and what are some of its consequences?
- What is disenfranchised grief, and how can it be addressed?
- How long does grief last?
- What kinds of help and support are available to those experiencing grief?
- How can employers aid employees who have suffered a loss?

What Is Grief?

Grief has a number of meanings. Here, as in Chapter 1, *grief* refers to a deep and poignant distress at the loss of someone close. *Grieving* is the process of trying to work through the pain caused by such a loss. Grief also can mean a yearning for the lost person, thinking repeatedly about past events, a sense of guilt, or even thoughts of suicide.

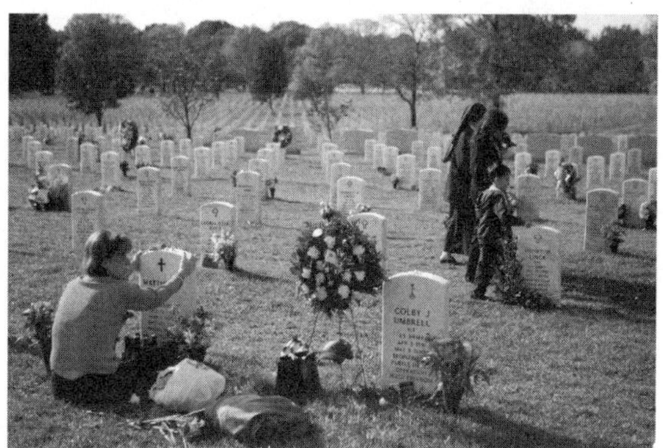

Mental health professionals characterize grief along five dimensions (Archer, 1999):

1. Grief causes stress reactions and physical changes, all of which can increase vulnerability to illness and make existing physical problems worse.
2. Grief affects perception and thought, both of which can lead to impulsive, and possibly harmful, decisions and increase accident risk.
3. Grief can cause a spiritual crisis, calling into question one's assumptions and values.
4. Recovery from grief is affected by family and community responses to loss.
5. Cultural heritage and existing support systems influence how stress is expressed and how a person copes with loss.

In some cases after loss, people are so overwhelmed by grief that adjusting to life and investing in relationships seems impossible. When this occurs, support from family, friends, clergy, support organizations, and counselors is crucial. The larger and stronger the support system, the more likely is a successful recovery.

Grief is different from bereavement or mourning. **Bereavement** is an objective state of loss, meaning if one experiences a loss, one is bereaved. Bereavement refers to the fact of loss, whereas grief is the subjective response to that state of loss.

Mourning generally means the social process, norms, behavior patterns, and rituals that publicly recognize bereavement. Wearing black or a black armband, sending cards and flowers, and attending memorial services, funerals, and graveside services are examples of mourning behaviors.

Gender Differences in Grieving

As summarized by Martin and Doka (2000), in most cases, men and women grieve differently:

- Widows are more likely to seek emotional support from others. Widowers more often turn to exercise, work, religion, creative expression, or alcohol.
- In dealing with the loss of a child, as a rule, mothers report more emotional distress than do fathers. Women tend to focus on emotion and seek support. Many men intellectualize their grief and focus on problem-solving strategies to adapt to the loss.
- After the loss of a parent, middle-aged sons are less likely than middle-aged daughters to experience intense grief, are less likely to have physical reactions to grief, and are more likely to use active approaches in adapting to loss.
- Differences between genders narrow as people age, perhaps because they become more androgynous.
- Differences in grieving also are affected by differences in social class, generation, and culture.
- Results from some studies have shown men to have better outcomes, others show women to do better, and still others show no significant difference or mixed results.

Patterns of Grief

The common notion that emotional grieving is more effective than non-emotional or cognitive/effective grieving has not been supported by clinical or research evidence. To avoid gender stereotyping in discussing types of grief, Martin and Doka (2000) use the terms *intuitive, instrumental,* and *dissonant* to describe basic patterns of grief that fall on a continuum.

Intuitive grievers, at one end of the continuum, feel their grief and express their emotions openly as they grieve—shouting or crying, for example. Intuitive grievers can be helped by self-help and support groups, or individual counseling, which allow them to vent their feelings.

Instrumental grievers, at the other end of the continuum, think and remember as they grieve and express grief by doing something related to the loss, by exercising or by talking about the loss. For example, a man whose daughter died in a car crash repaired the fence his daughter had wrecked, saying that it was the only part of the accident he could fix (Martin & Doka, 2000). Instrumental grievers are helped by **bibliotherapy** (reading self-help literature) and other cognitive and active approaches to coping with their grief.

Dissonant grievers experience grief a certain way, but they do not feel free to express it in compatible ways. A man might feel grief intuitively, for example, but consider it unmanly to express it emotionally. A woman might experience grief intuitively, but repress emotional displays in order to protect her family.

Where someone falls on the pattern of grief continuum also is affected by his or her culture. For instance, some Southern European cultures are emotionally expressive, whereas some Northern European cultures are stoic.

Young children, who might otherwise be supposed to fall near the intuitive end, will tend toward the instrumental if they are forced early in life to take on heavy responsibilities and become problem solvers.

Acute Grief

Acute grief is experienced in various ways (Lindemann, 1944; Osterweis, Solomon, & Green, 1984). Physical reactions include tightness of the throat, shortness of breath, headaches, dizziness, exhaustion, menstrual irregularities, sexual impotence, tremors and shakes, and oversensitivity to noise. Other symptoms (in order of typical occurrence) include depression, sleep disturbances, difficulty concentrating, weight loss, tiredness, and feelings of hopelessness. Mortality rates are higher in the first year after a loss, particularly for widows.

Emotions experienced in the wake of loss include anger, guilt, helplessness, sadness, shock, numbness, yearning, jealousy, and self-blame or, for some, a sense of relief or emancipation. Feelings such as sadness and relief can occur together.

Behavioral manifestations of acute grief include crying, withdrawal, avoiding or seeking reminders, searching, hyperactivity, and changes in other relationships. Cognitive manifestations include depersonalization, disbelief and confusion, inability to concentrate or focus, preoccupation with images or memories, dreams of the dead, or sensations of the person's presence.

Spiritually, grieving individuals try to find meaning in life and try to reestablish a sense of identity and order in their world. They may be angry with their God or struggle with their faith.

All these reactions to a loss are mediated by

- the unique meaning of the loss;
- the strength of the attachment;
- the circumstances of the loss (such as other crises);
- the experience of earlier loss;
- the individual's temperament and adaptive abilities;
- family support and other support systems;
- cultural and spiritual beliefs and practices; and/or
- general health and lifestyle practices.

Acute grief has been defined in various ways. Grief can be defined in terms of disease (Engel, 1961), which is consistent with the notion that definitions of disease are a social construct. For instance, epilepsy and certain mental illnesses were not regarded as diseases at other times or in other cultures. So, in disease terms, *acute grief:*

- has a clear onset in a circumstance of loss;
- runs a predictable course, beginning with an initial state of shock;
- includes a developing awareness of loss;
- has a prolonged period of gradual recovery;
- is influenced by psychological and social variables; and
- is universal and does not often require treatment.

In the psychological trauma model (Freud, 1917/2005), acute grief is a protective defense against the trauma of loss. To Freud, grief is a crisis, but one that likely will abate over time and usually does not require psychiatric intervention.

In the attachment model of grief (Bowlby, 1980), it is noted that attachment or bonding is a survival mechanism among social animals and is necessary for survival, given the length of infancy and dependent childhood. When the object of attachment (usually, a parent) is gone, crying, clinging, and searching are instinctual efforts to restore the lost bond. Also, by expressing distress, those in grief engage the support and protection of the family or community. If the loss is permanent, as in death, these behaviors continue until the bond loses its emotional meaning.

Bowlby (1980) noted that identification (finding a place for the dead person in one's sense of self) is an essential part of mourning. He concluded, however, that although mourners might identify with the dead person, psychopathology might be present if attachment to the dead person is prominent.

In more contemporary models (Klass, Silverman, & Nickman, 1996), grief is considered to be:

- a natural response to major transitions in life, not just death;
- a (painful) catalyst for growth, in which individuals reconstruct their sense of self, their spirituality, and their relationships to others and to the world;
- a bond to the dead person as a continuing but different form, after a loss.

Loss and Transformation

According to Schneider and Zimmerman (2005), grief is not only about coping, it also is about hope and its power to transform grief and loss and love into something that can help the griever move into a future made different by that loss. As such, the griever must find a way to reach beyond grief, to move into something different, and to find transformation through the process. These authors believe that three successive tasks are required for this transformation:

1. Discover what is missing, and what is no longer the same. To make these discoveries, safe places, or sanctuaries, are needed—which are not always easy to find and use. The discomfort of others caused by grief, and the everyday pressures of life, get in the way. Without a safe space to work, grief can turn into depression—or be misdiagnosed as depression. Completing the task of finding what's missing is necessary in order to move on to the next two stages.
2. Find out what is left or what can be restored. Shift the focus to attachments still there or that can be reassembled. Discover what is left, and then move on.
3. Finally, transform the loss, and make something new of the old—something more resilient, stronger, better than ever, or just different. Realize that change is the only constant in life.

Storytelling

Another way of dealing creatively with loss and grief is to construct a narrative account of the relationship with the dead person that can be told to others (Harvey, 1998). In the face of loss, people create stories and reconstruct memories. This process can help the bereaved make sense of the new world in which they live as well as to move on with their lives. This occurrence is true of a personal loss as well as of a national one, such as a terrorist attack or school killing.

People often attempt to explain what has happened with *attributions* (e.g., thoughts and words that seem to ask "Why?" or "Why is this happening?"). These attribution questions (and their answers) are combined with memories and feelings and concepts of the self to construct a new self-identity.

The effort to compose a coherent story to account for community grief is reflected in the continuously repeated media depictions of tragic national losses. Also reflected is the general desire to tell personal stories by, for instance, posting photographs and descriptions of dead loved ones on temporary shrines and memorials.

In Harvey's (1998) view, storytelling is an effective and long-lasting way to deal with the loss of a relationship, whether it is individual or collective. Because loss cannot be escaped, a story is constructed in an effort to understand it.

Spirituality

Many people believe that all humans are on a continual search for meaning (i.e., spirituality). In times of loss, to move forward, people must stop their everyday activities to reflect on the loss. By doing so, they might be pressed to find meaning in—and reason for—their loss, which might eventually lead to finding meaning for their lives overall.

When people find such meaning, they often believe that their loved one's life—and death—also had meaning. At that point, they have arrived at a more spiritual place for themselves than they had before. The emotional scar of the death is still there, but they might now have useful answers for the meaning of life (and death).

Continuing Bonds

Many people believe that grief involves eventually letting go of the dead person. But that might not be the case. In fact, many grieving survivors maintain a link or continuing bond that leads to a new relationship with the dead. This relationship changes over time but provides the griever with solace (Klass et al., 1996). For example, when actress Natalie Wood drowned, her daughter, Natasha Wagner, was a teenager. Natasha has said that she had to learn to have a relationship with someone who was no longer there (Nickman, Silverman, & Normand, 1998).

Until the beginning of the twentieth century, feeling a continuing bond with the dead was customary and expected in the West. Then Sigmund Freud (1917/2005) declared that grief freed mourners from attachments to the dead, so that when the work of mourning was completed, mourners were free to move ahead and become involved in new relationships.

Today, the current concept of continuing bonds has reintroduced the validity of a continuing attachment and relationship to the dead. But, to keep bonds alive, help is needed from support networks. Connections to the dead need to be legitimized. People need to talk about the dead, to engage in memorial rituals, and to realize that their grief is not a static process, but an evolving one.

A continuing bond does not mean, however, that survivors live only in the past. The dead are gone but continue to be with their loved ones, changing their daily, ongoing lives. The bond between the living and the dead changes and takes on new forms over time, but the connection is always there.

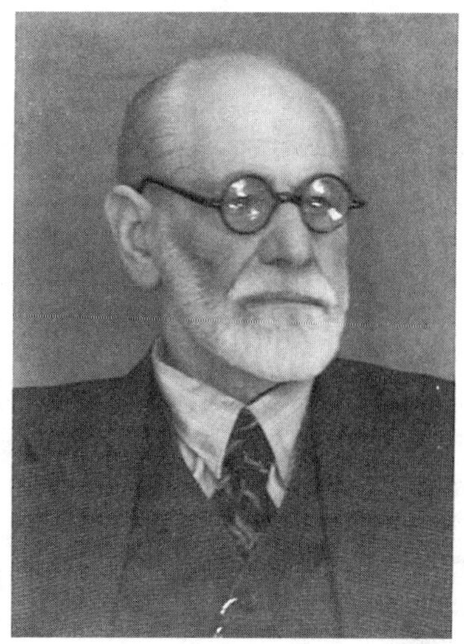

Anticipatory Grief

Advances in medical technology have brought the concept of **anticipatory grief** to the forefront. Death can be delayed, even when an illness is terminal. When the process of dying is extended, families and the patient find themselves grieving before death occurs.

The current conception of anticipatory grief (Rando, 1986) involves the dying patient, as well as the caregiver or family, and it involves more than just anticipated losses. It also redefines *decarthexis*, originally defined by Lindemann (1944), as a pulling away from the person. Instead, Rando calls it a pulling away from the expectations of a future with and for that person.

In this view, there are three types of losses in anticipatory grief:

- Past losses—opportunities not realized and experiences not repeated
- Present losses—deterioration of the dying person, uncertainty, and loss of control
- Future losses—economic changes, loneliness, and day-to-day life moments that will not come again

Stages of Anticipatory Grief

Anticipatory grief takes time to unfold and develop. Raphael (1983) suggested that the phases of anticipatory grief for both the dying person and those close to the person parallel the stages of actual bereavement suggested by Kübler-Ross (denial, anger, bargaining, depression, acceptance):

- Shock, numbness, disbelief, and denial
- Fear, anxiety, helplessness, and bargaining
- Anger, regret, resentment, sense of failure, feeling cheated, guilt, and depression
- Calm and acceptance
- Withdrawal by the dying person, as family/caregivers contend with conflicting desires to remain close and to draw away in order to lessen the upcoming pain of loss

Consequences of Anticipatory Grief

The consequences of anticipatory grief are not clear. Does it make post-death grief shorter and easier, as suggested by Ponder and Pomeroy (1996)? Or does it have adverse affects? Do the bereaved pull away from the dying person beforehand (Lindemann, 1944)?

Perhaps anticipatory grief actually helps. Many bereaved are able to set aside the past and make their peace with the dying person. Also, it gives the dying person time to wrap up unfinished business and take leave in an organized way.

Not much question remains regarding the very bad effect that anticipatory grief has on children losing a parent (Saldinger, Cain, Kalter, & Lohnes, 1999), but the effect on a parent losing a child is difficult to quantify. How much anticipatory grief for a parent is too much? An optimum amount seems not to exist (Pine & Brauer, 1986).

What about Alzheimer's disease and HIV/AIDS? The benefits of anticipatory grief are complicated by the uncertain nature of that experience. Uncertainties include how long the life of the afflicted will be, the effect of social stigma, the loss of cognitive ability and self-sufficiency, the progressive nature of the disease, the multiple losses that a caregiver has to face, and the eventuality that the caregiver might have to relinquish care of the patient to others (Walker, Pomeroy, McNeil, & Franklin, 1994).

Disenfranchised loss (Doka, 1989) describes a loss not recognized or validated by others (e.g., a homosexual relationship in most states or the lover of a person married to someone else). For those caring for an AIDS patient, for instance, anticipatory grieving can be greatly complicated by a lack of social acceptance of the dying patient.

Healthcare Professionals and Anticipatory Grief

Healthcare practitioners who are working with patients and caregivers experiencing anticipatory grief need to recognize the following (Walker, Pomeroy, McNeil, & Franklin, 1996):

- Anticipatory grieving does not necessarily involve pulling away.
- Over time, many losses occur.
- Anticipatory grieving occurs in stages.
- Anticipatory grieving involves working through unfinished business, for both patient and caregiver.

Practitioners must be aware of premature detachment and lessening communication between patient and caregiver. Caregivers should be encouraged to discuss their anger, fear, and loss. Ideally, a practitioner can help the caregiver continue hoping for the best, while, at the same time, let go of the dying person.

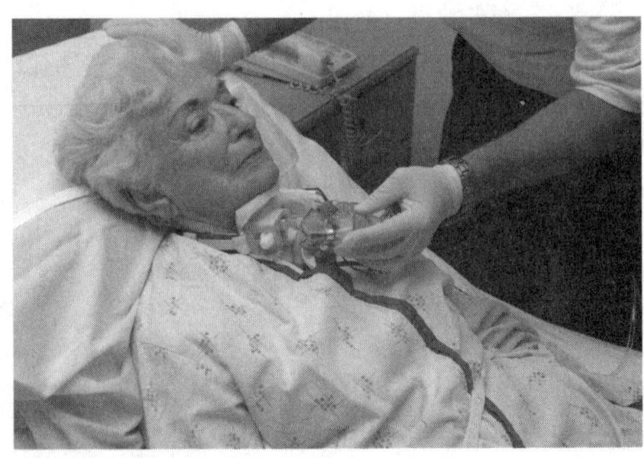

Disenfranchised Grief

Every society has norms that dictate how a bereaved person should behave, feel, and think; who legitimately can grieve for the loss; and who may receive sympathy and support from others. These norms often are embedded in formal rules—regulations and laws that specify who has control of the dead body, control of funeral rituals, and recognition as mourners. Normally, only immediate kin of the dead are accorded these privileges and allowances.

Yet people have many and varied attachments—to friends, roommates, nonrelatives, lovers, pets, reputation, job, even places and things. When such attachments are lost, by death or other departure, the individual may grieve, but alone, because the loss is not socially acknowledged. This is called **disenfranchised grief** (Doka, 1989).

Disenfranchisement can occur for a number of reasons, including the following:

- A relationship is not recognized because it is neither publicly recognized nor socially accepted (e.g., homosexual pairs in most states, nonmarital lovers, or close ties to others who are not kin).
- A loss is not acknowledged as a grief-bearing loss. Examples include perinatal loss (death of a newborn infant); divorce; the loss of a job or possessions; loss of reputation because of scandal, gossip, or arrest and incarceration; the physical and mental losses of aging; and even a teenager cut from a sports team.
- Disenfranchised grievers, such as the very old, the very young, and the mentally disabled, for instance, are excluded from those viewed as capable of grief.
- The circumstances of the death, such as suicide or AIDS, carry a social stigma.
- The cultural ways an individual grieves, such as stoicism or wailing, might fall outside the rules of a given society.

Disenfranchised grievers are not offered recognition from others, social sympathy and support, or such compensations as time off from work. (Company policies usually extend bereavement leave only to immediate family members.) Such individuals might then come to believe that their grief is inappropriate, leading them to have feelings of guilt or shame (Kauffman, 2002).

In a diverse society, however, disenfranchised losses can be acknowledged by a subculture. For example, the death of a gay lover might be recognized and supported within the gay community, if not by some others outside that community.

Also, grieving rules change over time. Younger people, for example, might be more supportive of the loss of one member of an unmarried couple than older people with more traditional views about marriage.

The Treatment of Disenfranchised Grief

The key to treating disenfranchised grief lies in analyzing empathic failure—the factors that limit support and thus generate disenfranchisement. Once the cause of empathic failure is analyzed, therapists can devise interventions that develop or compensate for the lack of support. These interventions can include individual or group counseling, support groups, expressive therapies, or the therapeutic use of ritual (Neimeyer & Jordan, 2002).

How Long Does Grief Last?

Even though there is no specific time period associated with getting over a loss, a typical period of grieving lasts from 6 to 18 months (Rando, 1983; Sanders, 1982–1983). Generally, according to these authors, certain feelings correlate with the time period following death. For example:

- Minutes to weeks: disbelief/numbness and yearning
- Weeks to months: withdrawal, preoccupation, anger, guilt, lack of motivation
- Months to years: resuming old roles, making new roles, re-experiencing pleasure, seeking companionship and the love of others

The following are signs that grief might be coming to an end (Sife, 1998).

- begins to look happier.
- becomes interested in starting new relationships.
- enjoys doing things that he or she liked to do before the loss.
- stops feeling guilty for having good days.
- allows happy memories to return, to coexist with the sad ones.
- realizes and accepts the reality that the loss did happen, that his or her feelings are a part of that loss, that life will never be the same again, and that he or she is a different person than before.

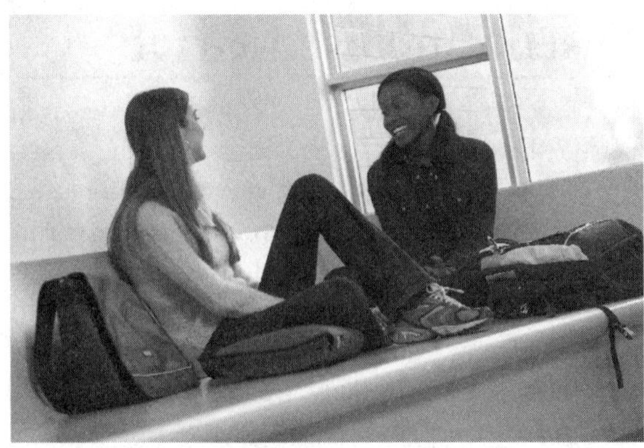

Group Help and Support

If help is needed in coming to terms with the death of a loved one, local support groups and grief counselors are trained and available for guidance. Many support groups are specific to a particular type of loss. People who attend meetings share their feelings with people who have experienced similar losses. Examples include survivors of suicide, or murder, or **sudden infant death syndrome (SIDS)**, the sudden and unexpected eath of a child less than one year old, as well as people who have survived the deaths of parents, children, or spouses.

Such groups are either self-help, in which survivors help and comfort one another, or counseling, in which a trained moderator or counselor presides over the meetings. In both self-help and counseling groups, meetings typically are held once a week in a safe, comfortable atmosphere.

Individual Grief Therapy

People experiencing grief symptoms often do not seek self-help groups or a grief counselor but rather seek individual counseling. Individual

My Grief Support Group

When my mother died last year, I just couldn't seem to get over it. I didn't know why, but I kept getting sadder and sadder. One day a couple of months ago, I just couldn't take it anymore and went to see the college counselor. She told me about an on-campus support group for people "like me." At that point, I thought I had nothing to lose, except me, so I went. That day I began to live again.

I love the people in my group. All of us have had a parent die. I believe that they are the first people to really understand how I feel. With them, I don't feel different anymore. We don't tell each other what to do; we just understand, and we are there for each other.

Last week, we wrote letters to our dead parents, thanking them for being our parents. Also we told them that we were angry that they left us. As I think about it now, that experience was exactly what I needed.

As new members enter our group, they sense that the old timers are happy. So, part of the reason that I want to continue in the group is to help the new people. That's one of the good things about this group—helping each other. I still miss my mother, but I'm not so sad all of the time anymore. I love my group.

grief therapy takes place over scheduled sessions, usually once a week to begin. Later, the sessions are less frequent. In these sessions, people are encouraged to talk to the therapist about their feelings of loss and about the person who has died. Many grieving persons have a difficult time expressing anger toward the dead person, and they need to be reassured by a counselor that these feelings are normal.

A family doctor, priest, or pastor can guide a grieving person to a therapist whose personality, credentials, style, and approach are suitable. Even so, the person might have to attend a session or two to decide if he or she is comfortable with the counselor. Changing to another counselor is sometimes necessary.

How an Employer Can Help

How an employer reacts to a death in an employee's family can help the grieving employee's recovery (Tyler, 2003). Employers should:

- ensure that bereavement policies are established.
- help the grieving worker communicate with colleagues.
- help coworkers express their sympathy.
- help the employee and supervisor deal with any productivity issues.

Policies and Procedures

An employer's most important task in helping employees overcome a loss is to make certain that there are policies and procedures in place for handling matters such as life insurance benefits, bereavement leave, emergency loans, leave-sharing, and condolence gifts. Also, employers can help employees and their families keep their end-of-life legal paperwork (e.g., wills, medical directives, powers-of-attorney, and funeral options) up to date so they do not have to deal with it while they are grieving. Employers also can do the following:

- Provide at least 1 week of paid bereavement leave. Provide an emergency loan program to help employees pay for funeral and related expenses.
- Immediately send an official condolence gift from the company.
- Treat all bereaved employees equitably. Employers should not send flowers to one employee and not to another.
- Streamline bereavement procedures so they can be completed quickly. One way is an e-mail system for notifying necessary administrative departments—HR, benefits, employee assistance program—about a bereaved employee.
- Offer a leave-sharing program through which coworkers can donate their unused personal time to a colleague in need.

Thoughtful Gestures

The following thoughtful gestures can be helpful to a bereaved employee:

- Serve as liaison between the bereaved employee and his or her colleagues. Ask the employee what to tell colleagues about the loss. Remember that some things are confidential (such as suicide) and not everybody needs to know the details of the death (Fitzgerald, 2007).
- Coordinate thoughtful gestures. Channel colleagues' desire to help their coworker into constructive avenues that offer compassionate support and practical assistance to the employee and family. Ideas include sending a fruit basket, cookies, flowers, or even a bag of paper plates, cups, napkins, and tissue for the endless stream of funeral visitors. Other ways to help include making meals, providing child care, or mowing the lawn.
- Spread out thoughtful acts over time. For example, writing a note or a card periodically shows ongoing support. And by all means, attend the funeral (Doka, 1996).

Return to Work

When the employee returns to work, have available an up-to-date resource list of community

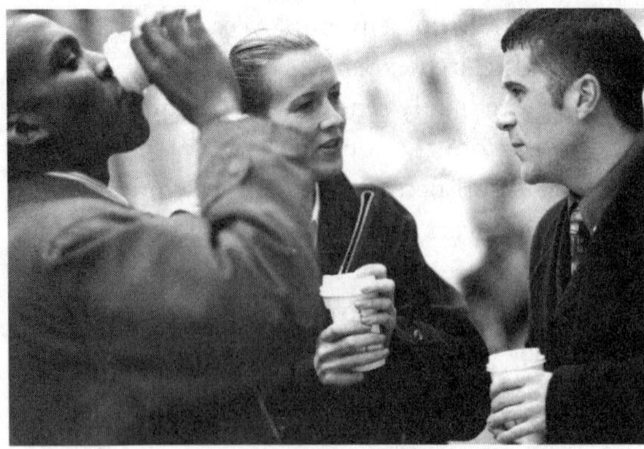

grief counselors and support groups. The employee might be overwhelmed and not know how to seek out resources. The employee also may not be able to work as efficiently as before the bereavement.

Set up a meeting between employee supervisor in which a bereaved person having difficulty can ask for help. Have regular follow-up meetings. Let the employee talk about the experience. Grieving takes time, so be flexible in allowing adjustments in schedule, workload, reassignments, and time off.

The ways an employer reacts to an employee's loss have far-reaching implications among the workforce. If coworkers see that the bereaved person is treated well, they will feel more confident about their employer.

SUMMARY

- In some cases, people are so overwhelmed by grief (deep and poignant distress at the loss of someone close) that adjusting to life and investing in relationships seems impossible.
- *Bereavement* refers to the objective state of experiencing a loss; *mourning* refers to the social process, norms, and so on, by which bereavement is publicly recognized.
- Differences in grieving are affected by differences in social class, generation, and culture.
- Intuitive grievers feel their grief and express their emotions openly; instrumental grievers think and remember as they grieve, expressing it by doing something related to the loss; dissonant grievers experience grief, but do not feel free to express it.
- Physical reactions to grief include symptoms such as tightness of the throat, shortness of breath, headaches, and dizziness.
- One way to deal creatively with loss and grief is to construct, and tell to other people, a narrative account (storytelling) of one's relationship with the dead person.
- Anticipatory grief refers to patients and family members grieving even before death occurs.
- Disenfranchised grief involves the griever grieving alone because the loss is not social acknowledged (e.g., homosexual relationship in many states or lover of a person married to someone else).
- Even though there is no specific time period associated with getting over a loss, a typical period of grieving lasts from 6 to 18 months.
- How an employer reacts to a death in an employee's family can help the grieving employee's recovery. Examples include sending flowers or food to the funeral home and helping the grieving worker communicate with employees.

ADDITIONAL RESOURCES

Books

Miller, J. E. (1996). *How will I get through the holidays?* Ft. Wayne, IN: Willowgreen Publishing. The author of this brief book offers 12 ideas for navigating emotionally charged holiday times, with a number of specific suggestions.

Roberts, B. K. (2002). *Death without denial, grief without apology: A guide for facing death and loss.* Troutdale, OR: NewSage Press. The former governor of Oregon tells the story of her husband's death from lung cancer, revealing in a very personal way how she mourned.

Zimmermann, S. (2003). *Writing to heal the soul: Transforming grief and loss through writing.* New York: Crown/Three Rivers. After the death of her daughter, Zimmermann found solace in writing about her pain. Drawing on experiences of her family and friends, she guides readers through writing exercises designed to stimulate reflection.

Movie

Away From Her. (2007). What happens to love when memory is gone? An affecting portrait of the dilemma of caring for (in both senses) an Alzheimer's patient.

Critical Thinking

Of all the ways of coping with loss and grief described in the chapter, which ones would work best for you? Why?

Class Activity

In groups of four to five students, research what employers in other countries offer employees who have had a loved one die. Each group should take a different country. Present your findings in a PowerPoint presentation.

References

Archer, J. (1999). *The nature of grief: The evolution and psychology of reactions to loss.* London: Routledge.

Bowlby, J. (1980). *Attachment and loss, Vol. 3: Loss: Sadness and depression.* New York: Basic Books.

Doka, K. J. (Ed.). (1989). *Disenfranchised grief: Recognizing hidden sorrow.* Lexington, MA: Lexington Books.

Doka, K. J. (1996). *Living with grief after sudden loss: Suicide, homicide, accident, heart attack, stroke.* Philadelphia: Taylor and Francis.

Engel, G. L. (1961). Is grief a disease? A challenge for medical research. *Psychosomatic Medicine, 23*(11), 18–22.

Fitzgerald, H. (2007). *Grief at work.* Washington, DC: American Hospice Foundation.

Freud, S. (2005). *On murder, mourning, and melancholia* (S. Whiteside, Trans.). London: Penguin Modern Classics. (Original work published 1917).

Harvey, J. (1998). *Perspectives on loss: A sourcebook.* Philadelphia: Taylor & Francis.

Kauffman, J. (2002). *Loss of the assumptive world: A theory of traumatic loss.* New York: Routledge.

Klass, D., Silverman, P. R., & Nickman, S. L. (Eds.). (1996). *Continuing bonds: A new understanding of grief.* Washington, DC: Taylor & Francis.

Kübler-Ross, E. (1969). *On death and dying.* New York: Touchstone.

Lindemann, E. (1944). Symptomatology and management of acute grief. *American Journal of Psychiatry, 101*, 141–148.

Martin, T. L., & Doka, K. J. (2000). *Men don't cry, women do: Transcending gender stereotypes of grief.* Philadelphia: Brunner/Mazel.

Neimeyer, R., & Jordan, J. (2002). Disenfranchisement and empathic failure: Grief therapy and the co-construction of meaning. In K. J. Doka (Ed.), *Disenfranchised grief: New directions, challenges, and strategies for practice.* Champaign, IL: Research Press.

Nickman, S. L., Silverman, P. R., & Normand, C. (1998). Children's construction of their deceased parent: The surviving parent's contribution. *American Journal of Orthopsychiatry, 68*(1), 126–141.

Osterweis, M., Solomon, R., & Green, M. (1984). *Bereavement: Reactions, consequences, and care.* Washington, DC: National Academy Press.

Pine, V. R., & Brauer, C. (1986). Parental grief: A synthesis of theory, research, and intervention. In T. A. Rando (Ed.), *Parental loss of a child.* Champaign, IL: Research Press.

Ponder, R., & Pomeroy, E. (1996). The grief of caregivers: How pervasive is it? *Journal of Gerontological Social Work, 27*(1/2), 3–21.

Rando, T. A. (1983). An investigation of grief and adaptation in parents whose children have died from cancer. *Journal of Pediatric Psychology, 8*(1), 3–20.

Rando, T. A. (1986). A comprehensive analysis of anticipatory grief: Perspectives, processes, promises, and problems. In T. A. Rando (Ed.), *Loss and anticipatory grief.* Lexington, MA: Lexington Books.

Raphael, B. (1983). *The anatomy of bereavement.* New York: Basic Books.

Saldinger, A., Cain, A., Kalter, N., & Lohnes, K. (1999). Anticipating parental death in families with young children. *American Journal of Orthopsychiatry, 69*(1), 39–48.

Sanders, C. M. (1982–1983). Effects of sudden vs. chronic illness death on bereavement outcome. *Omega: The Journal of Death and Dying, 13*(3), 227–241.

Schneider, J. M., & Zimmerman, S. K. (2005). *Transforming loss: A discovery process.* Phoenix, AZ: Integra Press.

Sife, W. (1998). *The loss of a pet.* New York: Howell Book House.

Tyler, K. (2003, September 9). Helping employees cope with grief. *HR Magazine, 48*, 54–58.

Walker, R., Pomeroy, E. C., McNeil, J. S., & Franklin, C. (1994). Anticipatory grief and Alzheimer's Disease: Strategies for intervention. *Journal of Gerontological Social Work, 22*(3/4), 21–39.

Walker, R. J., Pomeroy, E. C., McNeil, J. S., & Franklin, C. (1996). Anticipatory grief and AIDS: Strategies for intervening with caregivers. *Health and Social Work, 21*(1), 49–57.

Death-Related Tasks and Decisions

I bequeath my soul to God . . . my body to be buried obscurely.
For my name and memory, I leave it to men's charitable speeches,
and to foreign nations, the next age.
—FROM FRANCIS BACON'S WILL (1626)

Objectives

After reading this chapter, you will be able to answer the following questions:

- What is a will, how is one drafted, and what are the various forms it can take?
- What is probate, and how can it be avoided?
- What is a living trust and an AB trust?
- What is the estate tax?
- Are insurance death benefits taxable?
- What death benefits are available through Social Security?
- What benefits are available to veterans and their families?
- How is a death certified, and when is an autopsy performed?
- What happens if a person dies overseas?
- What are the various regulations and controversies regarding organ donation?

At one time or another, people should make a number of death-related tasks and decisions. Some of these are completed before death, and others occur after a death occurs. These tasks and decisions include making a will; making arrangements for a large estate to avoid probate; taking the estate tax into account, if necessary; obtaining life insurance; procuring social security survivor benefits and death benefits for veterans; certifying the death; making decisions about an autopsy; determining what to do if someone dies overseas; and whether or not to donate organs.

Wills

A **will** is a legal document made out by a person before he or she dies. In a will, exactly how a person's possessions are to be distributed is outlined. A will contains instructions from the will maker, or **testator**, about how to distribute the estate, which consists of all of one's possessions and valuables.

In most states, a testator must be at least 18 years old, be of sound mind, have at least two witnesses (three in Vermont), and have voluntarily specified the contents of the will.

People prepare wills for the following reasons:

- Give what they want to whom they want.
- Resolve possible disputes among the surviving relatives.
- Specify a guardian for surviving minor children.

In a **joint will**, two people make one will, each leaving everything to the other. Dictated in a will is what happens to property when the second person dies. A joint will has both pluses and minuses. This type of will typically prevents the survivor from doing something foolish or contrary to the wishes of the first spouse. However, it can tie up the property so that the survivor cannot make sensible decisions based on changed circumstances.

In a **conditional will**, specified conditions must be met after the testator's death for the will to be valid. For instance, an uncle might tell his nephew he will get his Porsche Turbo if he finishes college. If the nephew does not finish college, he doesn't get the car.

A will can be revoked and replaced by an entirely new will. Also, parts of the will can be changed, using a **codicil**, or appendix, to the will.

Some states accept **holographic** (handwritten) and **nuncupative** (oral) **wills**. A nuncupative will, however, typically is legal only under certain circumstances, for instance, from a dying soldier.

Do-It-Yourself Basic Will

If a person is under age 50 and the estate is not large enough for estate taxes, a basic will probably will suffice. As a person grows older and acquires more property, however, more sophisticated planning might be needed and professional advice sought ("Wills and Estate Planning," 2007).

Is a lawyer required to draft a will? It depends. It is a good idea to use a lawyer, but most people can draft a will (using appropriate reference materials) that takes care of such basics as leaving an unencumbered home, ordinary investments, and personal items to loved ones. A guardian for minor children, and for any property they inherit, should also be specified in a basic will. In a basic will, an **executor** should be named. An executor collects the property, pays debts and taxes, and then distributes what is left as specified in the will. The executor also notifies people and organizations of the death.

The will must be signed in front of two witnesses, who then countersign it in each other's presence. (As mentioned previously, Vermont requires three witnesses.) Although it is not necessary to use a notary, it can be helpful if a probate court would otherwise require an affidavit from, or the personal appearance of, the witnesses to prove a will.

A **guardian** is an adult given the legal right by a court to care for a minor or child's inherited property. A property guardian is called a *guardian of the estate*. One who can make personal decisions for a child, such as for physical, medical, and educational needs, is a *guardian of the person*. One person can be named as both. A court-appointed guardian for an incapacitated adult is usually called a **conservator**.

Death Without a Will

As many as two-thirds of Americans die without leaving a will. When a person dies without a will, the person is said to die **intestate**. In this case, each state has its own laws to determine how the person's possessions are to be distributed.

In the absence of a will, a person's estate goes to a probate court. State law will determine who gets the person's property, and a judge might decide who will raise any minor children. In most intestacy cases, property goes first to a spouse, then to the person's children and their descendants ("Wills and Estate Planning," 2007). If there are no descendants, it goes in order, to:

- parents
- siblings
- siblings' descendants
- grandparents
- parents' siblings
- parents' siblings' descendants

In the case of a same-sex couple who live in a state where same-sex marriage is not legal, the survivor will not inherit unless the state allows a registered domestic partner to inherit. At present, a domestic partner is allowed to inherit in Connecticut, Maine, and Vermont. U.S. states that recognize gay marriage (as of June 1, 2008) are California and Massachusetts. New Jersey offers same-sex civil unions the same rights as married heterosexual couples, and New York recognizes gay marriage of couples legally married in another state (Johnson, 2008).

If a person dies intestate with no identifiable heirs, the estate generally **escheats** (is legally assigned) to the government. In the United States, assignment of ownership of intestate property is specific to each state. (Information about how intestate property is distributed in each state can be found at MyStateWill.com.)

Probate

Probate is the judicial determination of the validity of a will. The probate process involves proving the will's authenticity; appointing an executor to handle the dead person's affairs; inventorying the dead person's property; paying debts and taxes; identifying heirs; and distributing the dead person's property according to the will or, if there is no will, according to state law.

Ways to Avoid Probate

Formal court-supervised probate of a will is a costly, time-consuming process that is best avoided if possible. A number of strategies are available to avoid having a large estate go to probate court. Some of these include payable-on-death bank accounts, gifts, retirement accounts, joint agreements, community-property agreements, the transfer of assets on death, and living trusts ("Wills and Estate Planning," 2007). All decisions about trusts, however, should be carefully considered and, in most cases, done with the advice of an attorney.

Bank Accounts.

Payable-on-death (P.O.D.) bank accounts serve as an easy way to keep money out of probate. To establish one only requires filling out a bank form naming a beneficiary. As long as the person is alive, the beneficiary has no rights to the funds. The account status and beneficiary can be changed at any time. To collect the funds, the beneficiary simply presents identification and proof of the account at the owner's death. In the case of a joint checking account, a P.O.D. designation only takes effect when the surviving spouse dies.

Gifts.

Giving away money or property can reduce an estate's value for probate purposes. Giving more than $12,000 to any one person in a calendar year ($24,000 for a married couple), however, requires filing a federal gift tax return, although no tax is due that year. A person can give away no more than $1 million over his or her lifetime. Anything above this amount requires payment of taxes.

Retirement Accounts.

When a retirement account, such as an IRA or a 401(k), is established, a beneficiary is named. After the account holder's death, the beneficiary can claim the money from the account custodian. Spouses inherit retirement accounts unless the spouse agrees in writing to another beneficiary. In community property states (Arizona, California, Idaho, Louisiana, Nevada, New Mexico, Texas, Washington, and Wisconsin), in the event of a divorce, a surviving spouse gets half of the contributions made during the marriage.

Joint Tenancy.

Joint tenancy property passes without probate to the surviving owner(s). Joint tenancy can work well for couples (married or not) who acquire valuable property together. In Texas, a separate written agreement signed by all joint tenants is required.

Joint tenancy has some potential drawbacks. A new joint owner can, for example, sell or mortgage his or her share or lose it to creditors. In addition, a gift tax return might need to be filed. A joint tenant to a bank account who was named to help manage a person's money may claim entitlement to keep the funds after the death. Obviously, it might be better to use a power of attorney to name someone to help manage things.

TENANCY BY THE ENTIRETY.

Tenancy by the entirety is similar to joint tenancy, but it is available only to married couples (or, in a few states, to registered same-sex partners).

COMMUNITY PROPERTY WITH RIGHT OF SURVIVORSHIP.

This process gives a surviving spouse automatic ownership of joint property without court proceedings. This arrangement is available in Alaska, Arizona, California, Nevada, and Wisconsin. In California, registered domestic partners can also benefit.

TRANSFER-ON-DEATH REGISTRATION OF SECURITIES.

These securities are similar to P.O.D. bank accounts. Based on the Uniform Transfer-on-Death Securities Registration Act, a person can name a beneficiary for stocks, bonds, or brokerage accounts without probate. When registering with a stockbroker or a company, the investor asks for ownership in "beneficiary form." The beneficiary is named on the ownership papers. After the investor's death, the beneficiary can claim the securities simply by providing proof of death and identification to the broker or transfer agent.

TRANSFER-ON-DEATH REGISTRATION FOR VEHICLES.

This registration is similar to the transfer-on-death registration of securities. It is available in California, Connecticut, Kansas, Missouri, and Ohio. A person can register a vehicle in "beneficiary form." The registration certificate shows the name of the beneficiary, who automatically owns the vehicle after the owner's death.

Revocable Living Trusts

Trust property is not counted as part of a probate estate (although it is subject to the federal estate tax), because the person owns the trust as a trustee, not as an individual. After the person's death, a successor trustee can distribute without probate the trust property to the heirs named in the trust. Because trust property is regarded as an asset, however, it does not protect against lawsuits.

Creation of a trust is similar to the drafting of a will. For a basic living trust, a declaration of trust is drafted. The person names himself or herself as the trustee. Then the person transfers ownership of the property to himself or herself in the capacity of trustee. The trustee names beneficiaries, including alternate (or contingent) beneficiaries. The trust must be signed in the presence of a notary public. Trust documents should be stored in a safe place, and the successor trustee should know where the trust is located.

Tax-Saving AB Trusts

Couples with more than $2 million in assets can avoid both probate and estate taxes with an AB, or credit shelter, trust. (The exemption will vary in years to come; see Table 11.1.)

How does an AB trust work? Each spouse leaves his or her property to the AB trust. When

HISTORY OF THE ESTATE TAX

In 1906, President Theodore Roosevelt proposed a federal inheritance tax ("United for a Fair Economy," 2007). The first estate tax was passed in 1916, with a graduated rate from 1% to 5%, and was applied to estates over $50,000, or approximately $850,000 in today's dollars.

During the 1930s, Congress raised the top estate tax rate to 70% on fortunes of more than $50 million, or $666 million in today's dollars. This tax raised 11% of the federal government's total revenue. The estate tax remained essentially unchanged until 2001, when Congress passed a tax bill that slowly phases the estate tax out until 2009, repeals it entirely in 2010, and then brings it back to life in 2011.

Table 11.1 EXCLUSIONS FOR ESTATE TAXES

Year	Exclusion
2007	$2 million
2008	$2 million
2009	$3.5 million
2010	Repealed
2011	$1 million

Source: Modified from the Internal Revenue Service Code §2000, Chapter 11, Estate Tax.

one spouse dies, the surviving spouse can make use of the trust property, but does not own it. Thus the property is not taxed as an estate when the second spouse dies, because the second spouse never legally owned it. In an AB trust, beneficiaries of the trust's property, usually their children, are named when the surviving spouse dies.

The Estate Tax

The **estate tax** (called the *death tax* by its opponents) is a tax based on the fair market value of an estate, minus deductions and exclusions. As a result, currently only the wealthiest 2% of all Americans are subject to an estate tax (Internal Revenue Service, 2007). In addition to the federal government, many states also impose an estate tax, with the state version called either an estate tax or an inheritance tax.

An estate generally consists of cash and securities, real estate, insurance, trusts, annuities, business interests, and other assets. This is the *gross estate*. The *taxable estate* is what is left after certain allowed deductions, such as mortgages and other debts, estate administration expenses, property that passes to surviving spouses, and donations to qualified charities. The most important deduction is the one for property going to the surviving spouse, because it can eliminate the federal estate tax.

Inherited property is assessed at **fair market value** at the date of death, which eliminates most or all capital gains if the heir sells the property before it appreciates. If any portion of an estate includes property inherited from someone else fewer than 10 years earlier on which estate tax was paid, there also may be an estate tax credit for that property.

After the taxable estate is determined, the value of **lifetime taxable gifts**—gifts given in the donor's lifetime—is added to this number and the tax computed. Such gifts are exempt, however, up to an annual amount of $12,000, or $24,000 for a married couple, per individual recipient. Also, a gift tax applies only on amounts given away that exceed a total of $1 million over a lifetime. The gift tax is simply intended to prevent avoidance of the estate tax by a person's giving away the whole of an estate just before dying.

The estate tax is then again reduced by the available unified credit, or exclusion (see Table 11.1). Presently, only net estates exceeding $2 million are subject to an estate tax. (**Unified credit** means that the estate tax and the gift tax are combined for purposes of calculating the exclusion.)

FAIR MARKET VALUE

The fair market value is the price at which the property would change hands between a willing buyer and a willing seller, neither being under any compulsion to buy or to sell and both having reasonable knowledge of relevant facts. The fair market value of a particular item of property includible in the decedent's gross estate is not to be determined by a forced sale price. Nor is the fair market value of an item of property to be determined by the sale price of the item in a market other than that in which such item is most commonly sold to the public, taking into account the location of the item wherever appropriate.—IRS Regulation §20.2031-1

ESTATE TAX EXCLUSIONS

Most relatively simple estates with a total value under a certain amount do not require the filing of an estate tax return. The ceilings change year by year, as shown in Table 11.1. (Note that the tax act was repealed for one year—2010—and then dropped back in 2011 to the year 2001 level.)

Estate Tax Return

Generally, an estate tax return is due 9 months after the date of death. A 6-month extension is available if requested prior to the due date and the estimated correct amount of tax is paid before the due date. An estate tax return should include copies or documentation of the following:

- The death certificate.
- The decedent's will and/or relevant trusts.
- Appraisals.
- Relevant documents regarding litigation involving the estate.
- Any unusual items shown on the return.

In many states, estate or inheritance taxes are also imposed. In some states the estate is exempt from state tax if it is exempt from the federal tax. In other states, an estate might be subject to state tax even though it is exempt from the federal tax.

Help might be needed with estate planning from professionals such as certified public accountants (CPAs) or enrolled agents (EAs). An EA is a tax professional who has passed an IRS test covering all aspects of taxation. Attorneys also should be included in estate planning, because CPAs and EAs cannot take care of probate matters and other situations that require a law license.

Insurance Death Benefit

An insurance death benefit is not taxable, unless the amount paid exceeds the benefit amount. If the benefit is paid as a lump sum, or not at regular intervals, then any amount over the benefit amount is taxable. For instance, if the death benefit is $150,000, and the insurance policy paid $200,000, tax is due on the extra $50,000. If the insurance is paid in installments, the benefit total can be divided by the number of years of payments, and that amount deducted from taxable income (WorldWideTax, 2007).

Social Security Survivor Benefits

In the case of a death, certain family members might be eligible for benefits from Social Security. Those eligible include a widow or widower, including those divorced; children (biological, grand-, step-, or adopted); and dependent parents (Social Security Administration, 2007). Age, year born, and the disability of survivors are the major factors in deciding eligibility.

How much a family will get from Social Security benefits depends on the average lifetime earnings of the deceased person. The Social Security statement, sent each year to every worker age 25 or older, provides an estimate of survivor benefits, as well as of retirement and disability benefits.

A small, one-time death payment is made upon death if the person had worked long enough. This payment can be made only to a spouse or minor children and only if they meet certain requirements.

Survivor's benefits should be applied for promptly. If the applicant is not already receiving benefits, a great many documents, as originals or certified copies, are required. If the applicant is already receiving retirement benefits as a spouse, only the death need be reported, and payments will be changed to survivor's benefits. If the survivor's existing benefits are based on the survivor's own work, the survivor will receive the higher benefit of the two. For this change, a death certificate and an application to switch benefits are required.

Generally, widow's or widower's benefits are lost at remarriage before age 60. Remarriage after 60 (or 50 if disabled) will not stop benefit payments based on a former spouse's work. At age 62,

My Story: The Best Inheritance of All

When I returned to my Tennessee hometown to attend my 40th high school reunion 20 years after my father died, I met some of my father's acquaintances as I went about checking out the lively downtown area. Many of the people asked, "Aren't you Morris's daughter?" Each and every one of them told me what a fine man my father was. Several of them told me in detail how he had positively influenced their lives. One man, who played basketball for my father 50 years ago, still had my father's picture on the wall. The man said that my father believed in him, and at the time, that was unusual. That man grew up to be an important political figure. To me, that was a finer inheritance than any material possession my father left me. I hope I leave my children the same type of inheritance.

benefits might be based on a new spouse's work, if those benefit are greater.

Life Insurance for Veterans

Military Service Group Life Insurance (SGLI) is a program of low-cost group life insurance, that was developed to provide insurance benefits for veterans and military service members who might not be able to get insurance from private companies because of the extra risks involved in military service or because of a service-connected disability (U.S. Department of Veterans Affairs, 2007a). SGLI coverage is available in $50,000 increments up to a maximum of $400,000. SGLI premiums are currently $0.07 per $1,000 of insurance, regardless of a member's age.

Service members with SGLI coverage can, upon being discharged, convert their full-time SGLI coverage to term insurance under the Veterans' Group Life Insurance program, or convert to a permanent plan of insurance with one of the participating commercial insurance companies. The SGLI Disability Extension allows service members who are totally disabled at time of discharge to retain their SGLI coverage at no cost for up to two years.

Death Benefits for Veterans

The spouse, dependent children, and dependent parents of dead veterans are offered a number of benefits by the Department of Veterans Affairs (DVA; U.S. Department of Veteran Affairs, 2007b). Benefits include compensation, vocational/educational counseling and assistance, work-study allowances, guaranteed home loans, and headstones/grave markers.

Dependency and Indemnity Compensation (DIC) is a tax-free monthly benefit paid to eligible survivors of a military service member. This benefit is paid for two years from the date it begins, but is discontinued earlier when there are no longer children in the family under age 18. A transitional benefit is added if there are children under age 18. Parents (biological, step-, adopted, or *in loco parentis*), whose child died in service or from a service-connected disability may be entitled to DIC if they are in financial need. Usually an application for DIC benefits is completed by a Casualty Assistance Officer and submitted on behalf of the survivors. The basic monthly rate is $1,067 for an eligible surviving spouse. The rate is increased for each dependent child; also, it is increased if the surviving spouse is housebound or in need of aid.

Survivors' and Dependents' Educational Assistance (DEA) pays a monthly education or training allowance to the spouse and children, aged 18 to 26, of a veteran who died of a service-connected disability. These benefits can be used for degree and certificate programs, apprenticeships, and on-the-job training. A spouse may also take a correspondence course. Remedial, deficiency, and refresher courses are approved under certain circumstances. Free professional, educational, and vocational counseling is available.

Three-quarters or full-time students enrolled in college degree, vocational, or professional programs can earn money while learning with a VA work-study allowance. The work done must be related to VA work and pays an hourly wage equal to the greater of federal minimum wage or state minimum wage. Some colleges and universities pay the difference between the amount the VA pays and the amount the school pays other work-study students.

A surviving spouse (who has not remarried) is eligible for a guaranteed home loan from a private lender. The loan may be used to build, buy, remodel, or refinance the home occupied by the spouse. A surviving spouse also may obtain a guaranteed interest rate reduction by refinancing an existing VA loan.

A *memorial certificate,* bearing the U.S. president's signature, wherein the service of honorably discharged dead veterans is recognized, is available from the VA. This certificate is for next of kin or other loved ones.

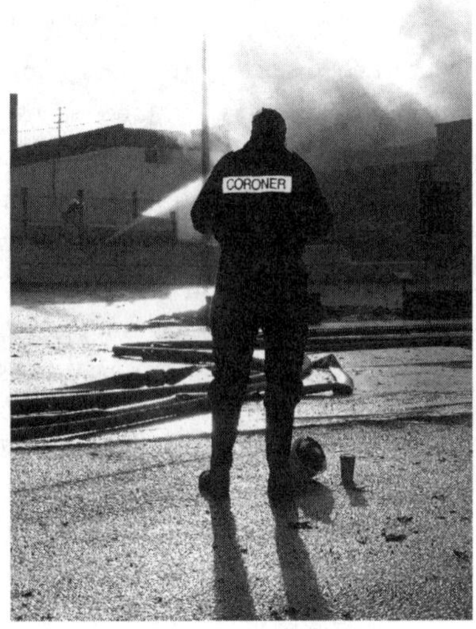

Death Certification

A death becomes official when it is certified by a physician on a death certificate. Certificates vary slightly from state to state, but name, sex, date of death, as well as the time, place, and cause of death are required (see Figure 11.1). Causes of death typically include heart attack, cancer, accident, suicide, murder, and AIDS.

Coroners and Medical Examiners

For a sudden or suspicious death, or one for which no physician has signed a death certificate, the cause must be established by a coroner or medical examiner. In most cases, **coroners** are elected officials who are not physicians, whereas **medical examiners** are usually medical doctors who are appointed. Deaths requiring action by a coroner or medical examiner include homicides, suicides, accidents, deaths on the job, deaths in government offices or prisons, deaths in hospitals or other healthcare facilities if sudden or the possible result of negligence, and deaths at home if no doctor was present. The examination consists of various chemical and biological tests and might include an autopsy, if required by law. The results are important for settling court cases and insurance claims.

HISTORY OF AUTOPSY

Autopsies began in Roman times, when they were done in criminal cases to determine the cause of death (Larson, 2007), but most cultures historically have resisted the dissection of a body (Lawrence, 2003). Thus, only legally required autopsies were performed, and only if ordered by a nonmedical coroner, and then only an external examination was allowed.

When dissection was introduced into medical training in late medieval times, it only could be performed on the bodies of executed criminals. When medicine was limited by the theory of humors (that the balance of fluids in the body determined health or disease), autopsies were not seen as revealing anything about disease. Then, in the eighteenth and nineteenth centuries, the correspondence of autopsy observations to disease in living patients became better understood. Even then, only the bodies of the poor who had died in hospitals were used (Lawrence, 2003).

Figure 11.1 STANDARD U.S. DEATH CERTIFICATE.

FORM VS NO. 1-A
(Rev. 5/02)

COMMONWEALTH OF KENTUCKY
CABINET FOR HEALTH SERVICES
REGISTRAR OF VITAL STATISTICS

116 ____________ FILE NO

CERTIFICATE OF DEATH

MUST BE TYPED

1. DECEDENT'S NAME *(First, Middle, Last)* | 2. SEX | 3. DATE OF DEATH *(Month, Day, Year)*

4. SOCIAL SECURITY NO | 5a. AGE Last Birthday *(Years)* | 5b. UNDER 1 YEAR *(Months)* *(Days)* | 5c. UNDER 1 DAY *(Hours)* *(Minutes)* | 6. DATE OF BIRTH *(Month, Day, Year)* | 7. BIRTHPLACE *(City/State or Foreign Country)*

8. WAS DECEDENT EVER IN U.S. ARMED FORCES? ☐ Yes ☐ No

9a. PLACE OF DEATH *(Check only one)*
HOSPITAL ☐ Inpatient ☐ ER/Outpatient ☐ DOA
OTHER ☐ Nursing Home ☐ Residence ☐ Other *(Specify)*

9b. FACILITY NAME *(If not institution, give street and number)* | 9c. CITY, TOWN, OR LOCATION OF DEATH | 9d. COUNTY OF DEATH

10. MARITAL STATUS Married, Never Married Widowed, Divorced *(Specify)* | 11. SURVIVING SPOUSE *(If wife, give maiden name)* | 12a. DECEDENT'S USUAL OCCUPATION *(Give kind of work done during most of working life. Do Not use retired)* | 12b. KIND OF BUSINESS/INDUSTRY

13a. RESIDENCE - State | 13b. COUNTY | 13c. CITY, TOWN, OR LOCATION | 13d. STREET AND NUMBER

13e. INSIDE CITY LIMITS? ☐ Yes ☐ No | 13f. ZIP CODE | 14. WAS DECEDENT OF HISPANIC ORIGIN? *(Specify No or Yes - If yes, specify Cuban, Mexican, Puerto Rican, etc.)* ☐ No ☐ Yes | 15. RACE – American Indian, Black, White, etc. *(Specify)* | 16. DECEDENT'S EDUCATION *(Specify only highest grade completed)* Elem/Secondary (0-12) College (1-4 or 5+)

17. FATHER'S NAME *(First, Middle, Last)* | 18. MOTHER'S NAME *(First, Middle, Maiden Surname)*

19a. INFORMANT'S NAME | 19b. MAILING ADDRESS *(Street and Number or Rural Route Number, City or Town, State, Zip Code)*

20a. METHOD OF DISPOSITION
☐ Burial ☐ Cremation ☐ Removal from State
☐ Donation ☐ Other *(Specify)* ____________

20b. PLACE OF DISPOSITION *(Name of cemetery, crematory, or other place)* | 20c. LOCATION – *(City, Town, or State)*

21a. SIGNATURE OF FUNERAL SERVICE LICENSEE *(Or person acting as such)* | 22. NAME AND ADDRESS OF FACILITY

23a. To the best of my knowledge, death occurred at the time, date, place and due to the causes stated

Signature and Title ____________________________

(MUST USE BLACK INK)

23b. DATE SIGNED *(Month, Day, Year)*

24. NAME AND ADDRESS OF PERSON WHO COMPLETED CAUSE OF DEATH (ITEM 28)

25. TIME OF DEATH | 26. DATE PRONOUNCED DEAD *(Month, Day, Year)* | 27. WAS CASE REFERRED TO MEDICAL EXAMINER/CORONER? ☐ Yes ☐ No

28. PART I. Enter the diseases, injuries, or complications that caused death. Do not enter the mode of dying, such as cardiac or respiratory arrest, shock or heart failure. List only one cause on each line.

Approximate interval between onset and death

IMMEDIATE CAUSE *(Final disease or condition resulting in death)* a. ____________
DUE TO (OR AS A CONSEQUENCE OF):

Sequentially list conditions, if any, leading to immediate cause. Enter UNDERLYING CAUSE *(Disease or injury that initiated events resulting in death)* LAST

b. ____________
DUE TO (OR AS A CONSEQUENCE OF):
c. ____________
DUE TO (OR AS A CONSEQUENCE OF):
d.

PART II Other significant conditions contributed to death but not resulting in the underlying cause given in Part I.

28a. If female, was there a pregnancy in the past 12 months? ☐ Yes ☐ No | 28b. Was an autopsy performed? ☐ Yes ☐ No | 28c. Were autopsy findings available prior to completion of cause of death? ☐ Yes ☐ No

28d. Did the deceased have Diabetes? ☐ Yes ☐ No | 28e. Was Diabetes an immediate, underlying, or contributing of or condition leading to death? ☐ Yes ☐ No

29. MANNER OF DEATH
☐ Natural ☐ Pending Investigation
☐ Accident
☐ Suicide ☐ Could not be determined
☐ Homicide

30a. DATE OF INJURY *(Month, Day, Year)* | 30b. TIME OF INJURY | 30c. INJURY AT WORK? ☐ Yes ☐ No | 30d. DESCRIBE HOW INJURY OCCURRED

30e. PLACE OF INJURY – At home, farm, street, factory, office building, etc. *(Specify)* | 30f. LOCATION *(Street and Number or Rural Route Number, City or Town)*

31. REGISTRAR'S SIGNATURE | 32. DATE FILED *(Month, Day, Year)*

Source: U.S. Department of Health and Human Services.

Autopsies

When a preliminary investigation of a dead body, or **corpse**, reveals the need to determine the cause of death, the corpse is brought to a **morgue** (place a dead body is kept until identified or until an autopsy is finished) and held until an autopsy can be performed. (The word *autopsy* means to "see for oneself.") The medical examination of a dead body is conducted to determine cause of death or, in some cases, the existence of and effects of a disease not identified when the person was alive. At this time, an opportunity exists to learn more to help in treating the living (Larson, 2007). This examination also is important for uncovering genetic factors for certain diseases.

In an autopsy, both the external and internal body is examined. After the organs have been examined and are no longer needed for further study, they are placed back in the body cavity and all incisions are closed. Funerals typically are delayed until the investigation is complete.

Autopsies conducted for medical reasons are performed by pathologists. A forensic autopsy is completed for legal reasons (suspicious, violent, and/or unexplained death, such as homicide, accident, or suicide). They may be performed or supervised by coroners or medical examiners. On occasion, it is necessary to exhume (dig up) a body for further investigation of the cause of death. Only courts can order the exhumation of a body.

A deceased person's family might request an autopsy to determine, for example, whether a genetic condition led to the death or whether medical malpractice was involved. Except when required by law, an autopsy can be performed only with the consent of immediate family members. Because a request to conduct an autopsy on a loved one can bring about conflicting feelings, effective communication is crucial.

Some religious groups (e.g., traditional Hindus) prohibit autopsies, considering it to be a violation of spiritual integrity. Islamic law forbids mutilation of a corpse. Orthodox Jews and traditional Christians are opposed to autopsy, an attitude that has lessened, but not gone away entirely (Lawrence, 2003).

In spite of their importance for medical research, the number of autopsies performed has declined over the past 20 years. One possible reason for the decline may be fear of malpractice claims by the physician who treated the person before death. Also, it might be that modern technology, in the form of CT scans and MRIs, provides the diagnostic information that previously only an autopsy could reveal (Larson, 2007).

Dealing with a Death Overseas

Travelers might think they are well prepared on a trip to a foreign country, but few know what to do if a traveling companion dies (Patterson, 2005). The following are useful tips in the case of the death of a U.S. citizen who dies overseas:

1. The nearest American embassy should be contacted immediately. The embassy should fax the necessary papers to the local funeral home or mortuary so the funerary process can begin. This procedure is especially urgent if the death has occurred just before a holiday weekend.
2. All the requirements of the American embassy for releasing the remains should be determined. The embassy might require that papers from the funeral home or crematorium be stamped by the embassy.
3. In the case of language barriers, an interpreter will be needed. The American embassy will, for a charge, help in this task.
4. A family member should have an up-to-date passport in case additional help and support are needed.
5. Being able to pay for unexpected, large funeral costs is essential. A friend or family member in the United States should have access to a large amount of cash that can be transferred, because a credit card may not work. For instance, one new widow discovered that her credit card did not fit into a

French credit card machine, and when she called American Express to use their travel medical protection plan, she was told to go to an American Express office to get a wire transfer of cash on the credit card. When she arrived, she was told, "Because he died, we canceled the card."

6. A widow or widower must show proof of marriage for funeral arrangements to proceed. This is a fairly universal requirement; thus, a marriage certificate should be carried with other travel documents.
7. Officials from the country where the death has occurred might require that police seal the coffin or box of ashes before allowing it out of the country.
8. Foreign mortuaries might not be willing to ship a metal box of ashes overseas, so be sure to use a wooden box, because airports do not allow a metal urn through security.

In summary, foreign travelers should take a marriage certificate, arrange for someone to send money transfers, know the location of the embassy and its policies, and designate a friend or relative who would be able to travel immediately to assist in an emergency. Travelers also should consider taking a notarized statement with them as they travel wherein it is shown that authority has been given to either a traveling companion or family member at home to make arrangements in case of death.

Organ Donation for Transplantation

Another important death decision is whether to donate organs. Organ donation has saved many lives. The organs most sought for transplantation are kidneys and livers. People also are on waiting lists for hearts, lungs, and pancreata. Donors can agree before they die to allow their organs to be taken for transplant.

For some organ transplants, such as a kidney, the donor is usually a living person, who might be a family member. Otherwise, organs are harvested from the body of a person who has been recently declared dead. Organs are kept viable for transplant by sustaining physiological functions in the body of the donor.

In the United States, about 75,000 people are on an organ transplant waiting list at any time. Each day about 60 people receive a donated organ, but 16 die because not enough organs are available. These high numbers have spurred debate about how to make enough organs available.

Rejection of the organ is the greatest obstacle to a successful transplant. The ideal candidate for a transplant is a patient who would die without it. The recipient's emotional stability and age also affect the success of the transplant.

A donor might specify that only certain organs can be harvested, or allow any body part to be taken. Organ donation instructions can be specified by completing a form such as the Uniform Donor Card (see Figure 11.2). In addition, a donor can specify on a driver's license the wish to be an organ donor. In emergency situations, a donor directive might not be clear-cut. Therefore, plans for organ donation should be discussed with family members in advance.

One reason potential donors or their families are reluctant to donate organs is their belief that all the body's parts should be together for a funeral. They typically question that if a part is

Figure 11.2 EXAMPLE OF AN ORGAN DONOR CARD.

MY COMMITMENT TO DONATE LIFE
UNIFORM DONOR CARD

I, ______________________ have spoken to my family about organ and tissue donation. The following people have witnessed my commitment to be a donor. I wish to donate:
☐ any needed organs & tissue ☐ only the following organs & tissue:
____

Donor Signature ______________________ Date ______

Witness ______________________ Date ______

Witness ______________________ Date ______

Source: From the National Foundation for Transplants.

missing, how can the body be put back together for a later existence? (Lock, 2001)

When an organ donor dies, a local organ-procurement organization will collect information about the donor and enter it into a program maintained by the UNOS (United Network for Organ Sharing) Organ Center, based in Richmond, Virginia. This program generates a list of potential recipients, ranked by physical compatibility between the donor and recipient, the health of the recipient, and how long the recipient has been waiting for an organ (Olson, 2007).

Half of persons offering organs are excluded because they have existing medical problems, such as cancer or infection. Of the 50% of potential donors with medically acceptable organs, half of the families refuse donation. The result is that there is only one organ donor out of 800 people who die in a hospital (Olson, 2007). On the bright side, organ donations are up. In 1993, 28% agreed to donate organs; in 2005, according to a Gallup Poll (Olson), nearly twice as many volunteered, or 53%.

Organ Donor Law Updated

The Uniform Anatomical Gift Act (UAGA) of 1968 was adopted by all 50 states and the District of Columbia. In the act, it was stated that a person can donate organs by signing a document that is witnessed. Before that act was adopted, the body of a person who died belonged to the next of kin [National Conference of Commissioners on Uniform State Laws (NCCUSL), 2007].

Because new medical technologies have caused an increase in the demand for organs, the UAGA was revised in 1987 to narrow the gap between supply and demand. Only 26 states, however, adopted the revision. Neither version of the act provided an allocation system for organs.

In the second revision of UAGA (2006), it is stated that a person can donate organs simply by signing a document, with no need for witnesses. This revision also encourages states (or some other entity) to create donor registries. These registries must be electronic and available around the clock. The 2006 UAGA revision also prevents families from changing or revoking donations—no one else can do so either, if the donor bars them from it (in a signed record or will, or in some circumstances, orally). Finally, if a person does not make known his or her wishes to donate, the new act provides for a priority list of people who can do that on behalf of the dead person. This list includes (1) agents acting under a healthcare power of attorney or other record; (2) adult children or grandchildren; or (3) a close friend.

Controversies Surrounding Determination of Death for Organ Donation

The ability to continue some bodily functions in a dead body to harvest organs for transplant, along with the increasing demand for them, has raised a number of ethical concerns about when a person can be safely declared dead before organs are taken.

The **dead-donor rule** is a term applied to organ retrieval. In the rule, it is written that vital organs should be taken only from deceased patients, and that living patients must not be killed by retrieving the organ (Younger, Arnold, & Schapiro, 1999). A violation of this rule, even with the prior consent of the donor or of his family or agent, is taken to be euthanasia, which is currently illegal (DuBois, 1999).

In the Uniform Determination of Death Act (UDDA; President's Commission, 1981), it is proposed that all states accept brain death, as well as circulatory–respiratory (CR) failure, as criteria for determining death, based on accepted medical standards. But the UDDA has been a source of controversy since it was first proposed.

First, some people argue that brain death is what defines death (Bernat, Culver, & Gert, 1981; Lamb, 1985). Because doctors usually wait at least 15 minutes after CR failure before declaring death, however, it is usually safe to assume that a patient is brain dead by then. If the heart is not beating, the need to avoid damage to organs requires a much shorter wait. To infer brain death from CR criteria requires, at normal temperatures, at least 10 minutes after CR functions are lost (Lynn,

1993). Thus, some people doubt that all organ donors are truly dead when procurement begins (Fox, 1993).

A second disagreement with UDDA is the importance of irreversibility, or in effect, bringing the dead back to life. Can it be done? Can it take place spontaneously (autoreversal)?

Finally, some people suspect that the UDDA is designed to permit organ donation, or, at the least, that UDDA is based on an underlying interest in organ procurement (Truog, 1997).

Against these objections to UDDA, DuBois (1999) argued that it is legitimate to declare death if the following circumstances are in place: when circulation and respiration have ceased; when these functions will not resume spontaneously; and that the physician should not resuscitate given proxies to withdraw life support. The 1993 Pittsburgh protocol for non-beating-heart deaths uses tests that seem to satisfy these criteria.

What American society is confronted with is the need to change the ancient objections to cutting into a dead body to harvest organs in order to help those who will die if they do not receive a donated organ. It is one thing to pass laws, establish guidelines, or create better procedures for allocation, but changes in general social attitudes are the crucial requirement if everyone who needs an organ to stay alive receives it in timely fashion.

Summary

- A will is a legal document completed before a person dies, which outlines how his or her life's possessions are to be distributed. In a joint will (or mutual will) made by two people, specifications are made whereby everything is left to the other. Also delineated in a joint will is what happens to the property when the second person dies. In a conditional will, conditions are specified that must occur after the testator's death to make the will valid. A will can be revoked and replaced or parts changed using a codicil or appendix. An executor of a will collects property, pays debts and taxes, distributes what is left, and notifies people and organizations about the death. A person who dies without a will is said to die intestate. In such cases, the estate goes to a probate court; state law will determine who gets the person's property; and a judge might appoint a guardian for any minor children.
- Probate is the judicial determination of the validity of a will. Gifts of money or property reduce an estate's value for probate purposes. Giving more than $12,000 to any one person in a calendar year ($24,000 for a married couple) requires filing a federal gift tax return, although no tax is due that year. A person can give up to $1 million over his or her lifetime without incurring tax liability. Following the death of a retirement account holder, beneficiaries of the account can claim the money from the account custodian. A surviving spouse is the beneficiary of a 401(k) account unless the spouse agrees in writing to another beneficiary.
- The estate tax (called the "death tax" by its opponents) is a tax based on the fair market value of everything a person owns or has an interest in on the day of his or her death, minus deductions and exclusions. The exclusion was $2 million in 2007. It goes up to $3.5 million in 2009, drops to zero in 2010, and then goes back to $1 million in 2011.
- Social Security survivor benefits depend on the average lifetime earnings of the dead person.
- The spouse, dependent children, and dependent parents of dead veterans are offered a number of benefits by the Department of Veterans Affairs.
- A death becomes official when it is certified by a physician on a death certificate. For a sudden or suspicious death, or one for which no physician has signed a death certificate, the cause must be established by a coroner or medical examiner. Coroners are usually elected officials who are not physicians, and medical examiners are usually medical doctors who are appointed. Autopsies done for medical reasons are performed by pathologists. A forensic autopsy

is conducted for legal reasons (suspicious, violent, and/or unexplained death, such as homicide, accident, or suicide).

- In the United States, about 75,000 people are on an organ transplant waiting list at any time. Each day about 60 people receive a donated organ, but 16 die because not enough organs are available. Organ donations can be made by completing a form, such as the uniform donor card, or specifying the information on the back of the driver's license.

ADDITIONAL RESOURCES

Book

Accettura, P. M., & Case, S. J. (2003). *Lost and found: Finding self-reliance after the loss of a spouse.* Farmington Hills, MI: Collinwood. This book offers a practical, step-by-step guide to navigating insurance forms, Social Security, retirement fund distributions, estates, and taxes for widows and widowers bewildered by their new financial landscape after a loss.

Rogers, S. (2003). *Grandfather Webster's strange will.* Unionville, NY: Royal Firemakers Press.

Movie

Melvin and Howard. (1980). This film is about the odd things that can happen when a rich man (Howard Hughes) dies intestate. This movie explores the life of someone (Melvin Dummar) who is essentially down and out most of the time, dreams of striking it rich, and goes to considerable fabricated lengths to achieve that goal.

CRITICAL THINKING

1. How would you respond to a family member who asked you, if you were a match, to donate a kidney?
2. How do you think you would feel about an autopsy being performed on your father or mother?

CLASS ACTIVITIES

1. Write a class will, being specific about what you, as a class, bequeath to the class taking this course the following semester.
2. Each class member should write a paper about his or her attitudes toward an after-life organ donation by a family member. If the writer has had experience dealing with organ donation, he or she can include a description of that. Discuss in class the various views expressed.

REFERENCES

Bernat, J. L., Culver, C. M., & Gert, B. (1981). On the definition and criterion of death. *Annals of Internal Medicine, 94*, 389.

DuBois, J. M. (1999). Non-heart-beating organ donation: A defense of the required determination of death. *Journal of Law, Medicine & Ethics, 27*(2), 126.

Fox, R. C. (1993). An ignoble form of cannibalism: Reflections on the Pittsburgh protocol for procuring organs from non-heart-beating donors. *Kennedy Institute of Ethics Journal, 3*(2), 231–239.

Internal Revenue Service. (2007). *IRS Code: Internal Revenue Code, Chapter 11, Estate Tax* (generally Internal Revenue Code §2000 and following, related regulations and other sources).

Johnson, R. (2008). Where is gay marriage legal? Retrieved August 28, 2008, from http://gaylife.about.com/od/samesexmarraige/a/legalgaymarriage.htm

Lamb, D. (1985). *Death, brain death and ethics.* Albany: State University of New York Press.

Larson, J. P. (2007). *Autopsy. Encyclopedia of medicine.* Retrieved May 17, 2008, from http://www.answers.com/autopsy?cat=health

Lawrence, S. (2003). *World of the body: The Oxford companion to the body.* New York: Oxford University Press.

Lock, M. (2001). *Twice dead: Organ transplants and the reinvention of death.* Berkeley: University of California Press.

Lynn, J. (1993). Are the patients who become organ donors under the Pittsburgh protocol for "non-heart-beating donors" really dead? *Kennedy Institute of Ethics Journal, 3*, 167–178.

National Conference of Commissioners on Uniform State Laws. (2007). *New revision to the rules governing organ donations approved.* Chicago: National Conference of Commissioners on Uniform State Laws. Retrieved May 17, 2008, from www.nccusl.org/Update/

Olson, L. C. (2007). *How brain death works.* Retrieved May 17, 2008, from http://www.howstuffworks.com/search.php

Patterson, B. (2005, February). Coping with the red tape of an overseas death. *International Travel News, 29*(12), 16.

President's Commission for the Study of Ethical Problems in Medicine and Biomedical and Behavioral Research. (1981). *Defining death: Medical, legal, and ethical issues in the determination of death.* Washington, DC: U.S. Government Printing Office.

Social Security Administration. (2007, August). *Survivors' benefits.* Publication No. 05-10084, ICN 468540. U.S. Government: Author.

Truog, R. D. (1997). Is it time to abandon brain death? *Hastings Center Report, 27*(1), 29–37.

United for a Fair Economy. (2007). *A history of the estate tax.* Retrieved May 17, 2008, from www.faireconomy.org/estatetax/ETHistory.html

U.S. Department of Veterans Affairs. (2007a). *Survivor benefits.* Retrieved May 17, 2008, from www.vba.va.gov/survivors/index.htm

U.S. Department of Veterans Affairs. (2007b). *Service members' and veterans' group life insurance.* Retrieved May 17, 2008, from www.insurance.va.gov

Wills and Estate Planning. (2007). Retrieved May 17, 2008, from http://www.nolo.com/resource.cfm/catID/FD1795A9-8049-422C-9087838F86A2BC2B/309/

WorldWide Tax. (2007). Retrieved May 17, 2008, from www.wwwebtax.com/income/life_insurance_proceeds.htm

Younger, S. J., Arnold, R. M., & Schapiro, R. (Eds.). (1999). *The definition of death: Contemporary controversies.* Baltimore: The Johns Hopkins University Press.

Chapter 12

The Funeral Business and Disposal of the Body

The dead don't care.
Only the living care.
—THOMAS LYNCH

Objectives

After reading this chapter, you will be able to answer the following questions:

- Is the need to ritualize death exclusive to humans?
- What are some of the various death rituals conducted in various parts of the world?
- What is a funeral, and what decisions need to be made regarding one?
- How is the funeral industry changing in the United States?
- What is cremation, and what factors affect whether cremation is chosen?

The Human Need to Ritualize Death

Humans, in general, struggle with the problem of defining themselves as being unique in nature. People used to think that the fact that humans communicate through language made them unique. Scientists have proven, however, that apes can communicate through sign language. Also, at one time, people believed that humans were distinctive because they made and used tools; later it became known that other species make and use tools. One human need does stand out, though; humans have an exclusive need to ritualize death and bury their dead.

Most religious traditions throughout history have included definite and elaborate rituals for handling the bodies of the dead. Today, funeral practices condense physical and social death, making death an event, rather than a process (Lock, 2001).

Funeral ceremony is a major subject in world literature (Gopnik, 2007). For example, in Homer's *Iliad,* it is not Achilles' wrath but Priam's desolation that truly moves readers, as he begs for the return of the mutilated body of Hector, his son. Sophocles' ancient Greek play, *Antigone,* is centered on the protagonist's demand for the burial of her dead brother. "It is the dead/ Not the living, who make the longest demands/

We die forever," said Antigone. In Shakespeare's *King Lear,* the mad king carries the body of his daughter, Cordelia, onstage and cries out his grief that she, only just before filled with stubborn life, is now as silent as stone. She was there and now she is not.

The Role of Religious Ritual in Celebrating Death

When a person dies, religious rituals are a way for people to express ultimate concern (i.e., concern for how humans relate to God) and to express feelings about dying and death (O'Connell, 1995). Religious expressions of ultimate concern include the Christian sacrament of the sick and the dying; the Jewish ritual of cleansing of the body; the Islamic ritual of wailing; the Hindu practice of offering rice or flour to the dead person's spirit; and the stylized lamentation, ritual weeping, shouting, and ceremonial fury of indigenous South Americans.

Religious traditions offer structured ways to celebrate, remember, and deal with the emotional and social burdens of dying and death. Religious ceremonies before death are opportunities for both patients and family members to compose themselves as they prepare for the end.

Persons who care for dying patients, especially patients coming from non-Western cultural and religious backgrounds, can enhance the quality of care by understanding when it is appropriate to incorporate religious milestones and symbolic events into a care plan. When responding to the death of a patient, nurses should approach the newly dead with propriety and respect as they prepare the body for transport, cleansing, and wrapping. Ritual enactment replaces routine practice and provides an organized and symbolically meaningful pathway to death and beyond.

Ancient Burial Traditions

Primitive people lived in a world of fear. Weather and life events, including birth and death, were attributed to divine powers or spirits. Because people were not able to see this spirit(s), they lived in fear. In an effort to make a truce with the spirits, primitive people devised ceremonies and rituals. The first burial customs were efforts to protect the living from the spirits who were believed to have caused the death (Rostad, 2000).

Fear of the dead is believed to have carried over into developing religious thought. In Biblical times, the dead were considered unclean. In an attempt to appease the spirits, sacrifices were offered to honor the dead.

Prior to being outlawed by the British, an ancient rite known as **suttee**, or widow burning, was practiced among Indian Hindus. The wife of a dead man was expected to dress in her finest clothes and lie down beside her dead husband on his funeral pyre, where she would be burned to death. The oldest son was responsible for lighting the fire.

Some of today's funeral customs, even the religious ones, have their beginnings in nonreligious rituals, such as the following (Rostad, 2000):

- Mourners wore different clothing—mourning clothes—to disguise themselves from returning spirits.
- The dead person was covered with a sheet because the dead person's spirit was believed to escape through the mouth. Sometimes, people would even cover the mouth and nose of someone who was dying, hoping to retain the spirits and delay death.
- People would keep watch over the dead in hopes that life would return (the source of the term "wake").
- Candles were lit so that the fire would devour spirits.
- Bells were rung in medieval times to drive away evil spirits.
- Flowers were placed around a coffin in order to gain favor with the spirit of the dead person.
- Funeral music began as ancient chants to calm the spirits.

Death Traditions Around the World

Although many death traditions are similar across cultures, most contemporary world religions mark death in different ways. The Hindus in India offer one example. Hindus believe that death is only one of a thousand such events that a person experiences over many lifetimes. The accumulation of good or bad *karma* (reaping what you sow) affects each life's rebirth (*reincarnation*) either favorably or unfavorably. In India, at death, male relatives carry the body to a river, where it is immersed for purification. Cremation follows to liberate the soul for reincarnation. If the heat of the fire is not sufficient to burst the skull, the eldest son of the dead person must crush it to release the soul. After cremation, the family (dressed in white) comes together for a meal and prayers. Friends visit for 13 days. The oldest son, considered the chief mourner, might shave his head as a mark of respect.

Immediately before a Buddhist in Thailand and other South Asian countries dies, the name of Buddha, the Buddhist god, is whispered into the dying person's ear in hopes of bringing good to the person after death. Immediately upon death, relatives begin wailing to express sorrow and to notify the neighbors. Monks, respected religious persons who live in monasteries, conduct the funeral rites and cremation. After the rites, a man carries a white banner on a long pole, leading the procession to the cremation grounds. After chants, people toss lighted candles into the dead person's coffin to begin the cremation.

Among Muslims, cremation is prohibited, and burial without a coffin is required so the body can decompose into the original four elements (earth, air, water, and fire). If possible, Muslims bury their dead within 24 hours. They believe that the soul departs at the moment of death. The dead body, wrapped in white material, is placed with the head facing right, toward Mecca, Islam's holiest city. At the burial, all the mourners participate in filling the grave with soil. The official mourning period is three days and might include a special meal to remember the dead (Gatrad, 1994).

Traditionally, most Christian mourners wear black, but wearing bright colors is becoming more common. Funeral services typically include readings from the Bible. Catholic funerals usually incorporate a funeral mass. This service represents the Last Supper that Jesus Christ shared with his Disciples before his death.

Orthodox Jews typically prepare the dead body for burial and remain with it continually until burial. Most Jews are buried in a cemetery, and some consider cremation a desecration of the body. Mourners might make a symbolic small tear (*keriah*) in their clothes to represent a broken heart. During the seven days of mourning (*shiva*), family members do not shave, bathe, wear makeup, use perfume, wear leather shoes, get haircuts, or engage in sexual relations.

The Maori of New Zealand place their dying in huts. After death, the body is nicely dressed and placed in a seated position for public viewing. Later, the hut and body are both burned. Mourners, wearing green leaves, cut themselves and give gifts to the relatives of the dead.

When death occurs in a family in China, all mirrors are removed from sight. This custom stems from the belief that if someone, a visiting mourner, for example, sees a reflection of the coffin in a mirror, that person soon will have a death in the family. As mourners arrive to visit, they enter the house through a door draped in white cloth.

Funerals

Have you ever thought about what kind of funeral service you want? Do you want a big or small funeral? Do you want people to send flowers? If so, what kind? Would you rather that people donate money in your name to a charitable organization instead of spending money on flowers? Do you want a religious service? What type of music do you want played? As you can see, a funeral can involve many decisions.

A **funeral** is a ceremony before burial that is held to honor the person who has died. A **funeral visitation**, also referred to as a *wake* or a *viewing*, is a time, usually a day or two before the funeral, when family and friends gather to be together and view the dead person. In most cases, funerals and funeral visitations are serious occasions, and many of the mourners are sad and might cry. Because friends and family members are sad that the dead

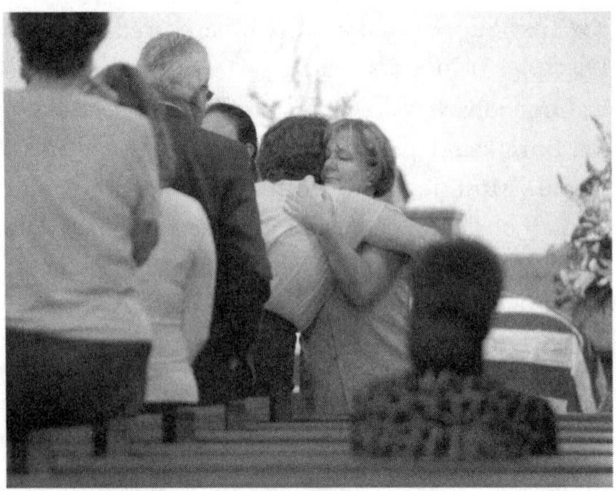

person is gone forever, many of them do cry. But sometimes they laugh, too. Feeling a great deal of love, they might tell funny stories as a way of remembering and honoring the dead person.

Many people do not know the right thing to say to someone who has suffered a loss. Actually, words are not always necessary. Many people also do not know how to handle the details of a funeral. That is the job of the funeral home director, who is responsible for conducting a funeral in such a way as to create good memories of the person who has died.

Questions & Answers

Question: I have been to three funerals, and all of them were too solemn. Does anyone ever have a different type of funeral? I want my funeral to be what I want.

Answer: The American funeral service is changing. Some funerals are very different from those in years past. Today, funerals are more about celebrating the life of the dead person than mourning his or her death.

Many people do not know it, but they are not required by law to use a funeral home to conduct a funeral. However, most people do not have experience with other providers, so they pick a funeral home because that is what they are familiar with, and they usually pick one that has been used by their family in the past and that is nearby (Federal Trade Commission, 2007).

In years past, people who made coffins for the dead decided to "undertake" more and more funeral details. Eventually they became undertakers, or funeral directors. At the funeral home, the funeral director and the funeral home staff are responsible for washing the body, draining the blood, and embalming the body. **Embalming** is the insertion of a liquid preservative into the veins of a dead person in order to postpone decay until after the funeral service. The purpose of embalming is to transform a corpse into a "memory picture" for family members. Embalming is not a legal requirement (Federal Trade Commission, 2007).

Embalming was first used in the United States during the Civil War when President Lincoln wanted Union soldiers' bodies preserved long enough to get them to their Northern homes for burial. Today, embalming has become common practice. The embalming process originated in Egypt. Embalming preserved the body for its eventual reunion with the soul—3,000 years later!

Questions & Answers

Question: I have heard that when funeral directors prepare a body for viewing they sometimes do some weird things. For example, I heard that they might remove the dead person's tongue to be able to close the mouth or that they might even break a person's arms or legs to fit the body into the casket. Do these things really happen?

Answer: Neither of the actions you asked about is true. No reason exists for funeral directors to do those things.

After embalming, the funeral director closes the eyes and mouth (most people die with their eyes and mouths open), dresses the body in clothes chosen by the family, applies makeup (even for males), and styles hair. (Sometimes a person's regular hairstylist comes to the funeral home to style hair.)

A funeral home director is on call 24 hours a day, 365 days a year. Moreover, few of them get rich. The size of the business, size of the community, and years of experience are factors affecting the funeral director's income.

Most funeral directors are honest, but some take advantage by inflating their prices, overcharging or doubling charges, or including unnecessary services (Federal Trade Commission, 2007). To protect consumers, the Federal Trade Commission enacted the Funeral Rule.

The Funeral Rule requires funeral providers to itemize prices and to give the customer a copy to keep. They also are required to provide descriptions and prices of all available caskets and burial vaults before showing any, because the average customer buys one of the first three caskets shown. And, in the past, it was not atypical for a funeral provider to show a customer the top-end, most expensive caskets first.

In keeping with the Funeral Rule, funeral directors also must allow the customer to select individual goods and services for a funeral, even if they are offering packaged funerals. If the customer chooses to buy a casket elsewhere, the funeral provider is not allowed to charge a fee to use it. A provider who offers cremations also must provide appropriate containers for the cremation and ashes. Because of the Rule, funeral directors also must be willing to rent a casket for viewing prior to a cremation (Federal Trade Commission, 2007).

Decisions to Be Made for a Funeral

One of the first decisions family members must make involves selecting a casket or a coffin. A **casket** is a box for burial. Sometimes the word *coffin* is used interchangeably with casket, although the two differ. Coffins usually are made of wood and have a familiar shape—octagonal, narrow, and wider at the shoulder. Caskets tend to be made of more durable materials, such as steel or bronze. They also can have gaskets to make them waterproof, but funeral directors cannot claim that they will preserve a body forever (Federal Trade Commission, 2007). Caskets can be expensive, but simple wooden coffins are not (Lynch, 1997).

Vaults or grave liners often are part of a traditional, full-service funeral. They are used to prevent cave-ins as the casket deteriorates. Liners, made of reinforced concrete, cover only the top and sides of a casket. A vault, made of steel or concrete, encloses the casket on all sides. Vaults and liners are not legally required, but some cemeteries require an outer container to prevent sinking of a grave (Federal Trade Commission, 2007).

Other funeral service decisions that must be made include the following:

- Burial or cremation? Overall, cremation is less expensive than burial. A casket is not required for cremation, and an unfinished wooden box or other container must be offered by the funeral provider (Federal Trade Commission, 2007).
- The type of funeral or memorial service (e.g., religious or nonreligious) and who will speak.
- Selecting **pallbearers**, the people (usually family and friends) who carry the casket at the funeral and burial.
- Choosing a place for the funeral or memorial service (church, synagogue, funeral home, or elsewhere).

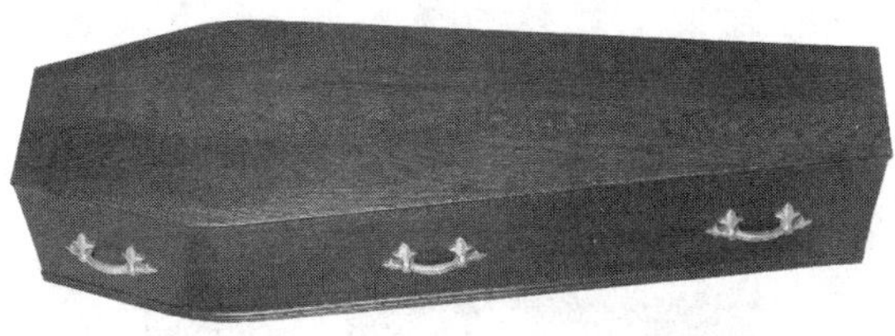

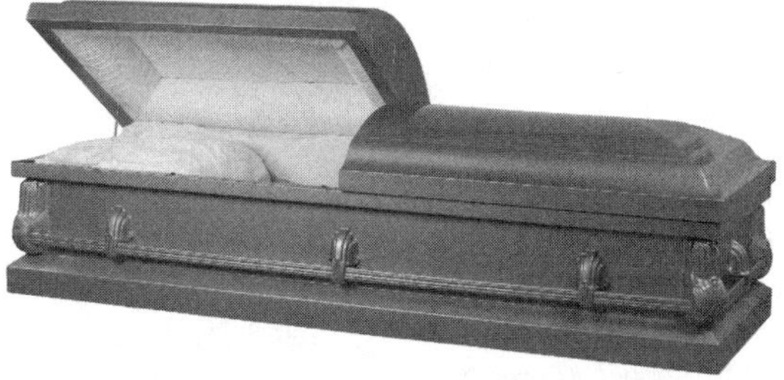

- Selecting the burial plot and the grave marker or tombstone. These costs are not included in the cost of a funeral. In choosing a cemetery plot, **mausoleum** (building for above-ground burials), or **columbarium** (from the word for dove cote; a structure of vaults lines with recesses for ash-bearing urns; also, the recess itself), be sure to determine all the costs and restrictions of the particular location. Also, ask if it includes perpetual care; if not, expect a separate fee for that.
- All veterans, their dependents, and some civilians engaged in military or public health service are permitted burial at no cost in a national cemetery. Some states also have state veteran cemeteries.

Children and Funerals

Children, even young ones, should be allowed to participate in funerals so that they can feel and express their grief over the loss of a loved one (Committee on Psychosocial Aspects of Child and Family Health, 2000). It is important, however, to prepare children for a funeral. This preparation should be appropriate to the developmental level of the child.

- A very young child should be accompanied by a trusted older person who can explain what is happening and be supportive.
- It might be important to break down the funeral process into briefer intervals so that the child can manage them.
- Older children, including adolescents, might wish to speak at the funeral or memorial service.
- Other forms of participation to express loss, such as drawing pictures, planting a tree, or putting a favorite object into the coffin, can be meaningful to the child.

After the Funeral

Burial takes place after the funeral service. In most cases, only family members and close friends attend. (If a person donates his or her body for medical study, the body is buried later, after use in medical training.)

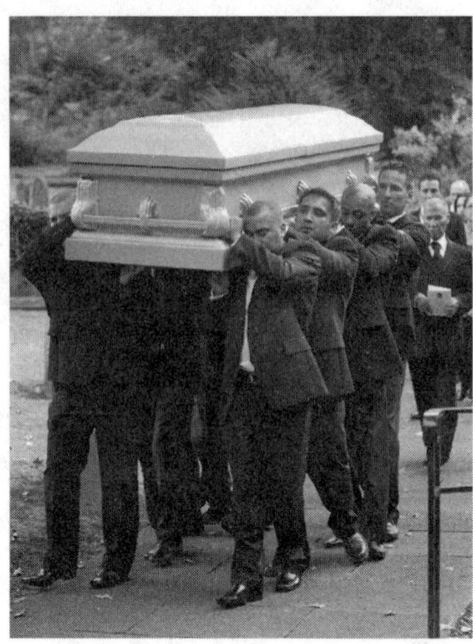

The burial place may be a **grave**, where the body is buried in the ground. A mausoleum is a building for above-ground burials.

An **obituary** is a newspaper account of the dead person's life. Some are simple, others might give details of the life of the dead.

Planning Ahead

Some people make their own funeral plans and pay the funeral director while they are alive (Federal Trade Commission, 2007). This process allows them to compare prices at several funeral providers, make choices, pay for the funeral costs when they have money available, and tell someone their wishes—saving loved ones from making

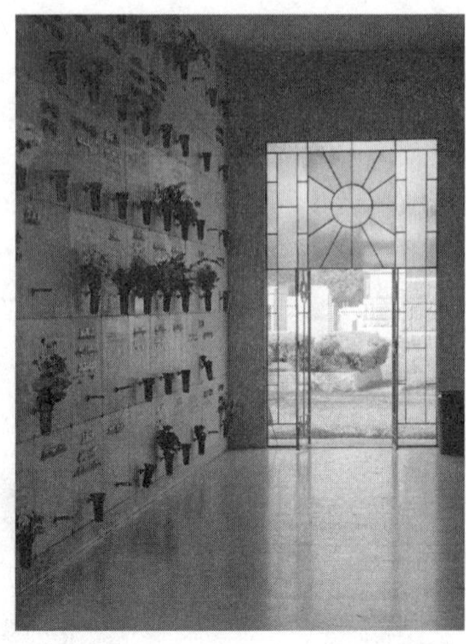

such difficult financial decisions while feeling weighed down by grief, a situation that often makes it difficult to make wise judgments. They can work directly with a funeral home or with one of a number of nonprofit funeral-planning organizations. One important decision to be made is the burial plot, tomb, or place to scatter ashes. This task is best done when one is not in a rush.

Memorializing a Life

People are remembered by a eulogy, the words spoken about them at a funeral, and/or an epitaph engraved on a tombstone.

If you walk through a cemetery, many monuments have "Beloved Mother" or "Beloved Father" inscribed on them. Some monuments have angels, hearts, crosses, or American flags engraved on them. In Victorian times, headstones had particular meanings (see Table 12.1).

Humor also is a way of memorializing a death—even on tombstones. For instance, many examples exist of epitaphs that are humorous, such as, "I Told You I Was Sick!" "Here lies Johnny Yeast/Pardon me/For not rising," and "She always said her feet were killing her but nobody believed her."

Table 12.1 VICTORIAN GRAVE-MARKER SYMBOLISM

Common Symbols on Monuments in Victorian-Era Cemeteries	Meaning
Angel blowing a trumpet	The day of judgment and call to the resurrection
Arch	Victory in death
Broken column	A life cut short
Candle with a flame	Life
Circle	Eternity has no beginning and no end
Crossed swords	Death in battle
Door/gateway	Entry into the afterlife
Dove	The Holy Spirit
Fish	Faith
Flame	Eternity
Hands	Departure
Hands holding a chain with a broken link	Death of a close family member
Heart encircled with thorns	The suffering of Christ
Ivy	Immortality, faithfulness
Lamb	Usually found on a child's grave: The Lamb of God, innocence
Lily	Purity
Lion	Guards the tomb against evil spirits
Pyramid	Eternity; it was believed that a pyramid-shaped tombstone prevented the devil from reclining on a grave
Rose	Love, beauty, hope
Rosebud	Normally found on the grave of a child under age 12
Triangle	The Holy Trinity
Upside-down flaming torch	The inverted torch symbolizes death, while the flame, which would normally be extinguished when the torch was turned upside down, symbolizes eternal life
Urn	Classical symbol of cremation
Wreath	Eternal life: no beginning or end; evergreen, so no death

Source: Brennan (2005).

IN LOVING MEMORY
OF
CHRISTOPHER HAMMOND

HERE LIES
THE BODY OF
JONATHAN BLAKE
STEPPED ON
THE GAS
INSTEAD OF
THE BRAKE

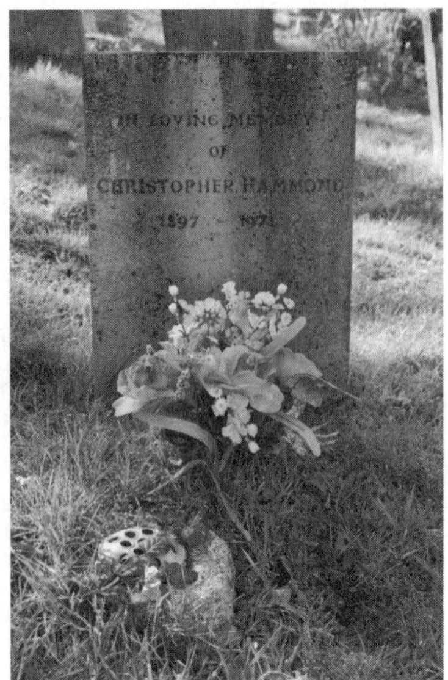

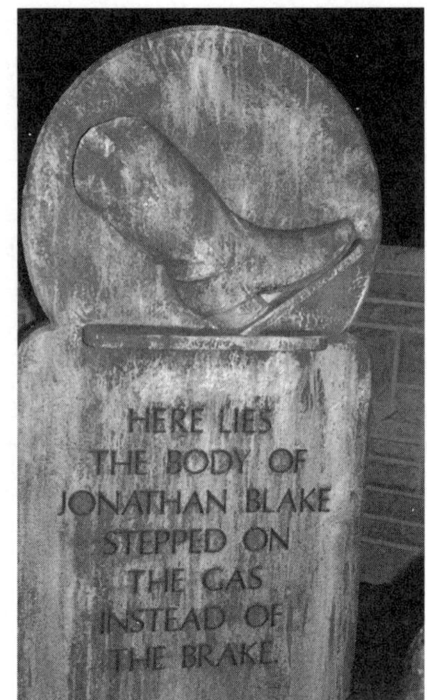

In addition to tombstone inscriptions, people might choose to remember a loved one by:

- planting a flower or tree
- writing a letter to thank the person or to resolve an issue.
- creating a mural about the person's life.
- placing a book in the library in the person's memory.
- writing a poem, story, or song about the person.
- making a video of memories of the person's life.

What's important is to appreciate the good feelings and positive lessons gained when remembering someone—and that goes for the here and now, as well as when someone dies.

National Memorials

A number of national memorials have been erected in honor of those who died during military service. One of the most profound and affecting is the Vietnam Memorial in Washington, D.C., designed by architect Maya Lin. A piece of black granite wedged in the earth, it carries all 58,175 names of those killed in the Vietnam war.

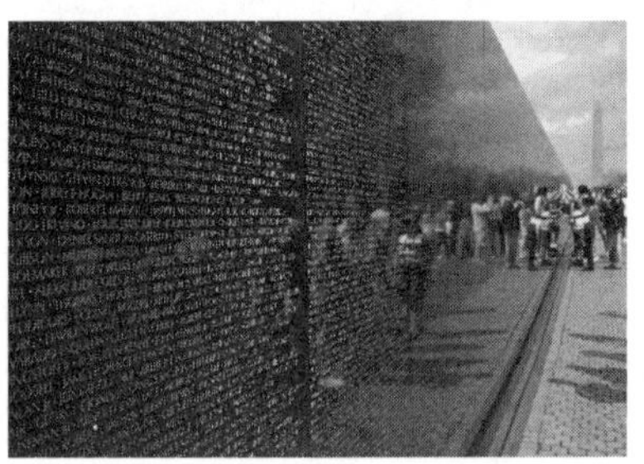

Military Headstones and Grave Markers

The U.S. Department of Veterans Affairs (2007) provides, when asked and at no charge, government headstones and grave markers for the graves of veterans anywhere in the world and for eligible dependents buried in state or national veterans' cemeteries. Flat markers are available in granite, marble, and bronze, and upright headstones are available in granite and marble. The style chosen must be consistent with monuments at the place of burial. Niche markers are available for identifying

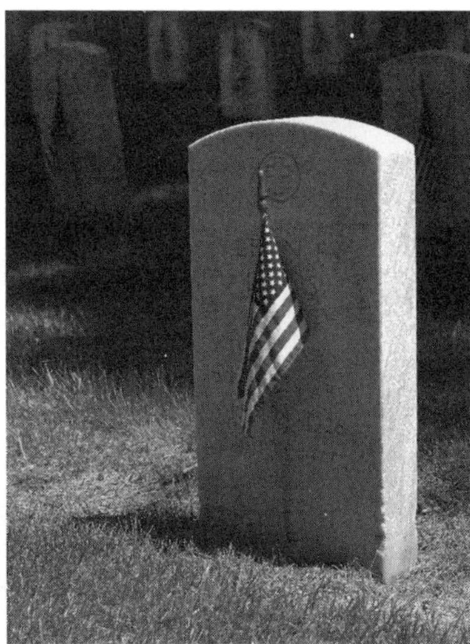

cremated remains in columbaria (recessed niches in a church wall) and memorial markers if the remains are not available for burial.

The New American Way of Death

Funerary practice in the United States has been changing. Funeral and burial expenses, as a percentage of GDP (gross domestic product), fell from 0.35% in 1960 to 0.15% in 1993. The cost of a funeral in 1993 was less than one-half the cost of one in 1960, as a percentage of per capita income. Most dramatic of all perhaps has been the rapid increase in cremation as compared to burial. In 1960, cremation was used in only 3.56% of American deaths. This amount increased to nearly 20% in 1993 and is projected to be more than 30% by 2010 (Gill, 1996).

This increase in cremation has affected the funeral business. As cremation rates have risen, many funeral homes have cut back on staff and the range of services, and they are not planning to reinvest in them. New cemeteries are now unwelcome in many communities. In the nineteenth century, residents gathered to celebrate a new cemetery. Today, protesters lobby legislators to prevent new or larger ones. Vandalism in graveyards has become a major problem.

Changes in funerary practices have been going on for a long time. In Puritan times, physical death meant decay. Few graves had permanent markers. Only the fate of the soul mattered. In the nineteenth century, funerals became more elaborate, but that practice began to fade by World War I. What might account for this decline? During the nineteenth century and up to World War I, Americans believed in progress and a long time line, and they thought they knew the general shape of things to come. Therefore, they could imagine a world beyond their death, so they believed it was meaningful to be memorialized after they died.

Since World War I, Americans have found it more difficult to foresee what life will be like after they have departed from the scene. Their departures are coming later in life, and at the same time, their ability to imagine a distant future has declined. As faith in a long-run future for the real world has faded, many Americans are turning to

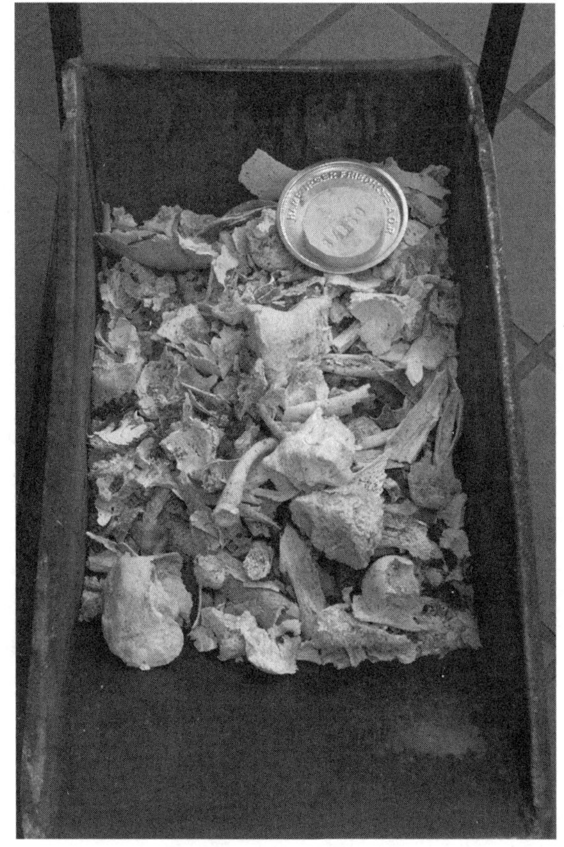

MY MOTHER'S EULOGY (BY LINDA LYSOBY)

In my mother's life, there are many things to talk about. Today, I choose to talk about her life by using three objects: a cup of tea, a puzzle, and a pair of socks.

As long as I can remember, my mother's house had the kitchen with the kitchen table as a center point. Besides a source of nutrition, the kitchen was a place where she gathered people. In particular, I associate her with tea—all kinds of tea—regular, flavored, and herbal. She used tea to sit down, calm down, pick yourself up, or just talk through a problem. I imagine that most of the people sitting here today can recall many times where her tea and her company warmed, comforted, and encouraged them. This habit and many others are things that I have incorporated into my life and have passed on to others. There are many things that can be, if not solved, then, at least, softened over a cup of tea.

My mother had many hobbies. One was putting together jigsaw puzzles, those large, boggle-your-mind, 5000 itty-bitty pieced jigsaw puzzles. My father made her a puzzle board so she could work on the puzzle, move it out of the way, and then come back to it again. She taught her kids, grandkids, and those she babysat how to do a puzzle. She approached her puzzles much like she did life, with the focus on structure and order and a little bit of trial and error. She taught us all to build the framework first, finding the straight-edged pieces that made up the border (finding a corner piece was a bonus). Next, we were taught to find the easy ones first and then keep going. "See if you can connect the colorful pieces and then build around that," she had said. As she taught children how to do a puzzle, she taught them many additional things:

- Patience
- Perseverance
- Structure/order
- Problem solving
- Persistence
- The need to sometimes walk away, return, and try again
- Spatial relations (she could tell if a piece fit without picking it up)
- The importance of keeping your mind challenged
- That there is a right way to do things
- A puzzle as a forum for conversation
- An appreciation that many individual things make up one whole beautiful picture

In later years, as physical limitations progressed, she stopped doing her puzzles. But in more recent months, we returned to puzzle making, this time in smaller versions, 50 to 100 pieces, usually animals. She amazed her family with her interest and ability to participate with us as this became a group activity. Sometimes she was still able to locate the correct piece by sight even though she was unable to physically pick it up. The glint that appeared in her eyes said it all when she realized that the piece she identified did fit.

And speaking of that glint in her eyes, those who know my mother know that she had a sense of humor and was sometimes a little ornery. She liked to tease, and she liked to laugh. She wore crazy socks. If you visited her, you couldn't help but notice the socks. She even wore them to the beauty parlor and doctor's visits, everywhere but church. She had Christmas socks, Halloween, Thanksgiving, and Valentine's socks; she had socks with stripes, Dalmatian-looking dots, and bright colors. In her final days in the hospital and hospice, she wore her Coca-Cola socks, her

(*continued*)

My Mother's Eulogy (by Linda Lysoby)

bright yellow taxicab socks, and her snowman socks. Today, she is wearing the Boston Terrier socks. Her ability to find fun and smile even in adverse times can be an inspiration to us all.

So, as we go forward from this day, it would make my mother very happy if we take forward a few lessons from her:

1. Many if not all of life's challenges can be, if not solved, at least softened over a cup of tea.
2. Patience, perseverance, and persistence can give you an appreciation that many individual things make up one whole beautiful picture.
3. Whatever your situation, approach life with a little humor and a glint in your eye.

The family invites all present to join us after the services for some food and, of course, tea and conversation as we celebrate my mother's life and the gifts she has given to us.

evangelical religion. All that matters then is immortality of the soul. Markers and monuments have once again become less relevant.

Is this trend good or bad? It might be good from the perspective of reducing the expense of a funeral, but new funerary practices suggest a deeper, more negative social shift in that our priorities have changed, notably with respect to the children and grandchildren who will live after us. Apparently, the only thing that matters to many of us is what happens in this world now. The temporal future after death is a blank. And children, more than the dead, appear to be the real sacrificial lambs of the modern-day decline in concern for the future.

Cremation

Cremation is the process of applying intense heat to the **remains**, which is the name given to a body after death. Sometimes, people leave instructions about their wishes regarding disposal of their remains. Oftentimes, people specify either cremation or burial in the ground as their preference. Others express a desire to be both cremated and buried afterward. If a person does not express his or her preference before death, one of the first questions that a family will need to answer after a loved one dies is, "What will we do with the remains?"

In a standard cremation, the **crematory** (the place where cremation takes place) is heated to 2,000 to 3,000°F. The body is placed in a container and then placed inside the crematory for about 80 to 90 minutes. Cremated remains, frequently referred to as *ashes*, are called **cremains**. Cremains usually weigh from 4 to 9 pounds and take up a space about the size of the inside of a baseball cap.

Because they are commonly referred to as ashes, many people believe that cremains are fine, gray ashes. Actually, cremains are whitish in color due to the calcium in bones. Also, cremains are not fine particles. Rather, they resemble coarse sand. (See picture on p. 137.)

Burning a dead body has been common practice for thousands of years. In Europe, cremations have been the primary method of disposing of remains since the Bronze Age. That's about 3,500 years ago, or 1,500 B.C. (Kroeber, 1927).

The first American cremations took place in the late 1800s, but the practice was slow to catch on. In 1876, the first crematory in the United States was built in Washington, Pennsylvania. In the 1960s, the percentage of U.S. cremations was 4%. In 1990 and 1995, the figures were 37% and 43%, respectively. In 2005, 46% chose cremation for themselves or their loved ones (Funeral and Memorial Information Council, 2005). According to this Council, the percentage of cremations is expected to jump to almost 50% by 2025. If this trend continues, America might have as many cremations as Japan (97%) or the Scandinavian countries (more than 65%; Cremation Association of North America, 2000).

Persons who favor cremation tend to be better educated and wealthier. Many Catholics mistakenly think that their religion does not allow it, but cremation has been allowed for U.S. Catholics since 1965. John F. Kennedy, the first Catholic president, was cremated. Two groups less inclined to choose cremation are African Americans and Baptists. Ceremonial funeral and burial services are very important to African Americans. Baptists shun cremation because it "destroys the body," which would make physical resurrection difficult.

As previously stated, changing attitudes toward cremation represent a challenge to the funeral home industry (Edmondson, 1987). Big funerals are decreasing in popularity, especially among the well educated and well-to-do. In Florida, cut-rate funeral services with cremation now cost as little as $355, and in 1980 a limited "direct disposal" license became available in Florida, which stimulated cremation as a business opportunity. One in five funerals now involves cremation, and start-up costs for a low-cost funeral business can be launched for less than $100,000 (Edmondson).

Religious Influences

Cremation always has been especially important for Asian Hindus and Buddhists. Buddhists believe that Buddha, their god, who was cremated, set the "right" way for body disposal. Buddha chose cremation because of his belief that the body is not needed after death, and that the spirit, which is needed for rebirth 49 days after death, cannot be destroyed by fire.

Ancient Hebrews considered burial to be the only proper method to dispose of remains. This belief influenced the early Middle Eastern Christians. Christianity, together with Middle Eastern Judaic and Islamic religions, curtailed the total acceptance of the long-held practice of cremation in Western Europe. Members of all of these groups believed that the body is the temple of the soul and, therefore, should not be destroyed by fire.

Today, Jews and Christians (except Latter-Day Saints, or Mormons) allow cremation. The world's 900 million Buddhists and Hindus continue to believe that cremation is a superior method of dis-

MY STORY: FAMILY TOGETHERNESS

For many years all of the people in my family who have died have been buried within our own family section in one of the local cemeteries. Recently, my parents said that only one plot remains in the cemetery section belonging to our family so that, if we want to stay together after death, we may have to consider cremation, and place our ashes in an urn, rather than burial.

Cremation? How could they even consider that? No one in our family has ever been cremated. I immediately wondered if cremation is even "natural" or "right." No one in our church has been cremated. At every casket burial I ever attended, the minister always said something about "from dust you came; to dust you shall return."

When I explained my concerns to my mother, she suggested that I search the Internet for information about cremation. Also, she told me that, instead of cremation, we could purchase another family plot in another close-by cemetery.

After searching the Internet, I found out some interesting things about cremation. I found out that people can still donate organs and that the ashes, or cremains, can be distributed among family members to be made into necklaces. Also, maybe if ashes are buried, dust-to-dust still applies.

I'm still not sure that cremation is what our family should do, but I believe that I should consider it. The most important thing I learned through this process is that our family could remain closer with side-by-side ashes rather than side-by-side caskets!

posing of remains. Muslims continue to oppose cremation. They believe that the dead, like the living, can feel pain. Also, Muslims believe that fire will be used exclusively by Allah (their god) to punish the wicked.

Besides the religious influences, the choice of cremation is affected by other influences, social, and psychological. Social influences include money, region of the country, personal values, ethnicity, or race. Psychological influences are one's thoughts and feelings.

Social Influences

In the United States, cremation is most popular in the Pacific and Mountain Regions and in Florida; it is the least popular in the South. This difference might be linked to religious preferences in those areas. The fewer numbers of cremations in the South is probably due to the influence of traditional Christian church groups. Also influencing more cremations on the West Coast and Florida is that greater numbers of elder retirees have moved there (Cremation Association of North America, 2000).

Another social influence regarding cremation is the expectation of convenience. Transporting an **urn**, a container that holds cremains, is easier and more convenient than transporting a casket. For example, a person who moves from the town where his or her loved one died can take along an urn, but not a casket.

Many people choose cremation because it is less expensive than traditional funerals. A traditional funeral typically costs $6,500 to $10,000. Cremation costs about $1,000 and up. Even though it makes sense to most people to be economical, funeral costs for loved ones are an emotional issue as well.

Psychological Issues

In American society, people often are judged by their material possessions, which include not only what they have, but their ability to buy things. In

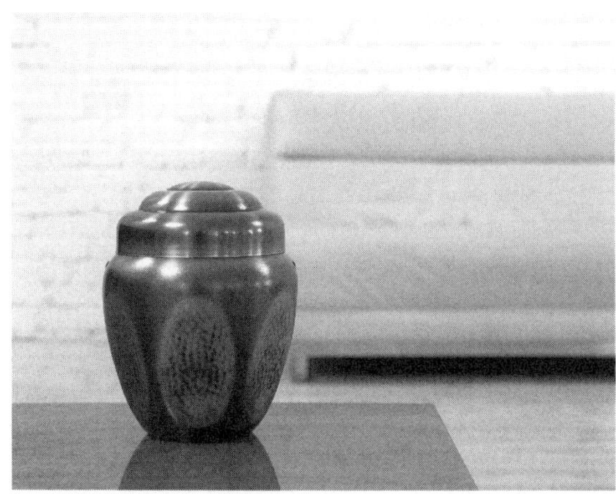

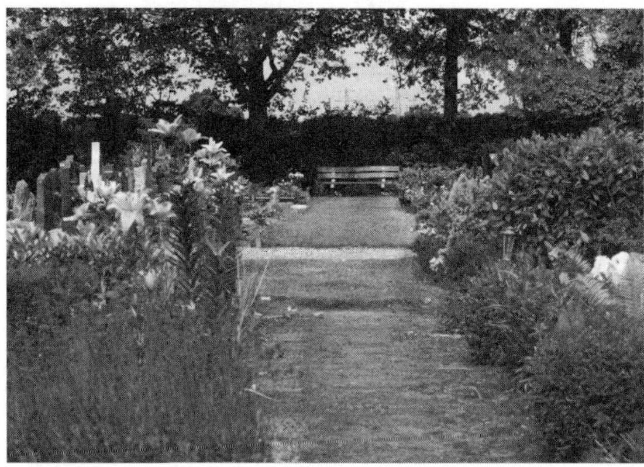

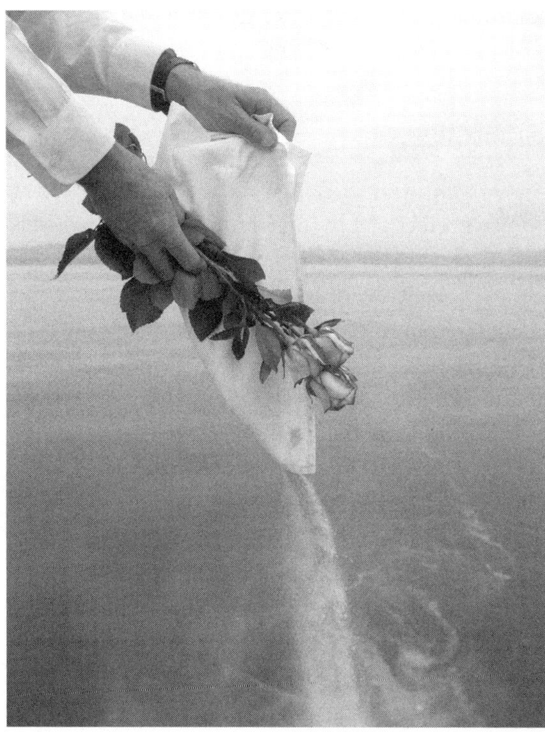

such a material culture, cremation might appear to be an unloving thing to do. For example, members of a church might not contribute to a college fund, but they might rally to contribute to a funeral.

Another psychological issue surrounding cremation is how important it is that a dead loved one be nearby. For example, cremains are frequently placed in urns displayed in a home. On the other hand, someone might find comfort in scattering cremains over the ocean or some other special place such as a memorial garden, for example. In memorial gardens, a permanent record, such as a bronze plaque engraved with the loved one's name, is usually provided. Also, cremains can be buried on family property without the involved legal procedures required to bury a dead body there. Another option for displaying cremains is a columbarium, a recessed niche in a wall, usually in a church, where an urn is placed.

A new trend with cremains is to incorporate them into keepsake jewelry. Cremains can be placed in pendants to hang from necklaces, for example. Many pendants can be made so that all family members can wear one. The remaining cremains are buried, scattered, or placed in an urn. Recently, a company in Chicago started offering diamonds formed from cremated remains (Blevins, 2002; Cremation Jewelry, 2008).

SUMMARY

- Primitive burial customs were efforts to protect the living from the spirits who were believed to have caused the death. Fear of the dead is believed to have carried over into religious thought.
- A funeral is a ceremony before burial that is held to honor the person who has died. A funeral visitation, also referred to as a wake or a viewing, is a time, usually a day or two before the funeral service, when family and friends gather to be together and view the dead person.
- At a funeral home, the funeral director or staff washes the body, drains the blood, and embalms the body. After embalming, the funeral director or staff closes the eyes and mouth, dresses the body, applies makeup, and styles hair. A funeral home director is on call 24 hours a day, 365 days a year.
- To protect the consumer, the Federal Trade Commission enacted the Funeral Rule. Among other things, it requires funeral providers to itemize prices and to give the customer an itemized copy of the expenses.
- Coffins are usually made of wood and have a familiar shape—octagonal, narrow, and wider at the shoulder. Caskets may be made of more durable materials, such as steel or bronze. A vault of steel or concrete can be used to enclose the casket on all sides.
- Children, even young ones, should be allowed to participate in funerals.
- An obituary is a newspaper account of the dead person's life.
- People are remembered by an eulogy, words spoken at a funeral, or by an epitaph engraved on a tombstone.
- A number of memorials exist to honor persons with military service.
- Cremation, which is generally less expensive than a conventional funeral with burial, is on the rise in the United States, but not everyone approves of it. Cremation is the process of applying intense heat to the remains. Cremated remains are called *cremains*.

ADDITIONAL RESOURCES

Books

Lynch, T. (1997). *The undertaking: Life studies from the dismal trade*. New York: W. W. Norton and Company. Literary and autobiographical musings on the significance of death and funerals are presented in this book, and they are interspersed with trenchant descriptions of the funeral process by a poet who is also a funeral director.

Mitford, J. (1963). *The American way of death*. New York: Simon and Schuster. This book offers the best-selling condemnation of the funeral trade in America.

Movie

Death at a Funeral. (2007). This movie is a comedy about a father's funeral in the family home.

Critical Thinking

1. List three reasons why you believe burial *is* an appropriate choice for your family.
2. List three reasons why you believe burial *is not* an appropriate choice for your family.
3. In what ways do you want people to memorialize your life?

Class Activities

1. As a class, visit a funeral home and ask the director to show you the casket room and the embalming room.
2. Visit a graveyard on your own and write a paper (to later share with the class) about what you saw. In your paper, describe what is written on tombstones in "family" burial plots and your feelings about being in the graveyard.

References

Blevins, J. (2002, November 3). Chicago entrepreneur's process turns cremated remains into keepsake diamond. *Knight Ridder/Tribune Business News*.

Brennan, M. (2005). Death and dying: Death is a biological certainty but the practices surrounding death and mourning are socially constructed. *Sociology Review, 14*(3), 26–29.

Committee on Psychosocial Aspects of Child and Family Health. (2000). The pediatrician and childhood bereavement. *Pediatrics, 105*(2), 445.

Cremation Association of North America. (2000). *Cremation statistics*. Retrieved May 19, 2008, from http://www.funeralplan.com/funeralplan/cremation/stats.html

Cremation Jewelry. (2008). *Keepsakes in pendant form are growing in popularity*. Retrieved May 19, 2008, from www.cremationjewelry.net

Edmondson, B. (1987). Please erase me, let me go. *American Demographics, 9*(6), 22.

Federal Trade Commission. (2007). *Funerals: A consumer guide*. Retrieved May 19, 2008, from www.ftc.gov/bcp/conline/pubs/services/funeral.shtm

Funeral and Memorial Information Council. (2005). *Wirthlin Report: A study of American attitudes toward ritualization and memorialization.* Retrieved May 19, 2008, from www.cremationassociation.org/docs/wirthlin-excerpt.pdf

Gatrad, A. R. (1994). Muslim customs surrounding death, bereavement, postmortem examinations, and organ transplants. *British Medical Journal, 309*, 521–523.

Gill, R. T. (1996). Whatever happened to the American way of death? *Public Interest, 123*(Spring), 105.

Gopnik, A. (2007, March 12). Remains of the days. *The New Yorker.* Retrieved May 19, 2008, from http://www.newyorker.com/talk/comment/2007/03/12/070312taco_talk_gopnik

Kroeber, A. L. (1927). Disposal of the dead. *American Anthropologist, 29*, 308–315.

Lock, M. (2001). *Twice dead: Organ transplants and the reinvention of death*. Berkeley: University of California Press.

Lynch, T. (1997). *The undertaking life: Studies from the dismal trade.* New York: Penguin.

O'Connell, L. J. (1995). Religious dimensions of dying and death. *Western Journal of Medicine*, *163*(3), 231.

Rostad, C. D. (2000). *The basics of funeral service.* Retrieved May 19, 2008, from http://www.wyfda.org/basics_2.html

U.S. Department of Veterans Affairs. (2007). *Survivor benefits.* Retrieved May 19, 2008, from www.vba.va.gov/survivors/index.htm

How Children and Adolescents View Death

I wish I were death: I would not let anyone die; I would let people live a wonderful life anywhere.
—SMALL BOY QUOTED TO E. KÜBLER-ROSS (1983)

Objectives

After reading this chapter, you will be able to answer the following questions:

- How do children view death and express grief?
- What do children say about death in their own words?
- How can parents and family, pediatricians, teachers, and bereavement centers help children cope with the death of a loved one or friend?
- How do adolescents view death and express grief?

Children look at death differently depending on how old and how emotionally and intellectually mature they are. Regarding death, children seek the reassurance of adults, which is not always forthcoming. Many adults think children should be shielded from the reality of death. Adolescents are interested in themselves; they usually view death in terms of how it affects them personally.

A Child's View of Death

Long before adults realize it, children are aware of death. Most young children are exposed to death on a regular basis. They see dead birds and dead animals lying by the roadside. They lose a pet, a grandparent, or worse, a parent or sibling. They hear about death in fairy tales and act out death in play. Also, they see a good deal of programming on television that includes death, real or imaginary.

Stories, Songs, and Games

Children are interested in how fairy tales deal with death-related events. In the original version of the story, Little Red Riding Hood and her grandmother are eaten by the wolf. The Big Bad Wolf in the Three Little Pigs dies in a pot of scalding hot water when he falls down the last chimney. Hansel and Gretel escape being shut in a hot oven, but the witch does not.

A large number of books for children and adolescents have death-related themes or explain

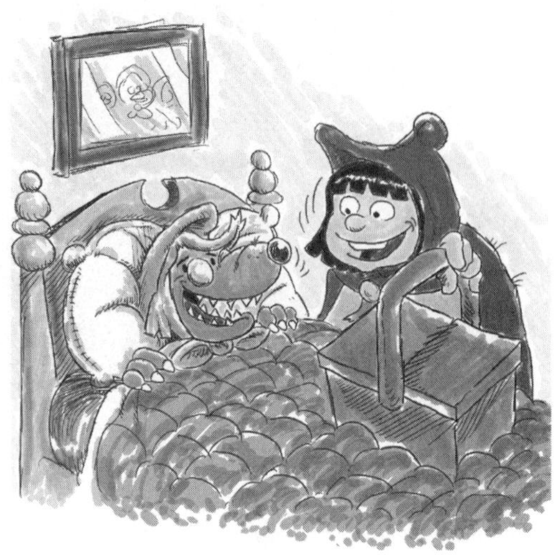

death (Seibert, Drolet, & Fetro, 1993). Books range from those about a dying leaf falling from its tree in the winter to stories that treat the death of a grandparent, parent, sibling, friend, or pet.

The lullaby "Rock-a-Bye Baby" is a song about a bough breaking and a cradle falling; the child's prayer "Now I lay me down to sleep" asks for protection from death and other hazards of the night; and the "Hearse Song," in its various versions, tells of worms crawling in and out of your dead and buried body.

Many childhood games involve death. Peek-a-boo is depicted as a game in which the entire world around a child suddenly vanishes, but then reappears, an act of resurrection or rebirth (Maurer, 1966).

The child who is "it" in tag chases and terrorizes others in the game. The touch of "it" claims a victim. In some versions, the victim must freeze until rescued by a child not touched by "it." Death is closer to the surface in a Sicilian version—a child plays dead and then jumps up to catch a "mourner."

The familiar childhood game of ring-around-the-rosie became popular during fourteenth-century Europe as a way for children to deal with the terrors of the Black Death (bubonic plague), one of the most lethal epidemics in history. The "rosies" referred to one of the symptoms of the plague, circular red marks on the skin. The game was performed as a slow circle dance in which "all fall down," and one child after another would drop. Children who played this game were aware that people all around them were falling victim to the plague (Opie & Opie, 1969).

Today, most children experience death through television, especially from animated cartoons. Through these cartoons, children come to think that bad people die because they deserve to die and that good people can come back to life.

Age-Related Concepts of Death

A child's concept of death differs by the child's level of maturation and age (Committee on Psychosocial Aspects of Child and Family Health, 2000; Didion, 2005; Jellinek, 2003; Nagy, 1948; Westmoreland, 1996):

- Up to age 2 or 3, there is no cognitive understanding of death. The loss of a parent or an other caretaker is perceived as abandonment.
- At ages 2 or 3 to 6, children might believe that death is similar to being asleep (and

SELECTED BOOKS FOR CHILDREN AND PARENTS DEALING WITH DEATH

- *The Dead Bird* by Margaret Wise-Brown (Addison-Wesley, 1958; ages 3 to 5)
- *Lifetimes: The Beautiful Way to Explain Death to Children* by Bryan Mellonie and Robert Ingpen (Bantam Books, 1983; ages 3 to 6)
- *When Dinosaurs Die: A Guide to Understanding Death* by Laurene Krasny Brown and Marc Brown (Little Brown, 1996; ages 4 to 8)
- *Accident* by Carol Carrick (Seabury Press, 1976; ages 6 to 8)
- *A Taste of Blackberries* by Doris B. Smith (Crowell, 1973; ages 8 to 9)
- *The Magic Moth* by Virginia Lee (Seabury Press, 1972; ages 10 to 12)

Source: Arnold and Gemma (1994).

Rock-a-Bye Baby

Rock-a-bye baby in the treetop,
When the wind blows the cradle will rock,
When the bough breaks the cradle will fall,
And down will come baby, cradle and all.

Now I Lay Me Down to Sleep

Now I lay me down to sleep.
I pray the Lord my soul to keep,
And if I die before I wake,
I pray the Lord my soul to take.

The Hearse Song

If ever you laugh
when a hearse goes by,
then you will be
the next to die.
They put you in
the cold, cold ground
with all your relatives
standing around.
The worms crawl in
The worms crawl out
The worms they crawl
all about.
The worms crawl in
The worms crawl out
They play pinochle
on your snout!

thus they fear falling asleep). The dead might wake up after a while, and a loved one who has died will return. Some children think someone is responsible for a death, perhaps themselves. They worry that someone else may die, a worry that can become an intense fear. Children at these ages picture death as a clown, a shadowy deathman, or a skeletal figure. They also typically think they can escape death if they are lucky or clever enough and can make their wishes come true by magical thinking (which can be true of adults as well).

- Between the ages of 6 and 9, children come to realize that death is final and irreversible,

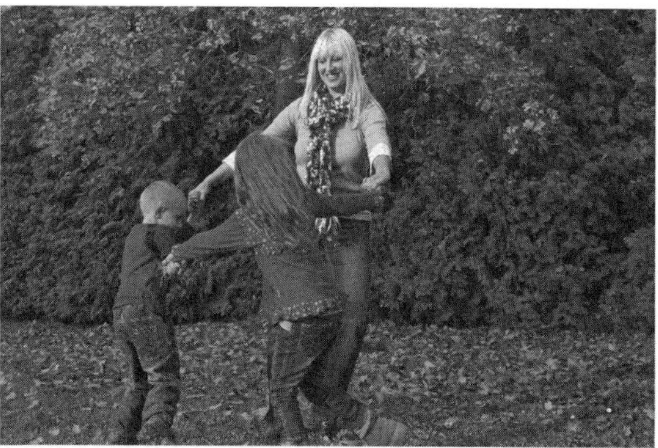

the dead stay dead. They become interested in what happens to the body after death, associating death with disintegration. They may see death as not affecting them, only other people; consequently, they found that the death of self or a loved one is difficult to understand. They frequently focus on themselves as the cause. For example, a child in this age group might cry and say, "I know it's my fault that Mama died. I told her that I hated her!" (Nagy, 1948).
- At age 9 or 10, children become aware that death is inevitable, universal, and personal. They realize that death comes to every person, animal, and thing, including themselves. They are more concerned, however, that a parent may die. They may develop a fear of death or appear indifferent. Sometimes they joke about death to conceal their feelings.

Childhood Grief

What about childhood grief? Sigmund Freud claimed in his essay, "Mourning and Melancholia" (1917/2005), that young children are not able to mourn, that resolving grief is too difficult for them. Grieving only becomes possible in adolescence. But children, even very young children, do grieve, though their grieving differs at different ages and often bears little resemblance to the mourning of adults.

- Very young children might become emotionally withdrawn or difficult to console. Their eating and sleeping patterns might change, and they might backslide on

milestones of maturation they had achieved (Jellinek, 2003).
- At ages 3 to 6, children typically believe that the dead loved one will return. They become angry when that does not happen. They also may believe they caused the death (Jellinek, 2003; Nagy, 1948).
- A child of 6 is just on the cusp of mastering the four essential attributes of death—that it has a specific cause, involves the cessation of bodily function, is irreversible, and is universal (Adler et al., 1997).
- Death can be the hardest to deal with between ages 9 and 12 (Harris, 1995). The child is no longer very young, so typically is reluctant to shed tears or sit on a lap. This child, though, is also not yet adolescent, with the sense of independence that comes with adolescence.
- Given appropriate adult support, most children are able to move on with their lives, without heavy psychological weather, at least for awhile (Christ, 2000).

Other Factors

Later research (Anthony, 1972) has confirmed that a child's comprehension of death develops along the lines described previously, but additional factors should be considered. These factors include the following:

- Level of maturation was found to be a better predictor of how a child views death than chronological age (Maurer, 1966).
- The influence of life experience is a mediating factor that deserves more attention (Deveau & Adams, 1995); what a child has gone through in life up to that point affects how the child views death.
- Children with potentially fatal physical conditions often reveal an understanding of death beyond their years (Bluebond-Langner, 1996).

After a Death

Children typically suffer the most acutely for at least 2 months following a loss. The suffering peaks at about 1 month. But up to one-third of children and adolescents feel intense grief from 6 months to a year later. Grief is an ongoing process that cannot be rushed (Jellinek, 2003).

Ward (1993) described four stages of emotional response during the period of time after a death. Children might move in and out of the following four stages during the grieving process:

1. Shock and disbelief: The child might withdraw from others and seem to be unusually calm, numb, or apathetic.
2. Denial: This stages begins usually in the first 2 weeks after the death and can last minutes, days, weeks, or months. A child might appear not to understand what has happened, behave as if nothing has happened, refuse to admit loss, or escape into fantasies.
3. Growing awareness: In this stage, a child may have difficulty dealing with unfamiliar, intense feelings. Such a child might:
   - exhibit anger at the dead person for leaving; at God for allowing the death; at medical services for not saving the dead person; at others for causing the death (e.g., a traffic accident); and/or at themselves for not preventing the death.
   - feel guilty about negligence toward the dead person; thinking they should have loved the person better, that their feelings about the death are not appropriate.
   - become depressed and feel inadequate and worthless.
   - feel anxious about changes and wonder how changes will affect their futures.
4. Acceptance: This stage usually comes in the second year. The child adapts to a new set of circumstances.

What Children Say About Death

"All children know intuitively about the outcome of their illness. Even little children will ask, 'Am I going to die?' Older children will write a poem or a page in their diary about it" (Kübler-Ross, 1983, p. 1).

The following anecdote demonstrates that young children believe that death is temporary. In autumn, when a mother's 4-year-old helped her bury a dog, the child said, "This is really not so sad. Next spring when your tulips come up, he'll come up again and play with me" (Kübler-Ross, 1983, p. 82).

After his grandfather died, one little boy wrote about it in school saying, "I wish this story was not true but it is. My mother's dad died, he is going to be cremated over a hot fire, his ashes are going to be spread over a cool lake. I wish I were death: I would not let anyone die; I would let people live a wonderful life anywhere. My mother's father always went fishing for beautiful trout in the lake that his ashes will be spread over. I wish he would never die. I wish I weren't sad" (Kübler-Ross, 1983, p. 67).

Another little boy, who was angry because no one was dying in order to give him a kidney so that he could live, said that any time he is quiet, the nurses are nice to him, but when he is mad they want to ship him over to the other hospital. The "other hospital" was University Hospital, "where children are sent when they need an operation or when they are dying."

"I hope I die when they don't expect it, so I can stay with my friends here," he added philosophically (Kübler-Ross, 1983, p. 70).

How Parents and Family Can Help

Loving reassurance from family members can help young children better understand and accept death. At appropriate times, extending for even years after the death, parents should ask the child about feelings or memories. By being asked, the child is given the opportunity to ask questions and reconsider the loss as he or she becomes more mature (Jellinek, 2003).

Family members can reassure a child that most healthy people will not die soon. They can talk openly about their own feelings, maintain a familiar routine, seek support from other adults in the child's life, and seek comfort from religious beliefs.

What Is Said to a Child Is Very Important

Because children take language literally, it is important that adults be careful what they say. Using direct, factual language in place of indirect or symbolic language is important to use with young children to eliminate fear and confusion (see Table 13.1).

For instance, parents should describe death as what happens when the body stops working and

Table 13.1 MEANINGFUL DEATH TERMS FOR CHILDREN

Instead of Saying	Say	Because
asleep	died	children may fear sleep.
in heaven (a belief)	died and/or buried (facts)	beliefs and facts need to be explained separately.
lost	died	children may continue to look for a "missing person." Also, if adults do not look for the person, the child might fear, "Wouldn't they look for me if I were lost?"
old	specific cause (e.g., heart attack)	an adult of any age seems old to a child.
passed away	died	vagueness encourages possible harmful imaginings to fill in gaps.
on a journey	died	children might come to fear trips.

cannot be fixed. They should not compare death to sleep, because the child might become afraid of sleep and also think that the dead person will "reawaken." Or if a child is told, "God loved your mother so much that He took her to heaven," the very young child is likely to think, "Why doesn't God love me?" If someone says, "Daddy went to sleep," the child might think, "Will I die when I go to sleep, too?" Or if the child hears, "Grandpa went on a long trip," the child might wonder, "Why didn't he take me?"

How Pediatricians Can Help

Children who have lost a loved one to death might experience shock and denial at first, then sadness and anger, lasting weeks to months. In the best result, the child comes to accept the death and readjusts to ongoing life. Pediatricians can help children and families with this adjustment.

Prolonged or severe behavior change signals the need for significant therapeutic intervention. The pediatrician should pay close attention to the child's behavior on the anniversary of the death, at holidays, or when other losses occur.

The child should be told about a death honestly and in language that is consistent with the child's concept of death. Children need reassurance that they did not cause the death, could not have prevented it, and cannot bring back the dead loved one.

A pediatrician can encourage discussion of reactions, thoughts, and feelings of family members, which increases mutual support and cohesion. The family also can be reassured that their showing such feelings as shock, disbelief, guilt, sadness, and anger is normal and helpful.

A bereaved parent or other close family member who shares feelings and memories (e.g., with pictures and stories) with a child reduces the child's sense of isolation. The ability to share, to rely on family members, and to engage in good communication helps a child and his or her family adjust in the long term (Committee on Psychosocial Aspects of Child and Family Health, 2000).

Things to look for that can help distinguish between expected responses to death, which will lessen or pass, and manifestations calling for professional intervention are listed in Table 13.2.

How Teachers Can Help

Some teachers might think they are protecting children from the pain of knowing death by discouraging discussion or misrepresenting what happens. These evasions only confuse and frighten children. Teachers can, and should, help students honestly deal with death.

Whenever possible, teachers should discuss death and grief with students before a loss occurs. Children gain more benefit from lessons about death before it happens. Although not every question a child has can be answered, teachers should be candid with students about the reality of death, including the whats and whys:

- Death is inevitable and natural
- Death is irreversible and permanent
- Being dead means that everything stops
- Living things do not die because the child had bad thoughts

Also, the teacher should:

- share his or her own feelings of loss and grief.
- be patient and understanding.
- listen when children need to talk, and acknowledge their feelings.
- explain funeral rituals, customs, and services.
- be aware of students' feelings of anger, fear, and guilt.
- expect children to try do their schoolwork, but be flexible with schedules and assignments.

Specific strategies a teacher can use include the following:

- Use journal writing to help children work through their feelings.
- Help students create a memorial book of writings, pictures, letters, or small mementos.
- Read or recommend books to children about death and grief. These stories

Table 13.2 Grief Manifestations in Children and Adolescents

Usual Behavior	Sign of Disorder*
Shock or numbness	Long-term denial and avoidance of feelings
Crying	Repeated crying spells
Sadness	Disabling depression and suicidal ideas
Anger	Persistent anger
Feeling guilty	Believing self is guilty
Transient unhappiness	Persistent unhappiness
Keeping concerns inside	Social withdrawal
Increased clinging	Separation anxiety
Disobedience	Conduct disorder
Lack of interest in school	Decline in school performance
Transient sleep disturbance	Persistent sleep problems
Physical complaints	Physical symptoms of the person who died
Decreased appetite	Eating disorder
Temporary regression	Disabling or persistent regression
Being good or bad	Being much too good or bad
Believing the dead person is still alive	Persistent belief that the dead person is still alive
Relating better to friends than to family	Promiscuity or delinquent behavior
Behavior lasts days to weeks	Behavior lasts weeks to months

*Should prompt investigation by a pediatrician.

Source: Committee on Psychosocial Aspects of Child and Family Health (2000).

demonstrate that grieving is a natural process and help students realize that all children experience fears, anxieties, and anger.

- Have a memorial service at the school so faculty and students can honor the person who died (Westmoreland, 1996).

How Bereavement Centers Help

Helping a child cope with the death of a loved one is among the toughest tasks anyone can face. Thus, bereavement centers have been established to help children. More than 160 bereavement centers exist around the country, allowing children to express their grief at the death of a loved one.

Because grief is slow to go away, children cling to their memories even as the years go by. According to Debby Shimmel, a volunteer at the St. Francis Center in Washington, D.C., they are afraid they will forget how their mother or father looked and how her or his voice sounded. She suggests that children can be helped by painting memories onto quilts or drawing pictures of their parents.

Stefanie Norris of the Good Mourning program in Park Ridge, Illinois, says that children sometimes draw a football stadium to show what they think heaven is like for their fathers. At the end of each 8-week group session, children hold a memorial for their dead parents—a more concrete memorial than a church eulogy—and more meaningful to a child. They wear something their parent wore or prepare a favorite dish.

Most important, bereavement centers provide a room where a child can vent anger. The Dougy Center in Portland, Oregon, includes a "splatter room," where kids throw paint. Most centers have some variation of the "volcano room," padded with foam and supplied with stuffed animals the children pummel into lint. Barney is said to be a teenage favorite (Adler et al., 1997).

The Adolescent View of Death

Grieving adolescents might feel especially vulnerable and believe that they have lost control of their lives. Their pain might resurface at major moments, such as a birthday or graduation. However, they are good at concealing feelings of depression from their parents (Jellinek, 2003).

The best way to handle grief, especially for adolescents, is to express feelings and share their sadness. Many of them share by creating memorials or expressing their grief in writing. This openness is very different from the accepted wisdom of a previous generation, when concealment and avoidance was the rule (Adler et al., 1997).

Adolescents also use various strategies to deal with awareness of their own mortality and fear of death (Piaget, 1973). For example, they:

- engage in risky activities for the thrill of survival.
- enjoy horror movies and other images of bizarre or violent death.
- enjoy playing computer games involving destruction of other beings.
- imitate death in appearance (e.g., wear black, wear white makeup, have garish tattoos).
- behave with so little affect as to seem already dead.

Taking risks (e.g., reckless driving, binge drinking, diving off high cliffs, trying dangerous drugs, fist fighting, using deadly weapons, engaging in extreme sports, performing feats of athletic endurance without proper training) can cause an adolescent to think that he or she is cheating death and earning social approval. The closer to the edge, the greater the thrill of defeating death.

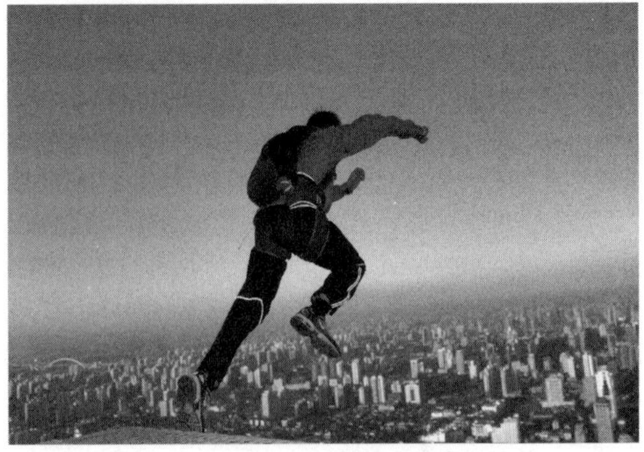

An adolescent also might choose to play with death-related objects in a more personal way. Examples include writing a last will and testament, for instance, or thinking about types of caskets, composing funeral music or poetry, creating morbid artworks, or exploring Internet sites that deal with death (Noppe & Noppe, 1996).

Helping a Bereaved Adolescent

If an adolescent who has experienced the death of someone with whom he or she is close exhibits the following signs, the young person might need additional help and support:

- Shows little energy
- Avoids friends
- Changes eating or sleeping habits
- Has no interest in favorite activities

The young person should be encouraged to talk. Be direct. Ask, "What's wrong? I'm concerned." Be considerate, and listen without judging. Don't pry; just ask "How are you doing?" Get the teen

"'The pain never goes away,' says Geoff Lake, who was 11 when his mother, Linda, died of a rare form of cancer. He is only starting to realize it, but at each crucial passage of life—graduation, marriage, the birth of children—there will be a face missing from the picture, a kiss never received, a message of joy bottled up inside, where it turns into sorrow. His sleep will be shadowed by ghosts, and the bittersweet shock of awakening back into a world from which his mother is gone forever.

"If he lives to be 100, with a score of descendants, some part of him will still be the boy whose mother left for the hospital one day and never came home. Every child who has lost a parent remains, in some secret part of his or her soul, a child forever frozen at a moment in time, crying out to the heedless heavens, as Geoff Lake did, when his mother died just days before his 12th birthday: 'Mom, why did you die? I had plans!'" (Adler et al., 1997, p. 58).

Books on the Death of a Sibling or Close Friend

- *Beat the Turtle Drum* by Constance C. Greene (Viking, 1976; ages 10 to 14)
- *Bridge to Terabithia* by Katherine Paterson (Crowell, 1977; ages 10 to 14)
- *Straight Talk About Death for Teenagers* by Earl A. Grollman (Beacon Press, 1993; ages 13 to 19)

Source: Arnold and Gemma (1994).

to talk, because talking about it is the best way to feel better.

Young females often are more willing to talk about how they feel; young males tend to bottle up their emotions, with the attitude of "Suck it up and get over it." But the feelings are going to come out in some way.

Many young males become angry and act out by being aggressive and picking fights, or they may isolate themselves, which is typical of depression. If possible, persuade the teen to play sports, go to a movie, or anything other than sitting and brooding.

Do not tell a grieving teen, "I know just how you feel," because no one knows exactly how another person feels. Make sure the teen knows that support is available (Sparling, 2006). If a teen threatens self-harm (cutting, using drugs, or talking about suicide), he or she needs professional help.

Death and the Student Athlete

In a society where the subject of death is avoided, student athletes are usually devastated by the death of a teammate or a coach. Because they spend more time with teammates and coaches than they spend with anyone else, it is similar to a death in the family.

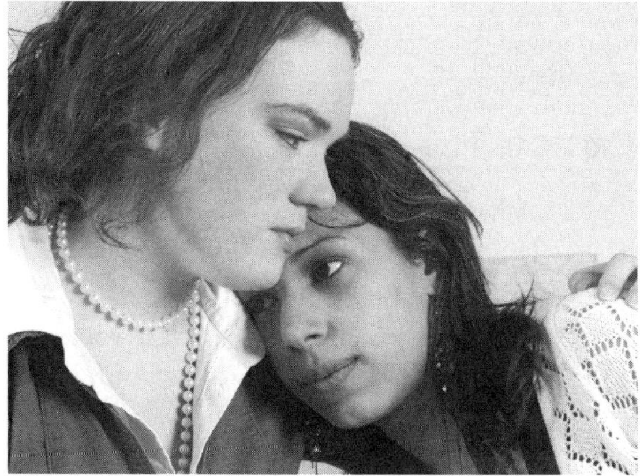

The athletic trainer or coach is someone who can help athletes deal with their sadness by communicating and providing unconditional support. The trainer or coach also can make it clear that grieving is not the same for everyone; it is an individual process. Just by listening, trainers and coaches let athletes know that grief is acceptable and healthy.

Athletic trainers and coaches also should create a place where grieving athletes can freely express their feelings, fears, and concerns without judgment from others, a place which allows others to offer support as well. Athletes who can express themselves physically and emotionally are better able to deal with their distress. Finally, assisting athletes to grieve helps them create the continuing memory of a loved one (Dunn, 1997).

Summary

- Most young children are exposed to death on a regular basis, including deaths in fairy tales, lullabies, games, TV cartoons, and sing-song rhymes. Children look at death differently depending on how old and how emotionally and intellectually mature they are.
- Children between the ages of 2 and 3 have no cognitive understanding of death. Up to age 6, children believe that death is similar to being asleep. About age 6, children come to know that death is irreversible; the dead stay dead. At age 9 or 10 children become aware that death is inevitable, universal, and personal.

- Children grieve, though their grieving differs at different ages, and often bears little resemblance to the mourning of adults. Young children process their loss a bit at a time. At ages 6 to 9 or so, they become fearful about their own death or the deaths of loved ones. Death can be the hardest to deal with at ages 9 to 12, in between childhood and adolescence.
- Level of maturation is a better predictor of how a child views death than chronological age.
- Children typically suffer the most acutely for at least 2 months following a loss, peaking at about 1 month, but they may feel intense grief from 6 months to a year later.
- Loving reassurance from family members can help young children better understand and accept death. Parents should ask the child about feelings or memories. Because children take language literally, it is important to use direct, factual language in place of indirect or symbolic language.
- Pediatricians can help children and families adjust to the death of a loved one, but prolonged or severe behavior change signals the need for significant therapeutic intervention.
- Teachers can and should help students deal with death honestly. Teachers should discuss death and grief candidly, and before loss occurs, if possible.
- More than 160 bereavement centers around the country allow children to express their grief at the death of a loved one by, among other things, providing a room where a child can vent anger without being admonished or punished.
- Grieving adolescents feel vulnerable. Major moments are especially difficult for them, such as a birthday or graduation. They conceal depression from their parents. Taking risks may make many adolescents believe that they are cheating death and earning social approval. A bereaved teen in need shows little energy, avoids friends, changes eating or sleeping habits, and has no interest in favorite activities.
- Student athletes are usually devastated by the death of a teammate or a coach. The athletic trainer or coach can help athletes deal with their sadness by communicating and providing unconditional support and creating a place where they can freely express their feelings, fears, and concerns.

ADDITIONAL RESOURCES

Books

Adams D. W., & Deveau, E. J. (Eds.). (1995). *Beyond the innocence of childhood: Factors influencing children and adolescents' perceptions and attitudes.* Amityville, NY: Baywood Publishing Co. This three-volume series discusses how adults can help children and adolescents deal with tragic circumstances such as the death of their pet, the terminal illness of a parent, their own struggle with a life-threatening disease, the accidental death of a sibling, or the suicide of a friend.

Buscaglia, L. (1983). *The fall of Freddie the leaf: A story of life for all ages*. New York: Henry Holt and Co. This story in this book explains that all living things are part of a natural cycle. As Freddie and his companions change with the passing seasons, Freddie learns from an older leaf, Daniel, that death is part of life, which prepares him for his own calm and peaceful experience as he falls from his branch with the winter's snow.

Seibert D., Drolet, J. C., & Fetro, J. V. (1993). *Are you sad, too?* Santa Cruz, CA: ETR Associates. In this book, suggestions for teachers, parents, and other care providers are presented for helping children deal with loss and death. A very good bibliography of children's books about death is included plus suggested readings for adults.

Movie

Dying Young. (1991). Recognizing his imminent death, a young leukemia patient makes the most out of the rest of his life.

CRITICAL THINKING

1. What would you say to a 5-year-old child whose father has died and who asks, "Is Daddy coming back?"
2. Describe the behavior(s) a friend would demonstrate in reaction to the death of someone to whom he or she was close that would prompt you to offer your support.

3. Describe what sorts of behavior would prompt you to immediately seek professional help on a friend's behalf who recently had experienced the death of a loved one.

Class Activity

Have the class role-play responses to the death of a close friend or family member. Class members should be paired. One student is the one in crisis, and the other plays a friend offering support. As the role-play proceeds, ask class members if the interactions seem helpful and appropriate and, if so, why. To follow up, class members should write about the responses that they thought were the most helpful (Sparling, 2006).

References

Adler, J., Wingert, P., Springen, K., Stone, B., King, P., Kalb, C., et al. (1997, September 22). How kids mourn. *Newsweek*, 58–61.

Anthony, S. (1972). *The discovery of death in childhood and after.* New York: Basic Books.

Arnold, J. H., & Gemma, P. B. (1994). *A child dies: A portrait of family grief.* Philadelphia: The Charles Press.

Bluebond-Langner, M. (1996). *In the shadow of illness.* Princeton, NJ: Princeton University Press.

Christ, G. H. (2000). *Healing children's grief: Surviving a Parent's Death from Cancer.* Oxford University Press.

Committee on Psychosocial Aspects of Child and Family Health. (2000). The pediatrician and childhood bereavement. *Pediatrics, 105*(2), 445.

Deveau, E. J., & Adams, D. W. (Eds.). (1995). *Beyond the innocence of childhood.* New York: Baywood.

Didion, J. (2005). *The year of magical thinking.* New York: Knopf.

Dunn, J. L. (1997). Helping athletes cope with grief. *Coach and Athletic Director, 66*(10), 12.

Freud, S. (2005). *On murder, mourning, and melancholia.* New York: Penguin Modern Classics. (Original work published 1917)

Harris, M. (1995). *The loss that is forever: The lifelong impact of the early death of a mother or father.* New York: Penguin Books.

Jellinek, M. S. (2003). The varying faces of grief. *Pediatric News, 37*(4), 21.

Kübler-Ross, E. (1983). *On children and death.* New York: Simon & Schuster.

Maurer, A. (1966). Maturation of concepts of death. *British Journal of Medicine and Psychology, 39*, 35–41.

Nagy, M. H. (1948). The child's theories concerning death. *Journal Genetic Psychology, 73*, 3–27.

Noppe, L. D., & Noppe, I. C. (1996). Ambiguity in adolescent understandings of death. In C. A. Corr & D. E. Balk (Eds.), *Handbook of adolescent death and bereavement* (pp. 25–41). New York: Springer.

Opie, I., & Opie, P. (1969). *Children's games in street and playground.* London: Oxford University Press.

Piaget, J. (1973). *The child and reality: Problems of genetic psychology.* New York: Grossman.

Seibert, D., Drolet, J. C., & Fetro, J. V. (1993). *Are you sad, too?* Scotts Valley, CA: ETR Associates.

Sparling, P. (2006). A friend in need: Help a pal by using tact and offering a sympathetic ear. *Current Health, 32*(6), 7.

Ward, B. (1993). *Good grief.* London: Jessica Kingsley Publishers.

Westmoreland, P. (1996). Coping with death: Helping students grieve. *Childhood Education, 72*(3), 157.

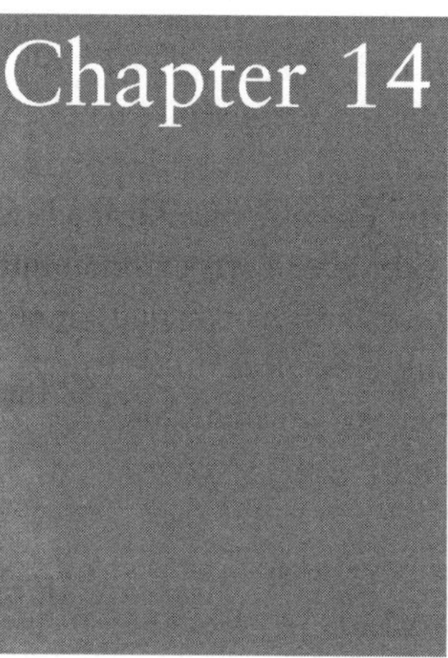

How Adults View and Represent Death

The weariest and most loathed worldly life
That age, ache, penury, and imprisonment
Can lay on nature is a paradise
To what we fear of death.
—SHAKESPEARE, *MEASURE FOR MEASURE*

Objectives

After reading this chapter, you will be able to answer the following questions:

- How have Americans' views toward death changed?
- What are some of the possible effects of media representations of death?
- What are four perspectives of death?
- What are the various social views of death?
- Do people respond differently when death occurs unexpectedly?
- What are people's fears regarding death?
- How does religious belief shape views toward death?
- What are the various forms of denial of impending death?
- How do people use humor to ameliorate their fears of death?

For most of the twentieth century, death was behind the scenes. The dying and the dead were confined to hospitals, mortuaries, and cemeteries. In general, in contemporary Western society, people wish to ignore death, typically saying someone has "passed away" rather than died.

Death and bereavement once were events that engaged the whole community. Now they are experienced largely by the immediate family. Social and religious rituals once helped give death meaning. Today, dealing with loss is left to the individual. This shift appears to have coincided with a decline in religious belief (Gorer, 1967).

The fragmentation of communities and the loss of family ties have removed the emotional and social supports that can help lessen the impact of death. People do not die at home, as a rule, and now the dying and dead are handled by institutions. Gone are the comforts of ritualized grief and mourning, such as preparing the dead at home and conducting a wake; ritualistic visits by family, friends, and neighbors; graveside ceremonies; and periods of formal mourning, including wearing black armbands and clothing (McLennan, Akande, & Bates, 1993).

How Have Americans' Views Toward Death Changed?

Americans are more interested in death and dying than they were earlier in the twentieth century. Media reports remind them daily of death: AIDS, wars, natural disasters, the prevalence of cancer, chronic illness, death by individual violence—and terrorism.

The attack on September 11, 2001 came as a shock to most Americans, who historically had been protected by the Atlantic and Pacific oceans from direct attacks on civilian targets. Such devastation occurs more or less regularly in other parts of the world, where people do not react with the same widespread hysteria, disbelief, and paranoia (in media reporting, at least) as have Americans to 9/11.

Many Americans have been disturbed by the number of deaths of American soldiers in Iraq—a number that now exceeds the number who died in 9/11. This coincidence has helped lose a majority of public support for the war, but the deaths in Iraq happened over time, and combat deaths are not unfamiliar to generations who grew up with World War II and Vietnam. The upshot of 9/11 for Americans has been more surveillance of everyday gatherings in public places in the United States and chronic fear of a recurrence.

Effects of Media Representations of Death

In general, Americans have become desensitized to the realities of death. Moreover, they appear ill-equipped to deal with death when it happens to those they know or to whom they are close. The frequent portrayals of violence and death on TV and the movies and news, which, except for news reports, usually do not include showing the emotional aftermath for survivors, have caused many Americans to become desensitized to death (Browne & Pennell, 1998). This desensitization leads many viewers to think that death is an end in itself, without real consequence (Carr, 2005). By age 15, most people in the United States have seen 13,000 murders on television and in film, along with the same number of deaths in news stories of violent death in war and disaster (Bordewich, 1988).

The proliferation of modern-day scenes of torture, bloodletting, and gruesome injury might be driven by the popularity of the thrillers in which they are featured. These scenes also might be a product of the increasing violence seen in real human society (Carr, 2005).

Violence on Television

"If it bleeds, it leads," is a well-known journalistic catchphrase, characterizing the decisions of most print and television news organizations. Almost everyone in the United States has one or more TV sets. Pervasive media images of war, violence, accidents, murders, and the deaths of missing children obviously affect people's feelings and thoughts about death.

News reports on TV and in print are influenced by fame or celebrity, and reports of death might linger regarding the public perception of that person, good or bad, rather than simply of the event. Also, TV reporters at death scenes always seem to want to show someone, a relative or neighbor, breaking down emotionally.

Cartoons on television seem to have a similar effect on children. Characters are repeatedly smashed, deformed, and killed—but do not die. Those once "dead" spring up and head into more mayhem.

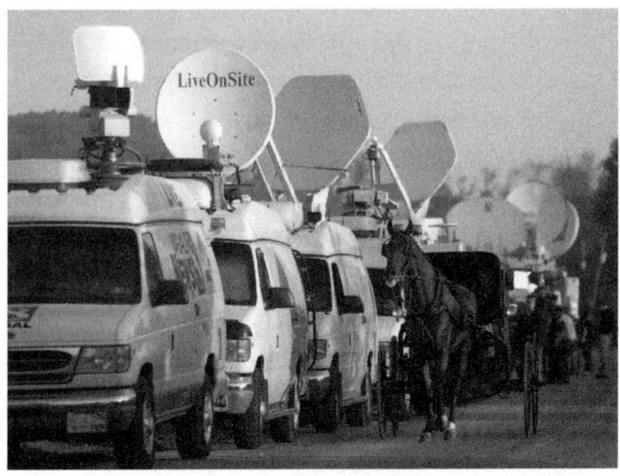

Realistic Film and Television

Death in the movies, up until 1970, was taboo except for the villains, who died as punishment for their evil deeds. Then Hollywood began making movies about the death of leading characters, as in *Love Story, Philadelphia,* and *Saving Private Ryan.*

TV followed suit, most notably with episodes that accounted for the real deaths of actors playing significant characters, such as Mr. Hooper, the storekeeper on *Sesame Street,* and the father played by John Ritter in *Eight Simple Rules for Dating My Teenage Daughter.* TV documentaries have been used to present the deaths of cancer patients and death itself, as in *On Our Own Terms: Moyers on Dying* and *With Eyes Open,* companion shows on PBS hosted by Bill Moyers. HBO launched a successful drama series called *Six Feet Under,* which was set in a funeral home. Public displays of emotion following the death of Diana, Princess of Wales, and the approximate 3,000 who died on 9/11, alongside the popularity of serious television programs about death, suggest a public level of interest in death unseen in earlier periods (Brennan, 2005).

Music

Music always has been a powerful emotional medium for expressing feelings about death. Much gospel and church music includes images of death, for example, "When the Saints Go Marching In," "Will the Circle Be Unbroken?" and "Precious Memories."

Examples of popular music featuring death themes include Elton John's "Candle in the Wind," which was written about the death of Marilyn Monroe and later sung by him at Princess Diana's funeral; Holly Near's song, "The Letter," which concerns the death of a friend dying from AIDS; Snoop Dogg's song about urban homicide, "Murder Was the Case"; and Eric Clapton's song, "Tears in Heaven," in which he mourns the accidental death of his young son (Insel & Roth, 2002).

A well-known use of funeral music is the celebrated New Orleans jazz band that typically follows a funeral procession to the cemetery. This band plays a version of a *dirge,* a musical form long associated with funeral processions and burials.

Classical music has a long history of lyrics with death themes. Berlioz, Mozart, and Verdi, among others, have written Requiem Masses (Mass for the Dead). Poulenc, in his opera, *Dialog of the Carmelites,* ends with a chilling scene of nuns singing a quartet, a trio, a duet, and finally a solo as they go, one by one, to the gallows.

Laments are a musical expression of ceremonial leave-taking. For example, the playing of bagpipes at a clan funeral in Scotland, and the Hawaiian chants called *mele kanikau*, are sung to celebrate memories of shared experiences with the dead (DeSpelder & Strickland, 2005).

Literature

Through sharing stories and poems about death, which is a part of medical training, medical staffs learn ways of helping people, and eventually their patients, deal with death and dying. Expressing feelings of loss through stories and poems also helps dying people and their loved ones (Bowman & Richard, 2004).

Literature about death can be profound and can affect ruminations on life and death. One of best examples of this is the short story, "The Dead," by James Joyce. Set at a family Christmas party, Joyce presents the congeniality, warmth, and love at such a party, and he very convincingly presents images of those who are gone to serve as reminders that the shadow of death is never far behind the living. The Joyce story ends with an image of snow falling across Ireland, over graveyards as well as over the houses where people were currently living. As the party guest, Gabriel Conroy, drifted off to sleep, "His soul swooned slowly as he heard the snow falling through the universe and faintly falling, like the descent of their last end, upon all the living and the dead."

Death Perspectives

According to Russell (1999), there are at least four distinct perspectives on life and death:

- The first perspective is *ecological*. In this perspective, a person views all forms of life, including humans, as equal in value and importance. Death is viewed as a necessity to complete the cycle, to provide the earth with resources for new life. This view assumes no afterlife.

- The second perspective is *humanistic*. In the humanistic perspective, human life is viewed as more important than other forms of existence. Other than that difference, this perspective is similar to the ecological perspective. For example, in both perspectives, the belief is that death is the end of consciousness. Humanists do believe that they "live on," but through other people remembering their contributions and accomplishments.
- In the Western *religious* perspective, all forms of life are believed created by a supreme being. Eternal life is possible. In this perspective, death should be celebrated, on the assumption that the person who has died will live after death in heaven, if the life lived was a righteous one.
- The *reincarnation* perspective is more common in Eastern religions than in the West. In this perspective, existence is continuous, spanning many lifetimes. Death is simply entering another life. Each life has a unique purpose, with selflessness as the ultimate goal.

Social Views of Death

Death and dying, until recently, had replaced sex as a taboo topic of conversation. Lately though, sociology has begun to look at how social meaning is formed with respect to death. Although death is a biological event, what leads up to and follows death is socially constructed. Once viewed in religious and spiritual terms, death has become a medical and scientific phenomenon (Brennan, 2005).

In contrast to the fixed religious patterns of many past funerals in America, funerals today often are customized by the dead and his or her family, who might choose pop music and personalized readings, sometimes in combination with choral hymns and religious verses. In other words, people now seem to prefer more cheerful send-offs.

This change explains what happened after Diana, Princess of Wales, died in 1997. There was a mixture of rituals during her funeral service; for example, a military gun carriage carried the coffin, and Elton John sang at her funeral service, which was contrasted with the majestic surroundings of Westminster Abbey, the traditional burial site of poets and kings (Kear & Steinberg, 1999).

In public, people gathered in large mourning crowds, and the reticent Queen herself was persuaded to address the nation and come out to observe the funeral procession. A huge sea of flowers was placed around Kensington Palace, along with shrines here and there of toys and personal memorabilia. Definitely, death is no longer taboo.

Unexpected Versus Expected Death

When someone dies of old age, it is considered expected and even natural. The person has had time to make plans for his or her funeral, and loved ones have had time to plan for life without their loved one.

When a person dies without warning, however, the death is unexpected. Unexpected death due to accident, murder, suicide, or sudden heart attack or illness typically makes grieving more painful for family members than death after a long illness. In the case of sudden death, the people left behind do not have time to say goodbye.

Whether the dying person is male or female might affect preference for a quick or delayed death. Kastenbaum (2004) explained that when a woman is terminally ill, she is more concerned for the fate of her family after her death than for herself. For example, she may wonder if her children will be okay or if her husband can manage the household without her. If so, she is likely to want to live longer, even if she is in pain. In contrast, Kastenbaum explained that a terminally ill husband/father might think that if he cannot continue to work and support his

DEATH AND THE BOOMER GENERATION

In a few years, the baby boomer generation is going to enter the prime perishing years—and turn dying into a form of self-expression. Examples of such self-expression include the following:

- San Francisco has a Zen hospice, in which "death companions" or "midwives of death" are trained.
- The Paradise Memorial Crematory outside Scottsdale, Arizona, offers a Cremation Cam, with Internet broadcasts of cremations—but not including inside the oven, fortunately.
- On www.ObitDetails.com, obituaries can be posted, and on www.plan4ever.com, families can converse in memorial chat rooms.
- Celestic Inc. will send cremains into space for about $12,500. In San Francisco, fierce competition has erupted for burial plots with a water view, at family plot prices over $100,000. Dying has become something that might need a real estate agent.
- And then there is the new look in coffins. A Dallas firm called Whitelight can, with digital printing technology, put any mural on a casket. Are you a golf nut? You can have Fairway to Heaven, a golf course scene. Or you can have zebra stripes in honor of that African safari you never took.

Not only are baby boomers expected to bankrupt the Social Security system and give every state the profile of Florida or Arizona, they are likely to have afterlife crises—rather than a midlife crisis—trying to make sure their very souls are self-actualized (Brooks, 2000).

family, which he frequently equates with being a "real man," he would rather die quickly.

Fear of Death

Oftentimes when people say that they fear death, it is not death itself they fear, but the physical and psychological processes of dying. The physical fear of dying is actually the fear of pain. Psychological fear is letting go of people and things loved—and, because many people die alone on the late shift in a hospital or nursing home, dying alone.

Death anxiety seems generally to be higher in females, African Americans, and the young and middle aged and lower for religious believers and those who are mature and have self-control (Wass & Neimeyer, 1995). Rasmussen and Brems (1996) found that psychosocial development appears to be the stronger predictor of lessened anxiety than age, but the combination of the two significantly decreases death anxiety.

In general, older people are less afraid of death than younger people. Young people who are religious are least likely to be afraid of death. Greater fear is found in people who hold no particular religious beliefs, as compared to those who are either religious or nonreligious (Kalish, 1985).

Even if they fear death, young people probably believe that it is too far away to give it much thought. Elderly people are usually resigned to, or accepting of, impending death. Ferrini and Ferrini (2000) suggested that middle-aged people fear death more than those of other ages. Part of their fear may be due to realizing that after their parents die, they are next.

Fear of Not Dying Well

In the past, people feared death because it often came unexpectedly and prematurely. They consoled themselves with the thought that the dead loved one would go to a better place—an afterlife, either in heaven or in reincarnation (Kearl, 1996). Now, many people in their later years fear, not death, but becoming like Tithonus in Greek mythology, continuing to deteriorate, but not die—becoming totally dependent, having no

THE MYTH OF TITHONUS

The Greek myth of Tithonus is a parable about what can happen to people who want to live forever. Aurora (Eos), the Greek goddess of the dawn, falls in love with Tithonus, a mortal youth, and persuades Jupiter to grant him everlasting life—but forgot to ask for youth. He becomes old and feeble, and although she loses interest in him, she keeps him around. Eventually, she confines him to his chamber, where he chatters endlessly. Finally, taking pity on him in his wretched state, Aurora turns him into a grasshopper. In Greek mythology, the grasshopper is immortal, and grasshoppers chirrup ceaselessly, like demented old men.

control over themselves, being without dignity, living in an institution, and using up the money and sympathy of family members.

The worst fear for most elderly is to become a victim of Alzheimer's disease, a disease characterized by physically alive victims who otherwise might as well be dead (the sad fate of former president Ronald Reagan). Of Americans aged 85 and older, 42 percent have Alzheimer's, compared with 2 percent at age 65 (Alzheimer's Association, 2007). Thus, dying well now means being able to control when and how death comes.

Types of Death Fears

Humans fear the process of dying, the unknowns of death, and of not being. Some people fear death because they do not know what will follow bodily death. For example, Christians who believe in an afterlife might fear the Day of Judgment and possible punishment for what they did wrong or did not do right in an earthly life.

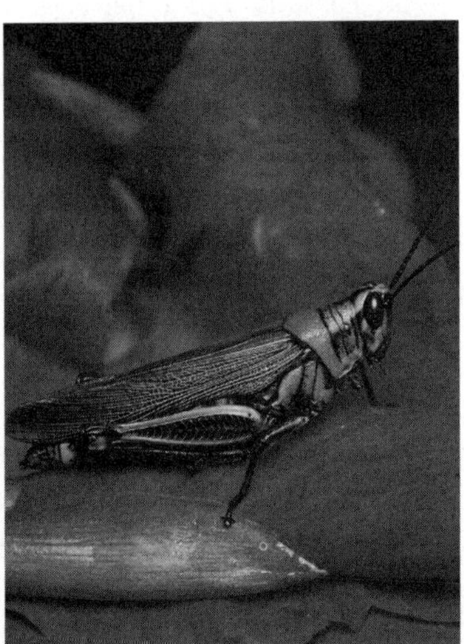

Many people fear the unknowns associated with death, because they need to be in control. Even if they have well-formed beliefs concerning death and its consequences, as well as beliefs about afterlife, some people might fear that they are mistaken about these beliefs.

The ultimate anticipatory anguish of which humans are capable may be the fear of simply not being. As Shakespeare's Hamlet so famously says,

> To be, or not to be: that is the question: . . .
> But that the dread of something after death,
> The undiscover'd country from whose bourne
> No traveller returns, puzzles the will
> And makes us rather bear those ills we have
> Than fly to others that we know not of.

Reducing Anxiety About Death

One way to reduce anxiety about death among nursing home residents who have a terminal illness is to allow them involvement in decisions about treatment (Brown University, 1990). Asking them to complete a document to provide answers about questions such as CPR, transfer to a hospital, antibiotics, tube feeding, and respirators has been found useful. Kept with medical records and intended for caregivers, the document applies only if the individuals are terminally ill and cannot speak for themselves. Surrogate decision-makers are named in the document. A physician is required to sign the form, along with the resident, to make sure that he or she understands the resident's wishes and that the physician is in agreement with those wishes (see Chapter 8).

My Story: How I Got Over My Fear of Death

Ever since I can remember, the thought of dying has been so scary for me. I think it started when Dad told me that Grandpop, who had just died, was sleeping. For years, I was afraid even to go to sleep. I really never told anybody about those fears, because I assumed I couldn't "do" anything to make fear go away.

In health class one day, the health instructor said that it was natural, but not necessary, to fear death. Well, I already knew that it was natural! But how could it be both natural and unnecessary? She said that fearing death was natural because people typically fear the unknown. She told us that if we understood the naturalness of death, though, we also might find that fearing it was not necessary. I could not imagine that she could explain away the fear of death, but I was interested.

The teacher began by explaining that death was just a natural life process—like one of the natural seasons in a year. "Death—a part of life?" we questioned. She told the class that probably none of us had been afraid when our spring season (our childhoods) became summer season (our teen years). She had a point, because most of us were pretty eager to become teens!

Next, our health professor asked the class to consider if we believed that it would be safe for us when our summer turned into early and late fall (adulthood and old age). After discussion, my classmates and I agreed that the fall of our lives would be okay and maybe even fun. "These safe changes," she said, "are natural changes. Why, then, should you be afraid of death, at the end of the final season—the winter—of life?"

Before that class, I had not heard death described as changes of seasons. I think my death is a long way away, and I think that, like the health instructor said, "It will get here in its own perfect season." Somehow, that thought has helped ease my fears about death, and I didn't have to "do" anything; I just needed to think differently.

Death and Religion

Death's apparent lack of meaning creates anxiety about the meaning of one's existence in the world. When someone dies, those left behind must come to grips with such questions as "What is the meaning of life?" The more important question might be, "What is the meaning of my life?"

At times when the search for significance becomes primary, religious traditions can give meaning to existence. The dying process thus becomes a religious rite of passage, and the place where someone dies becomes sacred, be it home, hospital, or battlefield (O'Connell, 1995). Religious belief also can offer an eternal afterlife. Death is not an end, but a beginning (Brennan, 2005).

Religious belief also can provide a reason for human suffering by offering redemption as a reward; for example, suffering is the price paid for deliverance from eternal sin and damnation. Religion, thereby, for these believers, can offer an escape from the seeming meaninglessness of death (Berger, 1969).

Denial of Impending Death

The dying, and their families, commonly deny that death is near. They want to live, so they refuse to accept the prognosis of death. Denial can help with initial coping, but it also keeps the dying process from being peaceful. Denying impending death can encourage futile treatments and postpone or prevent patients and families from organizing financial matters, completing advance directives, resolving personal issues, and saying goodbye (Rousseau, 2000).

Most dying patients do finally resolve their feelings and accept that they have a terminal disease. But, in the meantime, physicians caring for terminal patients must deal with patient denial. The following are some tips for evaluating physician behavior toward the dying patient who appears to be in denial:

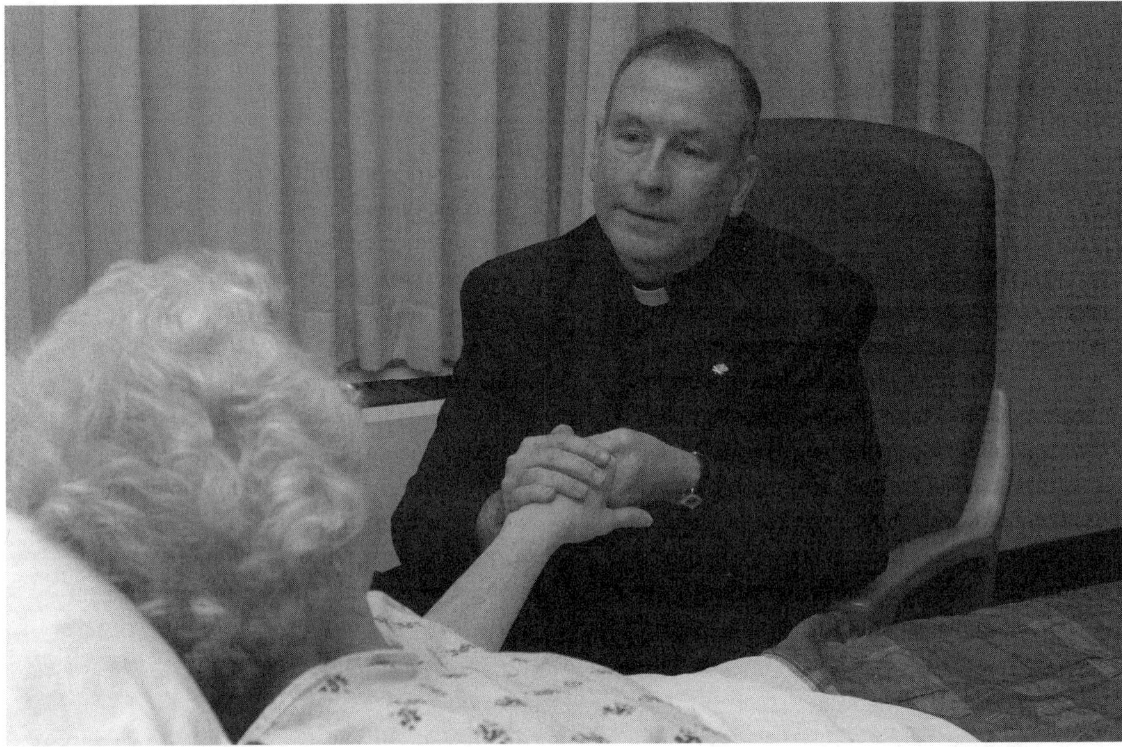

- Is the patient in denial? If so, should anything be done about it?
- Diagnosing denial is subjective and depends on an assessment of the patient's views and values, individual desires, and cultural, ethnic, and family influences.
- Rather than denying, the patient might disagree with the diagnosis or treatment and express a desire for autonomy, control, and better quality of life.
- If denial is adaptive and does not affect the patient's willingness to ask for help, the physician should ignore it.
- If denial interferes with daily activity and medical therapy, the physician should address it—but be tolerant and compassionate in doing so.

Recommended ways for physicians, nurses, social workers, and other medical staff to discuss end-of-life issues with patients or their surrogate decision makers (SDMs) and their families (Balaban, 2000; Buckman, 1992):

- Sit down with the person and/or family member in a private place.
- Begin by introducing everyone.
- Ask "How are you feeling today?" or "I know you're not feeling well, but perhaps we could talk for a few minutes."
- Find out what the person knows about the illness.
- To show interest and active listening, repeat in paraphrase what is said.
- Determine how much the person wants to know, and give it, but do not offer too much information at one time or use confusing medical terms.
- Reinforce and clarify information often.
- Explain the therapeutic choices.
- Respond empathetically to the person's feelings and reactions.
- Discuss treatment recommendations if asked.
- Encourage questions.
- Arrange a follow-up visit.

Denial can be beneficial or harmful. It can alleviate emotional distress and give patients time to absorb the idea of impending death and to complete life tasks. But if denial interferes with an

Death Denial and Consumerism

Here's a whole new spin on the expression, "Shop till you drop." Who would have thought that conspicuous consumption might be an expression of a fear of death? Humans are avaricious; enough is never enough, so history can be seen from one angle as one giant shopping spree. Plundering and acquiring went on for a long time before the first shopping mall was built. Humans also are the only animals who are aware that they are going to die. According to Kasser and Kanner (2003), the desire to feel good and somehow avoid dying can, in some cases, reinforce the urge to splurge.

Two personality disorders appear to characterize compulsive acquisition: materialistic value orientation (MVO) and acquisitive desire (AD). Sometimes, buying a Jimmy Choo isn't just about the shoe. People with MVO have doubts about their self-worth, their ability to cope effectively with challenges, and their safety in a relatively unpredictable world. They report lower subjective well-being and a lower quality of life. Adolescents with MVO report lower self-actualization and vitality, as well as more depression and anxiety. They are lower in social productivity and general functioning and higher in conduct disorders. MVO in college students is positively associated with narcissism, physical symptoms, and drug use and negatively associated with self-esteem and quality of relationships.

Examples of AD include the bank president who had a gold-plated toilet installed at company expense next to his private office or the school superintendent who was discovered to have a Caribbean island condo for "business meetings." These individuals' neurotic greed gets so far out of hand that they get caught. They are usually diagnosed as having a narcissistic personality disorder: self-aggrandizement motivated by extreme reaction to failure.

orderly dying process, medical staff needs to deal with it to allow a dignified and peaceful death.

Humor

Humor can help people cope with painful situations. It helps people confront their fears and gain a sense of mastery over the unknown. Finding humor in death, putting it in a conventional light, relieves some of the anxiety that accompanies awareness of one's own mortality. Individuals who encounter death on their jobs, as emergency services personnel do, sometimes use humor to distance themselves from horror as well as to rebound as a team rather than feel their individual grief after traumatic incidents (DeSpelder & Strickland, 2005).

Humor also is used to soften the news of a death. A hospital intern announced one day, "Guess who's not going to shop at Wal-Mart any more?" This expression became a standard way for staff at that hospital to announce a death.

For people who are seriously ill, humor can offer a way to cope with the effects of a shattering diagnosis. Humor does not necessarily make the situation better, but it can serve a protective psychological function and help people keep their equilibrium.

Humor can be social glue that helps people empathize with others (Peniston-Bird & Summerfield, 2001). In situations involving interactions between patients and healthcare providers, humor is "one of the great tools of reassurance on the hospital ward" (Francis, Monahan, & Berger, 1999). After a death has occurred, humor can comfort survivors as they recall the funny, as well as painful, events of a loved one's life.

Humor functions in several ways with regard to death (Peniston-Bird & Summerfield, 2001). As such, it:

- raises consciousness about a taboo subject and offers a way to talk about it.
- presents an opportunity to rise above sadness, providing a release from pain and

THE MARX BROTHERS AS THERAPY

A famous example of the power of humor to help someone deal with serious illness is the experience of the journalist and writer, Norman Cousins (1979). Told that he had little chance of surviving a crippling and life-threatening collagen disease, Cousins developed a recovery program incorporating mega doses of Vitamin C along with a positive attitude and laughter induced by Marx Brothers films.

Cousins made the discovery that 10 minutes of genuine belly laughter had an anesthetic effect that provided at least 2 hours of pain-free sleep for him. After the pain-killing effect of laughter wore off, he watched the film again and, most often, it led to another pain-free interval.

promoting a sense of control over a traumatic situation, even if nothing can be changed.

- is a great leveler; it treats everyone alike and sends the message that there are no exemptions from the human predicament.
- binds others together and encourages a sense of intimacy, which helps people face what is unknown or distressing.

SUMMARY

- Most Americans have become desensitized to the realities of death, mainly because of news coverage and TV programs. Therefore, many are ill-equipped to deal with death when it happens to someone they know or to whom they are close.
- Death in the movies, up until 1970, was taboo, except for the villains. Then Hollywood began making movies about the death of leading characters. TV followed suit, with realistic programs and documentaries dealing with death. Music, both popular and classical, has always been a powerful emotional medium for expressing feelings about death. Literature about death can be profound and affect ruminations on life and death.
- Four perspectives on life and death are: (1) ecological, in which all forms of life, including humans, are viewed as equal in value and importance, and there is no afterlife; (2) humanistic, in which human life is viewed as more important than other forms of existence, but there is no afterlife except in the minds of others; (3) the Western religious perspective, in which all forms of life are believed created by a supreme being, and there is life after death; and (4) reincarnation, in which existence is continuous, spanning many lifetimes.
- Funerals today are often customized by the dead person (before death) and his or her family (before and after the person dies).
- When someone dies of old age, it is expected and even considered natural. When a person dies without warning, grieving can be more painful for the people left behind, who did not have time to say goodbye.
- Death anxiety seems generally higher in females, African Americans, and the young and middle-aged and lower for older people, religious believers, and those who are mature and have self-control. People used to fear death because it often came unexpectedly and prematurely. Now, many in their later years fear continuing to deteriorate, but not die. The worst fear for many elderly is to become a victim of Alzheimer's disease.
- Dying well means being able to control when and how death comes.
- One way found to reduce anxiety about death among nursing home residents is by allowing them to make decisions about treatment.

- Patients who are dying, and their families, commonly deny that death is near.
- Humor can help people cope with death. Humor treats everyone alike, binds people together, and encourages a sense of intimacy.

Additional Resources

Books

Albom, M. (1997). *Tuesdays with Morrie.* New York: Doubleday. A young man visits an older, dying friend. In this book, it is revealed how the older man, Morrie, dealt with his impending death and what the young man, Mitch, learned from him.

Wanzer, S., & Glenmullen, J. (2007). *To die well: Your right to comfort, calm, and choice in the last days of life.* Cambridge, MA: Da Capo Press. This book explores how patients and their families can work with physicians to control the manner of dying.

Movie

Saving Private Ryan. (1998). This movie involves a story about soldiers trying to save another soldier's life as they struggled with the risks involved as well as how they, and the man they tried to save, viewed life and death.

Critical Thinking

1. What type of death do you wish for yourself—unexpected or expected?
2. What type of death do you wish for your loved ones?
3. Explain the differences between, or similarities in, your answers to these questions with those of your classmates.

Class Activity

1. As a class, watch *Saving Private Ryan.* Discuss with your classmates: "Were the struggles to save the man's life was worth it?"

References

Alzheimer's Association. (2007). Alzheimer's disease facts and figures. Retrieved May 27, 2008, from www.alz.org/alzheimers_disease_facts_figures.asp

Balaban, R. B. (2000). A physician's guide to talking about end-of-life care. *Journal of General Internal Medicine, 15,*195–200.

Berger, P. (1969). *The social reality of religion.* London: Faber & Faber.

Bordewich, F. M. (1988). Mortal fears: Courses in "death education" get mixed reviews. *Atlantic Monthly, 261.*

Bowman, K. W., & Richard, S. A. (2004). Cultural considerations for Canadians in the diagnosis of brain death. *Canadian Journal of Anesthesia, 51,* 273–275.

Brennan, M. (2005). Death and dying: Death is a biological certainty but the practices surrounding death and mourning are socially constructed. *Sociology Review, 14*(3), 26–29.

Brooks, D. (2000). *Bobos in paradise: The new upper class and how they got there.* New York: Simon & Schuster.

Brown University. (1990, December 8). Ethical and legal issues in long-term care: Food for futuristic thought. *Long-Term Care Letter, 2*(24), 1–3.

Browne, K., & Pennell, A. (1998). *The effects of video violence on young offenders.* London: Home Office Research and Statistics Directorate.

Buckman, R. (1992). *How to break bad news: A guide for health care professionals.* Baltimore: Johns Hopkins University Press.

Carr, T. K. (2005). *Introducing death and dying: Readings and exercises.* Upper Saddle River, NJ: Prentice-Hall.

DeSpelder, L. A., & Strickland, A. L. (2005). *The last dance: Encountering death and dying* (7th ed). New York: McGraw-Hill.

Ferrini, A. F., & Ferrini, R. L. (2000). *Health in the later years* (3rd ed). New York: McGraw-Hill.

Francis, L., Monahan, K., & Berger, C. (1999). A laughing matter? The uses of humor in medical institutions. *Motivation and Emotion, 23*(2), 155–174.

Gorer, G. (1967). *Death, grief, and mourning.* New York: Doubleday.

Insel, P. M., & Roth, W. T. (2002). *Core concepts in health* (9th ed). New York: McGraw-Hill.

Kalish, R. (1985). *Death, grief, and caring relationships.* Pacific Grove, CA: Brooks/Cole.

Kasser, T., & Kanner, A. D. (2003). *Psychology and consumer culture: The struggle for a good life in a materialistic world.* Washington, DC: American Psychological Association.

Kastenbaum R. J. (2004). *Death, society, and human experience* (8th ed). New York: Pearson.

Kear, A., & Steinberg, D. L. (1999). *Mourning Diana: Nation, culture and the performance of grief.* New York: Routledge.

Kearl, M. C. (1996). Dying well: The unspoken dimension of aging well. *American Behavioral Scientist, 39*(3), 336–361.

McLennan, J., Akande, A., & Bates, G. W. (1993). Death anxiety and death denial: Nigerian and Australian students' metaphors of personal death. *Journal of Psychology, 127*(4), 399–408.

O'Connell, L. J. (1995). Religious dimensions of dying and death. *The Western Journal of Medicine, 163*(3), 231.

Peniston-Bird, C., & Summerfield, P. (2001). "Hey, you're dead!": The multiple uses of humour in representations of British national defence in the Second World War. *Journal of European Studies, 31*(123), 413–435.

Rasmussen, C. A., & Brems, C. (1996). The relationship of death anxiety with age and psychosocial maturity. *The Journal of Psychology, 130*(2), 141–144.

Rousseau, P. (2000). Art of oncology: Death denial. *Journal of Clinical Oncology, 18*(23), 3998–3999.

Russell, R. D. (1999). *Death perspectives.* College class presentation at Southern Illinois University Carbondale.

Wass, H., & Neimeyer, R. A. (1995). *Dying: Facing the facts* (3rd ed). Washington, DC: Taylor & Francis.

Chapter 15

Suicide and Death by Violence

The thought of suicide is a great consolation:
by means of it, one gets successfully through many a bad night.
—Friedrich W. Nietzsche

Objectives

After reading this chapter, you will be able to answer the following questions:

- What are the risk factors for suicide?
- How does suicide vary by gender and age group?
- What are warning signs to indicate that someone is considering suicide?
- What are the causes of suicide?
- What are some of the myths surrounding suicide?
- How can suicide be prevented?
- How are survivors affected by a suicide?
- How are first responders affected by traumatic death?
- Why do people become violent?
- How are victims affected by violence?
- How can businesses prevent workplace killings?
- How do people deal with the violent death of a loved one?
- How can violent behavior be stopped or prevented?
- What instances of political assassination have occurred in U.S. history?
- How can people avoid being victimized?
- What are some of the causes of terrorism?

The death of someone by suicide or violent act, such as murder, is abrupt and shocking. As such, it leaves most people reeling, wondering why and how it might have been prevented. In this chapter, the factors, causes, and precursors to self-destruction and the behaviors that lead to violent death are explored.

Suicide

Each year in the United States, about 32,000 people, or 87 a day, commit **suicide**, the intentional taking of one's own life (from the Latin *sui caedere*, "to kill oneself"). In 2004, the suicide rate was 11 suicide deaths per 100,000 people. Up to 25 suicides are attempted for each one completed (National Institute of Mental Health, 2007).

NATIONAL SUICIDE PREVENTION LIFELINE

Anyone in crisis who needs help right away can call a toll-free number that is available 24 hours a day, every day. That number is 1-800-273-TALK (8255)—the number of the National Suicide Prevention Lifeline. The service is available to anyone. You may call for yourself or for someone you care about. All calls are confidential.

Suicide is a major public health problem, but understanding suicidal behavior is complex. Some risk factors vary with age, gender, or ethnic group and occur in combination or change over time. Most suicide attempts are expressions of extreme distress, not simply bids for attention.

A person who is suicidal should not be left alone. The person should be encouraged to seek immediate help from his or her doctor, the nearest emergency room, or 911. The person should not have access to firearms or other potential tools for suicide, including unsupervised access to medications. Keep in mind that people who are suicidal require the care of trained professionals.

Risk Factors for Suicide

The following are risk factors for suicide:

- Depression and other mental disorders or a substance-abuse disorder (often in combination with other mental disorders). More than 90% of people who die by suicide have these risk factors (Moscicki, 2001).
- Stressful life events, in combination with other risk factors, such as depression. Suicide and suicidal behavior, however, are not normal responses to stress. Nevertheless, many people who have these risk factors are not suicidal.
- Prior suicide attempt.
- Family history of mental disorder or substance abuse.
- Family history of suicide.
- Family violence, including physical or sexual abuse.
- Firearms in the home, the method used in more than half of suicides (Miller, Azrael, Hepburn, Hemenway, & Lippmann, 2006).
- Incarceration.
- Exposure to the suicidal behavior of others, such as family members, peers, or media figures (Moscicki, 2001).
- Changes in brain chemicals called neurotransmitters, including serotonin. Decreased levels of serotonin have been found in people with depression, impulsive disorders, and a history of suicide attempts. Also, decreased levels of serotonin have been found in the brains of suicide victims (Arango, Huang, Underwood, & Mann, 2003).

Risk Factors for Nonfatal Suicide Attempts

Risk factors for nonfatal suicide attempts include the following:

- For adults, depression and other mental disorders, alcohol abuse, cocaine use, and separation or divorce (Kessler, Borges, & Walters, 1999; Petronis, Samuels, Moscicki, & Anthony, 1990).
- For youth, depression, alcohol or other drug-use disorder, physical or sexual abuse, and disruptive behavior (Petronis et al., 1990; U.S. Department of Health and Human Services, 2001).

Gender and Age Differences

More women attempt suicide, but men succeed more often. Four times as many men die by suicide (six times as many in the 20–24 age group). The most common suicide methods are firearm, poison or drug overdose, and suffocation. More men use guns; women are more likely to use poison (including drug overdose). Half of all suicides reported in 2001 of women worldwide occurred in China (De Leo, 2007).

Suicide rates increase with age. In 2004, suicide rates were as follows for white men per 100,000 population (National Institute of Mental Health, 2007):

- 8.2 for ages 15 to 19
- 12.5 for ages 20 to 25
- 14.3 for ages 65 and older
- 17.8 for ages 85 and older

Suicide Among Youth

Adolescent suicide is a major public health problem (Bridge et al., 2003). In the United States, each year nearly 2,000 young people aged 15 to 19 commit suicide. By the end of the twentieth century, automobile accidents were the leading cause of adolescent death, followed by suicide (Mishara, 2007a). Each suicide leaves behind surviving family members, friends, and acquaintances who must cope with the loss. There are 6 to 10 survivors for each suicide (McIntosh, 1989), resulting in 12,000 to 20,000 new survivors of adolescent suicide each year.

In the United States, five times as many males aged 15 to 25 commit suicide as do females, although many more females attempt it and do not succeed (Mishara, 2007a). What accounts for this difference? Adolescent males use violent and lethal methods. In addition, males are more likely to keep problems to themselves and not confide in others or use mental health services. Male stereotypes and role expectations also might contribute to this difference.

Events that trigger teenage suicide include academic pressure, alcohol and other drugs, loss of a relationship, depression, and moving from one place to another. Although academic pressure appears to be related to suicide among college students, it is not a simple correlation. For example, many undergraduates who committed suicide had a high grade point average, but believed that they were performing below their own or their parents' expectations. A student may explain a near-fatal suicide attempt by saying, "My Dad had bragged on me so much that I couldn't let him down!"

The risk of suicide increases with excessive drinking. Adding the loss of a relationship through rejection, separation, or death raises the risk even more. The loss of a valued relationship (e.g., death of a parent or breakup of a love relationship) is one of the most common triggers of youth suicide. Breakups, including saying goodbye because of changing where you live, weaken the support system so critical for young adults.

Some characteristics of families of suicidal youth include (Leenaars & Wenckstern, 1991):

- rigid rules;
- poor communication patterns;
- "smother love" that does not encourage independence;
- patterns of dysfunction (e.g., alcoholism, divorce, absent parent, and mental illness).

In 2003, 20% of adolescents had a friend who had attempted suicide. For both males and females, knowing a friend who has attempted suicide is a significant predictor of moving from suicidal thought to action. Being part of a cohesive friendship group is important for decreasing the incidence of suicide, especially among females (Bearman, 2004).

Teens who are friends with a teen who commits suicide are at greatest risk of developing MDD (major depressive disorder) within the first month after the suicide. After the first month, the incidence declines to levels matching teens who have not had the same experience. Background factors that tend to predict the onset of MDD are a past history of alcohol abuse, a family history of MDD, interpersonal conflict and loss within the family, and similar conflict with friends (Bridge et al., 2003). Because the risk of MDD is highest at the outset, young people identified as having a family history of MDD, whose last contact with the victim occurred within 24 hours of the death or who feel accountable for the death, need to be monitored closely, especially during the first few weeks after the death.

Adults often suppose that children are blissfully unaware of suicide and, therefore, never contemplate it or talk about it, which is not true. As early as age 7, children know what suicide is and discuss it with each other. They know if someone in their family has committed suicide, even if adults try to conceal it, and they see it depicted or threatened on TV and in soap operas and cartoons. Even so, children usually regard suicide as taboo until age 12 (Mishara, 2007b). After that, the dangerous adolescent fascination with suicide can kick in.

Suicide Among the Elderly

Although suicide is a serious problem for all ages, elders commit more suicides than other age groups. Suicide rates for men and women age 75 and older are three times that of youth under age 25, a trend that is steeper for males (De Leo, 2007). Elders 85 and older have a suicide rate more than double the national average, and elderly men have the highest suicide risk. Depression, alcoholism, poor physical health, and loss of a relationship (divorce or death) are common precursors of elder suicide.

Yet, since 1970, rates of elderly suicide have declined in Western countries, especially among U.S. Caucasian males (around 50%). Reasons suggested are improvements in social services, political and social activism, attitudes toward retirement, economic security, and improved psychiatric care (De Leo, 2007).

Effective treatments are available for geriatric depression. Drug therapy and several versions of psychotherapy—interpersonal, brief psychodynamic, problem-solving, and cognitive–behavioral therapy—can reduce symptoms of depression. When these psychotherapeutic treatments are described in detail to them, older adults prefer psychotherapy to drugs (Scogin, 2007).

Like other age groups, elders frequently provide clues prior to suicide. Many people leave suicide notes—although not all farewell notes are left by people who commit suicide. One man who died of cancer left a goodbye note stuffed among his things where he knew that his wife would find it.

In addition to a farewell in writing, people who leave this world sometimes give verbal signs. For example, an older person who is planning suicide might question, "What's the point of going on?" He or she also may give away valued possessions and stockpile pills or buy a firearm.

Warning Signs

Contrary to what many think, talking about suicide will not increase its likelihood of happening. Many suicides could be prevented if someone identified a person at risk and referred him or her for appropriate help. Warning signs that a person is considering suicide include the following (American Foundation for Suicide Prevention, 2008):

- Depression
- Self-neglect
- Neglect of home, finances, pets
- Loss of appetite
- Giving away prized possessions
- Changing a will
- Drinking to excess
- Verbal suicidal statements
- Previous suicide attempts

Causes of Suicide

Many people believe that suicide is a sinful or criminal act or a weakness manifested in the person committing it. More likely, suicide is caused by psychosis or depression and is viewed as an escape, subintentional, or a cry for help.

Psychotic suicide is associated with a delusional state of mind. In this type of suicide, the person has no conscious intention to die; he or she is engaging in self-punishment by self-destruction. For the depressed, "hopeless-feeling" suicidal victim, alcohol or drug abuse is frequently involved.

Escaping physical or mental anguish is sometimes a reason for suicide. For example, a cancer or AIDS patient might end his or her life to avoid suffering. Some people call this type of suicide a "rational suicide," based on the person's desire to escape pain. Some escape suicides are related to expectations. For example, a young person might believe, "I give up. I'll never please my parents/myself."

Subintentional suicides involve a person hastening death unconsciously. This type of suicide victim "lives on the edge," taking unnecessary, unwise risks.

Questions & Answers

Question: My friend's dad committed suicide after suffering with cancer for 2 years. I don't know what to say. Should I just say nothing?

Answer: Your friend can be greatly comforted by the words, "If you need me, I'm here for you." Those words are always ok.

A person using suicide as a *cry for help* is likely trying to force a change. In this case, the goal is not death, but the elimination of a problem: "I can't go on like this; I might as well kill myself." Even if a person is just trying to get sympathy, any suicidal statement is potentially deadly.

Suicide Myths

Suicide is surrounded by a number of myths. Many times, these myths prevent a person from getting the help he or she needs. Review the following list of some common suicide myths and note which ones you might have believed:

- *People who talk about suicide do not commit suicide.* Almost three-fourths of people who eventually kill themselves give some hint ahead of time. This myth encourages people to ignore cries for help.
- *Suicidal people are fully intent on dying.* Although some people who attempt suicide ultimately do it, most do not. Most people who intend to commit suicide can have their minds changed right up to the minute before. A suicide attempt does not necessarily mean that a person wants to die.
- *Only people in a certain economic class commit suicide.* People in all income brackets commit suicide.
- *Asking people about suicide will encourage suicide attempts.* The reverse is true; many lives have been saved by open communication about suicide.
- *Only crazy people commit suicide.* Some suicides are due to obvious mental disorders, but rational people can feel overwhelmed by circumstances and try to commit suicide.

Suicide Prevention

Many suicides can be prevented. Kindness can go a long way in preventing suicide. Specific guidelines for preventing suicide include the following (Kastenbaum, 2004):

- A suicidal statement or intent should be taken seriously.
- Do not issue a provocation to suicide. In other words, do not "dare," "belittle," or "joke" about the issue.
- Do not judge. It is not helpful for a potentially suicidal person to hear that it is "wrong."
- Know what resources are available in the community, such as in schools, religious groups, mental health centers, or crisis centers.

Psychotherapy can help prevent suicide. Cognitive and dialectical behavior therapy has reduced the rate of repeated suicide attempts by 50% during a year of follow-up (Brown et al., 2005; Linehan et al., 2006). (**Cognitive therapy** emphasizes substitution of desirable patterns of thinking for maladaptive or faulty ones; **dialectical behavior therapy** focuses on helping a patient develop skills for coping with everyday life crises.)

The medication clozapine has been approved by the Food and Drug Administration for suicide prevention. This medicine, however, is limited to people with schizophrenia (Meltzer et al., 2003).

Older adults and women who die by suicide are likely to have seen a primary care provider in the year before death; thus, primary-care providers' ability to recognize and treat risk factors might help prevent suicide among these groups (Luoma, Pearson, & Martin, 2002).

Community programs geared to help prevent suicide should include (Knox et al., 2004):

- ongoing communication about suicide;
- destigmatization for seeking help for a mental health problem;
- training of everyday gatekeepers.

Suicide Survivors

Probably the most devastating grief is felt by survivors of someone who commits suicide (Doka, 2007). The emotional suffering and decision to die by the person committing suicide implies rejection and desertion. These facts, along with society's negative reactions to suicide, typically make the post-suicide experience especially difficult for family members and friends of the person who committed suicide. Less emotional support is available for suicide survivors, and they experience more in the way of physical illness, depression, and anxiety, believing they might have precipitated the suicide or could have prevented it (Cain, 1972).

Suicide has a powerful impact on its survivors. For example, survivors of gunshot suicides can recall smelling the lingering odor of gun powder and finding tissue and bone fragments of the victim. Even after using a professional cleaning service, they find it necessary to clean the area again. Many describe experiencing mental images, dreams, or flashbacks of the death scene. Some describe vividly recurrent episodes in which they relive the experience of discovering the victim's body. Following these episodes, they reported being totally exhausted and unable to go back to their daily activities (Van Dongen, 1990).

The suicide survivor's feelings of guilt and shame often go unrecognized. Shame and guilt are not easy to tell apart. Someone who feels shame focuses on a defect in self-image, whereas someone who feels guilt focuses on the act and its consequences.

Another, more intense emotion among suicide survivors is anger at the dead person for perceived desertion and abandonment and for not having accepted help. Survivors also might feel anger that the suicide victim has deprived the survivor of a shared future and has left the survivor to deal with all of the legal and financial problems. Anger also may be directed against health professionals for failing to prevent the suicide (Lester, 1990); at society for its negative attitudes toward suicide; at the social network of the person who committed suicide for withdrawing; and, with religious people, at religion, for failing to give comfort. There also may be anger at God for His having "let" the suicide happen.

Because suicide often carries a stigma, family members might react to it with silence, secrecy, and even denial. Children react to suicide with nearly the same feelings as adults, but they behave differently, clinging and whining, regressing in development, and developing unrealistic fears and anxieties. Even so, even young children should be told the truth about the suicide. Otherwise, children and young adolescents might have terrible fantasies of guilt (Dunne-Maxim, Dunne, & Hauser, 1987). Adolescents might withdraw and isolate themselves socially or become truant, delinquent, and openly aggressive.

Patient suicide is not an unusual occurrence for hospital workers and therapists. Kahne (1968) estimated that 25% of psychiatrists experience a patient suicide and 22% to 51% of private-practice therapists have those experiences. Kleespies, Penk, and Forsyth (1993) found that about 11% of psychology interns have experienced a patient's suicide attempt.

Therapists react to a patient suicide much the same way as do other survivors, along with self-doubts about professional competence and fear of litigation. For psychiatrists, long experience typically lessens feelings of guilt and loss of self-esteem.

In-hospital suicide provokes the same feelings and reactions among health personnel as in private-practice therapists: shock, numbness, denial, guilt, insecurity, and so on. Other patients are frequently angry at the staff for not preventing the death, or they identify with the dead person and assume responsibility for the death.

Van Dongen (1990) found that many survivor families identified the family physician as the key individual to initiate follow-up care. Unfortunately and typically, many physicians do not seem to know how to help surviving family members.

Adult survivors of suicide are most commonly helped by joining a group consisting of other survivors of a suicide. The objective is to provide mutual comfort and support and a place to talk about the suicide and its effects and how to deal with it. Suicide survivor support groups are offered by suicide prevention centers, crisis service centers, and community health centers.

Death by Violence

"To millions of Americans, few things are more pervasive or more frightening than violent crime" is a quote you might have seen in a media report (Donatelle, 2002). You might think that this quote came from one of today's media reports. In fact, it is taken from an 1860 Senate report on crime. Obviously, Americans' concerns over violence are not new. As in years past, violence can strike anyone at any time.

The term **violence** is used to define behavior that brings about injuries or death. These injuries can be both unintentional (accidents) and intentional (intending to cause harm, as in rape or homicide).

On an average day in America, 53 persons die from **homicide**, the act of one human killing another. What country you live in indicates how likely you are to be murdered. A person is most likely to be murdered in South Africa and least likely to be murdered in Japan. The United States ranks eighth (Fox, Levin, & Quinet, 2004).

Homicide is legally differentiated by intent. The following are different forms of intent followed by an example of each (Fox et al., 2004):

- First-degree murder: Woman decides to kill her husband to get his insurance money.
- Second-degree murder: Man kills wife during argument over how to discipline children.
- Felony murder: Young man starts a fire at home to collect house insurance money, not realizing that his wife, who died in the fire, was home.
- Voluntary manslaughter: Man kills his wife when he finds her spanking their child with a belt.
- Involuntary manslaughter: While putting on lipstick while driving, woman slams into a tree, killing her husband who was in the car with her.
- Misdemeanor manslaughter: As a prank, young woman yells "fire" at a movie theater and her boyfriend dies trying to escape.
- Justifiable homicide: Wife kills her husband as he is trying to kill her (considered self-defense).

Emergency Responders and Death

Police, firemen, and EMTs are involved with traumatic death throughout their careers. Most of the death scenes they face result from suicides, homicides, or accidents. Police officers frequently are the first people on the scene.

People sometimes get the impression that emergency responders are not affected by death. Yet many of them must see a counselor to deal

Death Investigator

Marilyn Schwartz (2003) said that after 12 years as a death investigator, she still could not remove herself emotionally from a violent or accidental death. Schwartz explained that there was "nothing fair" about these types of death. Sometimes, after looking at the scene, she knew what the last few minutes or hours for the person were like. Many times, she was unable to get the scene out of her head.

Schwartz revealed that many people bond with her after she gave them the news that their loved one was dead. Others never want to see her again. Said Schwartz,

> The murdered woman's family is very gracious with how they respond to my apologies about not being able to give them more information. . . .They thank me and comment on what a god-awful job I have. Agreeing, I tell them they are in my heart. They say they will pray for me. I feel inadequate in the face of their faith (p. 3).

Questions & Answers

Question: When police or other emergency responders arrive at a fatal car accident, what's the hardest thing for them?

Answer: The death scene itself usually is not as difficult for them to face as informing families about the death. Most times, families want to see their loved ones, who might not be recognizable due to traumatic injuries.

with the emotions surrounding their experiences with on-the-job deaths.

Some police officers specialize as death investigators. Their job is to document and identify the cause and manner of death. The investigator asks, "Who was this person?" "How did he die?" "Why did he die in this manner at this time?"

Why Do People Become Violent?

A damaged childhood can be the source of psychopathic violence. In this progression, people go through five psychological stages:

1. Hurt as a small child without recognizing it.
2. Not reacting to suffering with appropriate anger.
3. Showing gratitude to parents for their "good intentions."
4. Forgetting everything.
5. In adulthood, venting stored-up anger onto others or against self.

As children, psychopaths often were beaten to eliminate obstinacy, defiance, and natural exuberance. Parents manipulated the child and then rationalized that it is for the child's own good. The use of humiliation was used to destroy the child's self-confidence. To suppress crying and feeling, parents rewarded stoicism and self-control. Childhood excitement was a vice, and life was to be inhibited (Miller, 1983).

Consistent with Miller's findings, Gilligan (1997), from his work in prisons, concluded that violent criminals are subjected to violence without love, both physical and verbal, from their early childhood. As a consequence, as children they are not able to establish any love of self and they come to feel only shame, humiliation, bitterness, and rage. Such shame kills the self, resulting in the inability to feel anything.

According to Gilligan (1997), ritualistic murder and the other acts of violence these children, or these once-children, commit are triggered by intolerable feelings of shame. Doing something violent diminishes the intensity of that shame and substitutes pride. Violent criminals not only seem unfeeling, they are unfeeling. Many go to their death by execution with indifference. What lies below their rage is a frustrated childhood need to be loved.

A paradox of violent behavior is evident in the battered women's shelter, a fairly recent social development. Before shelters were created, about as many husbands killed wives as wives killed husbands. Now that women can leave an abusive relationship, twice as many husbands kill wives. Why? According to Gilligan (1997), such husbands feel homicidally threatened by a wife's leaving them because they are, without knowing it, dependent on their wives and are like infants who would die if their mothers left them.

Victims

Every child in America has been affected by violence, although many children have been exposed to violence primarily through television. The average young person in America watches 28 hours of television each week and has seen 16,000 simulated murders and 200,000 acts of violence by the age of 18 (Brown & Bzostek, 2003).

For a young child, the home is the primary place to be the victim of violence. The homicide rate for children from birth to about 15 months is higher than for any age group until age 17. Of deaths resulting from child abuse in 2001, 85% were children under age 6 (Paulozzi & Sells, 2002).

Bullying is a form of violence. Sixth graders are more likely bullied than any other grade through grade 12. Fighting is a problem for middle school students as well. More than 73% of these middle

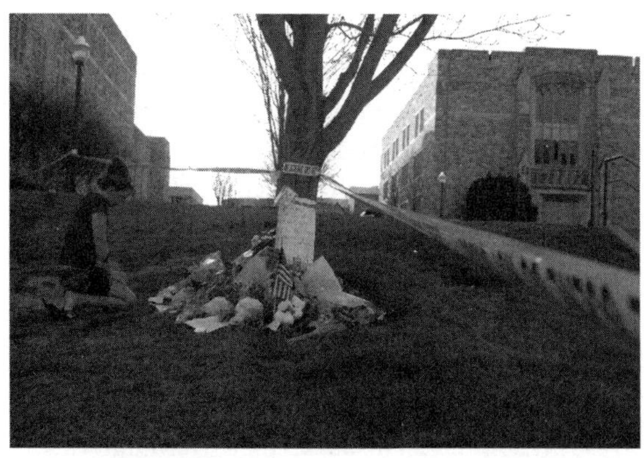

school students reported being in a physical fight (Centers for Disease Control, 2007).

School Shootings

In the last few years, killings have swept across American schools and colleges. In a number of these school shootings, bullying and revenge appear to be common motives. Bullying behavior, once considered a "childhood rite of passage," is currently playing out more as homicide.

Some reasons for violent behavior spill over into schools. These reasons include poor parenting, ineffective welfare systems, availability of weapons, racism, gang growth, violence on television, bullying, hate crimes, and drug involvement.

No matter where Americans live, chances are their children are going to school with troubled children, particularly boys, capable of shooting to kill. As a result, children are afraid to go to school, teachers are afraid of their students, and parents fear for their children's lives (Garbarino, 1999).

Violent teenagers follow specific patterns of behavior and give recognizable warning signals. The warning signs to look for are lack of connection, masking emotions, withdrawal, silence, rage, trouble with friends, hypervigilance, and cruelty toward other children and even animals.

Many boys who turn violent carry a deep-seated sense of shame, based on their experiences of abandonment, victimization, abuse, and powerlessness. Children who see themselves as poor are more likely to feel like outsiders—devalued, shamed, and enraged. They invest considerable energy in defenses to repress and deny these emotions and memories. Minor insults to their self-esteem lead to a powerful reawakening of these repressed feelings, and the violent response helps them to repress and deny them again.

In childhood, the causes for this kind of behavior stem more from parent and family issues than from peer modeling and social pressures. Thus, intervention by the family is crucial.

Workplace Killings

In the past two decades, school shootings have been more highly publicized, but there have been many more incidents of homicide in the work-

The Virginia Tech Shooting

The deadliest shooting rampage in American history occurred on the campus of Virginia Tech University in Blacksburg, Virginia, on April 16, 2007. Thirty-three people were killed in two separate attacks.

At about 7:15 A.M., two people were shot and killed in a dormitory. Nearly 3 hours later, 31 others were shot and killed across campus in a classroom building where some of the doors had been chained by the killer. Among the dead was the gunman, later identified as student Cho Seung-Hui.

On April 20, 1999, the most highly publicized school attack came in Columbine, Colorado, where 2 teenagers killed 12 fellow high school students and a teacher before killing themselves. The shooting at Virginia Tech occurred in the same week 8 years later.

Source: New York Times, April 16, 2007.

place. In 1986, a soon-to-be fired letter carrier killed 14 and wounded 6 fellow postal workers before killing himself. He was the first in a number of post office killings, which caused the term "going postal" to enter the vernacular. The rise in such workplace killings has led to increased efforts by firms to identify potential killers and to know how to respond to such events after they happen (Green, 2007).

The signs to look for among workers who might "go postal" are frequent absenteeism, withdrawal or outbursts of anger, and a marked decline in work performance. The assailant is most often a white male over 30 who has recently experienced a suspension, demotion, or firing and who wakes up one morning and decides to take out his anger with a gun (*Terror Nine to Five*, 2004).

Companies are advised that a coworker or supervisor who notices signs of trouble in a person should pass that information to the human resources department. Psychologists typically are called to evaluate the employee, and if he or she appears to pose a threat, help for that person is sought. The employer might grant a medical leave wherein the employee is not brought back until a mental health professional determines that he or she no longer poses a threat.

The layout of the workplace also can reveal potential problems. For example, a firm might have good security at the front, but have unsecured outside smoking and eating areas through which someone can enter the building.

Employers should have a plan in place beforehand to protect employees against workers who might display violent behavior. The plan should include orderly evacuation of the immediate area, notification of law enforcement, and containment of the affected area. Employees need to be trained about what to do until law officers arrive. When a shooting begins, it goes fast, and there is no time to figure out what to do.

How Does One Deal With the Violent Death of Another?

How does someone deal with the trauma of losing a loved one to death by violence? According to Rynearson (2001), the survivor might use narratives to retell the story, to make sense of a violent death. The story eventually moves from remembering the death to remembering how the loved one lived. Such narratives usually fall into one of the following forms:

- *Reenactment*: The survivor cannot stop thinking about what happened.
- *Remorse*: The survivor should have been able to save the lost one.
- *Retaliation*: The survivor will avenge the death.
- *Protection*: The survivor will prevent another family tragedy.

Most people move through this process without professional help. Those who cannot are generally those who suffer from psychiatric illnesses, who have suffered childhood abuse or neglect, and who have lost a child to violent death.

The lack of rituals and social conventions might deter loved ones from storytelling and, therefore, dealing effectively with a violent death. People are generally not comfortable listening to stories of pain, confusion, and anger. Support systems dwindle quickly as friends and family find that they cannot "fix" things. Not being heard might attach people more firmly to their story, and they might then be unable to move forward to a new story. Rynearson (2001) encourages therapy in a family context, where family members reconstruct their stories together.

Survivors of the Virginia Tech Shooting

At first, many student survivors of the shooting at Virginia Tech (see box) thought that they needed to get away. Most of them came back, feeling that they could cope better in a familiar setting. Seeing TV reruns of the event, and pictures of the gunman, made it even more difficult for students to deal with the aftermath.

Some students did not think they could continue with their schoolwork, so they were relieved when the university gave them the choice of leaving campus and taking a grade for work to date.

Others believed that getting back to a school routine and being around familiar faces would help.

Many students spent time at a makeshift memorial on the campus, not returning to their rooms until they were exhausted enough to sleep. The emotions of some students vacillated between anger and guilt, and a few of them confessed that the incident shook their belief in God (Madhani, 2007).

How to Prevent or Stop Violent Behavior

The following ideas might be useful in preventing or stopping violent behavior:

- A solid mentoring relationship can help a young person mitigate the effects of abandonment and loss and help build a sense of having a meaning in life, someone who cares about him/her, and the potential to achieve (Garbarino, 1999).
- Stable living and home environments, stable parenting figures, and stable routines help children feel safe in the world and feel that they are cared for, protected, and able to predict what will happen around them.
- Boys should be taught to recognize and cope with their own feelings. Then, they can identify others' feelings and develop the empathy that helps them control antisocial behavior. Also, boys should be helped to develop skills and to foresee themselves having a future.
- Children and adolescents need to be educated to provide them with more options in life. Also, through education, these youth can be taught about the world and about how to make more and better decisions on their own.
- Getting guns off the streets, out of homes, and away from teenagers' hands is important.

Political Assassination

The murder of a political leader has both public interest and a private, family interest. A few prominent U.S. figures who have been assassinated and their assassins (in parentheses) include (Kastenbaum, 2004):

- Abraham Lincoln in 1865 (John Wilkes Booth)
- William McKinley in 1901 (Leon Czolgosz)
- John F. Kennedy in 1963 (Lee Harvey Oswald)
- Martin Luther King, Jr. in 1968 (James Earl Ray)
- Robert Kennedy in 1968 (Sirhan Sirhan)

In addition, presidents Garfield (1881), Roosevelt (1912), Truman (1950), Nixon (1974), Ford (twice in 1975), and Reagan (1981) were the targets of assassination attempts.

Gender Differences in Death by Violence

Young men are more likely to be victims of violent crime, and females are more likely to become victims of domestic violence. Six of every ten females in the United States will be assaulted by husbands or lovers at some time in their lives (National Center for Injury Prevention and Control, 2006). On average, more than three women are murdered by their husbands or boyfriends every day (Bureau of Justice Statistics, 2003).

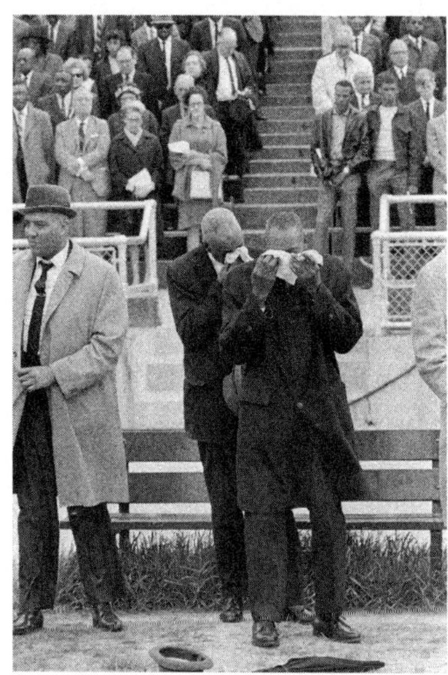

The Perpetrators

Males are more likely than females to be the perpetrators of violent crime. When a weapon is used (gun, knife, or club of some sort), a gun is the most often chosen weapon. Although more young African American men are arrested for gun violations than other groups, most homicides (contrary to popular mythology) are not racially motivated. Almost all murder victims are killed by members of their own race (e.g., most white murder victims killed by other whites) (Crissman & Parkin, 2003)

A **hate crime** is a crime committed against another person for reasons of that person's race, national origin, religion, sexual orientation, or disability. About 10,000 hate crimes are reported every year. Racial bias accounts for about half of all hate crimes, followed by religion, sexual orientation, and national origin. Many hate crimes are associated with racist and homophobic fringe groups, and most perpetrators of hate crimes are males under the age of 20 (Leek, 1999).

Avoid Being a Victim

Violence affects many people directly and/or indirectly. A person cannot prevent all violent acts from occurring, but a person can reduce his or her chances of being a victim of a violent crime. To reduce the likelihood of becoming the victim of violent crime, consider the following tips:

- If you walk or jog, vary your route and use only well-lit areas.
- If you have a cell phone, program it with emergency numbers.
- After dark, do not walk alone.
- Tell friends your class schedule, thereby creating a buddy system.
- Be sure that the doors and windows of your dorm room, apartment, or house have sturdy locks, and use them.
- Be alert when using an ATM, and do not display large amounts of cash.
- Report weapon-carrying behavior to university officials.
- Do not let anyone (repairmen, police officers, and others) into your dorm, apartment, or house without identification.
- If you have a vehicle, park in well-lit areas.

Terrorism

Terrorism is the systematic use of violence or the threat of violence, especially as a means of coercion. Today, the United States, and indeed the entire world, seems like a terrorist battleground. Before the events of September 11, 2001, Americans were shaken by the bomb that killed 168 people and demolished the Federal Building in Oklahoma City on April 19, 1995. In addition to terrorist acts in the United States, Americans see TV images of terrorist suicide bombings in various parts of the world on an almost daily basis. Unlike the terrorist organizations of times past (Merrill's Raiders, the Mafia, the Ku Klux Klan), modern-day terrorists are willing to sacrifice their own lives.

The numbers of deaths caused by terrorism can be numbing. It can become an unfortunate part of everyday life, as it has become in Iraq and Afghanistan. Children in other parts of the world, for example, incorporate the results of terrorist activity into their regular lives. In Israel, a favorite costume during the Purim holiday (similar to Halloween in the United States) is a replica of the Zaka uniform. Zaka is a volunteer organization

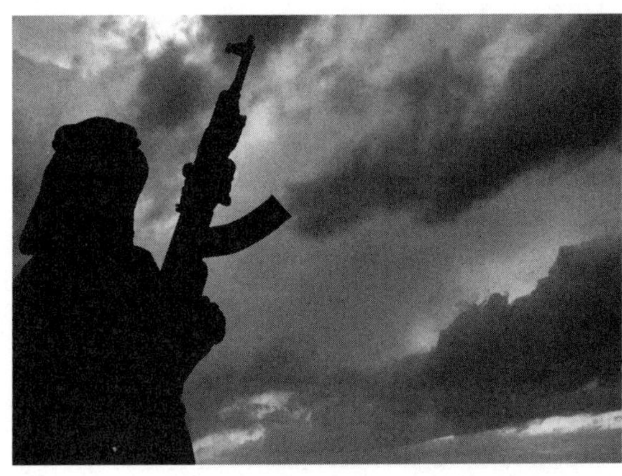

THE 9/11 TERRORIST ATTACKS ON THE UNITED STATES

On September 11, 2001, approximately 3,000 Americans died in Washington, D.C., New York, and Pennsylvania when Middle Eastern terrorists flew passenger airplanes into the World Trade Center, the Pentagon, and into a field in Pennsylvania. Among the many heroic attempts in Washington, D.C., New York, and Pennsylvania to save people that day, Lisa Beamer wrote about her courageous husband's last recorded remarks when he and others tried to save everyone aboard the skyjacked Flight 93 that crashed into a Pennsylvania field. To finalize the plan to attack the terrorists, he asked his co-conspirators aboard, "Are you guys ready? Let's roll!" (Beamer & Abraham, 2006).

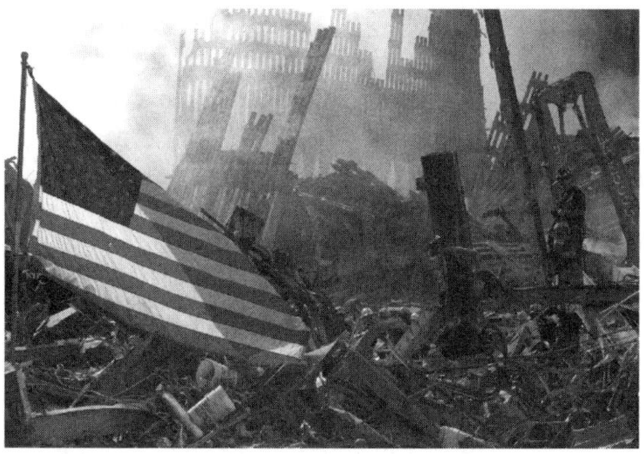

dedicated to ensuring proper burial according to Jewish rituals. In the immediate aftermath of a terrorist attack, Zaka members search for body parts, so as to bring back as much of a body as possible for burial (Galai-Gat, 2004).

Terror often is unleashed against people who share the same experiences and live in the same land, but who are perceived as "different" in some significant way, usually religious. Most German Jews, for example, were law-abiding and patriotic, but when Hitler came into power, Germans who were Jewish were killed or shipped to concentration camps and killed there. Terrorism is frequently preceded by ostracism, implying that "our people are human; others are less human." Many of the bloodiest reigns of terror have been carried out by people who were convinced that only their religion was true, so other religions had to be destroyed (Kastenbaum, 2004). Others were political. Some of the most destructive terrorist operations have been planned as "rational" ways to achieve political objectives. Stalin killed 12 million Russians so that he could achieve his economic and political aims.

Despite all the carnage and disruption it causes, terrorism ultimately fails. It does so because no society of humans can survive with terrorism rampant in its midst.

When sudden tragedy happens, people typically remember for the rest of their lives where they were and what they were doing. Most of your parents and grandparents can tell you exactly where they were on November 22, 1963, when they were told that President Kennedy had been assassinated.

September 11, 2001, may be as etched in your mind. In one TV news account, a New York City sixth-grade teacher, whose students personally watched one of the twin towers of the New York Trade Center collapse, gave her class the date and the time and told them that this day was one that they never would forget. Where were you on September 11, 2001?

SUMMARY

- Each year in the United States, about 32,000 people, or 87 a day, commit suicide. Up to 25 suicides are attempted for each one completed. Risk factors for suicide vary with age and gender and might occur in combination or change over time.
- More women attempt suicide, but men more often succeed. Men are more likely to use a gun to commit suicide, and more

women are more likely to use poison (including drug overdose). Suicide rates increase with age.

- In the United States, each year nearly 2,000 young people between the ages of 15 and 19 commit suicide. There are 6 to 10 survivors for each suicide, resulting in 12,000 to 20,000 new survivors of adolescent suicide each year.
- Teenage survivors of a suicide are at greatest risk of developing MDD (major depressive disorder) within the first month after the suicide.
- Many suicides could be prevented if someone identified a person at risk and referred him or her for appropriate help. Warning signs of suicide include depression, self-neglect, neglect of home, finances, pets, loss of appetite, giving away prized possessions, changing a will, drinking to excess, verbal suicidal statements, and previous suicide attempts.
- *Psychotic* suicide is associated with a delusional state of mind. *Escaping* physical or mental anguish is sometimes a reason for suicide. *Subintentional* suicides involve a person hastening death unconsciously. A *cry for help* person is likely trying to force a change.
- Many myths about suicide exist, but the thing to remember is that all threats of suicide should be taken seriously. One emotion among suicide survivors is anger at the dead person for perceived desertion and abandonment, for not having accepted help, for depriving the survivor of a shared future, and for leaving the survivor with legal and financial problems.
- Because suicide often carries a stigma, family members might react to it with silence, secrecy, and even denial.
- *Violence* is behavior that brings about injuries or death. On an average day in America, 53 persons die from homicide. Homicide is legally differentiated by intent: first- and second-degree murder; felony murder; voluntary, involuntary, and misdemeanor manslaughter; and justifiable homicide.
- A damaged childhood can be the source of psychopathic violence.
- The average young person in America watches 28 hours of television each week and has seen 16,000 simulated murders and 200,000 acts of violence by the age of 18.
- In the last few years, killings have swept across American schools and colleges. Some reasons cited for violent behaviors spilling over into schools include poor parenting, ineffective welfare systems, availability of weapons, racism, gang growth, violence on television, bullying, hate crimes, and drug involvement.
- Violent teenagers follow specific patterns of behavior and give recognizable warning signals: lack of connection, masking emotions, withdrawal, silence, rage, trouble with friends, hypervigilance, and cruelty toward other children and even animals.
- The rise in workplace killings has led to increased efforts by firms to identify potential killers.
- Dealing with the trauma of losing a loved one to death by violence often is helped by using narratives to retell the story in order to make sense of a violent death.
- Young men are more likely to be victims of violent crimes, whereas females are more likely to be victims of domestic violence. On average, every day, 3 women are murdered by their husbands or boyfriends.
- To prevent becoming a victim of a violent crime, take sensible precautions, such as varying your route and using only well-lit areas when you take daily walks.
- Terrorism is the systematic use of violence or threat of violence, especially as a means of coercion. Terror often is unleashed against people who share the same experiences and live in the same land, but who are perceived as "different" in some significant way, usually religious.

Additional Resources

Books

Garbarino, J. (1999). *Lost boys: Why our sons turn violent and how we can save them.* New York: Ballantine Books. A psychologist explores adolescent violence, identifies the risk factors for potentially violent children, and offers proven methods to prevent the development of aggressive behavior.

Gilligan, J. (1997). *Violence: Reflections of a nation.* New York: Vintage Books. The United States is more violent than any other democracy and economically developed nation. Based on the author's 25 years of working in the Massachusetts prison system, the thesis of the book is that violence springs from hidden shame and that how our society responds causes further shame and shaming, thus creating more violence. This view is especially significant during a time of rising moralism and righteousness in the body politic.

Jones, L. (1998). *Our America.* New York: Washington Square Press. Based on more than a hundred hours of taped National Public Radio interviews with two high school students, the author of the book provides a frank look at their Chicago neighborhood, where many boys do not expect to live past age 20. Gunfire is so prevalent that they describe ducking bullets from daily fusillades as though they were dodging a rainstorm. Says one, "In Vietnam, them people came back crazy. I live in Vietnam, so what you think I'm gonna be?"

Noel, B., & Blair, P. D. (2000). *I wasn't ready to say goodbye: Surviving, coping, and healing after the sudden death of a loved one.* Milwaukee, WI: Champion Press Ltd. Outside the publicized tragedies of air crashes, terrorist bombings, and school shootings, many families and individuals suffer the losses of sudden death. Tapping the personal histories of both authors and numerous interviews, the authors show grieving readers how to endure, survive, and grow from the pain and turmoil surrounding the sudden loss of loved ones.

Movie

Gandhi. (1982). This movie is the story of the life of Gandhi, who introduced to India and eventually to the world the doctrine of nonviolent resistance—a concept he acquired from the study of the writings of Henry David Thoreau.

Critical Thinking

1. What troubles you most when you hear that someone has committed suicide?
2. What steps would you take to ensure that school shootings decline?

Class Activities

1. Divide the class into teams to debate the pros and cons of suicide.
2. Plan and implement a campus-wide Violence Prevention Week program, which can consist of making presentations or designing posters to display across campus. Some ideas for programs or presentations include the following:
   - Rape awareness and education
   - Crime prevention techniques
   - Conflict resolution services
   - Bullying behavior education

References

American Foundation for Suicide Prevention. (2008). *Warning signs of suicide.* Retrieved May 27, 2008, from http://www.afsp.org/index.cfm?page_id=0519ec1a-d73a-8d90-7d2e9e2456182d66

Arango, V., Huang, Y. Y., Underwood, M. D., & Mann, J. J. (2003). Genetics of the serotonergic system in suicidal behavior. *Journal of Psychiatric Research, 37,* 375–386.

Beamer, L., & Abraham, K. (2006). *Let's roll!: Ordinary people, extraordinary courage.* Carol Stream, IL: Tyndale House Publishers.

Bearman, P. S. (2004). Suicide and friendships among American adolescents. *American Journal of Public Health, 94*(1), 89–95.

Bridge, J. A., Day, N. L., Day, R., Richardson, G. A., Birmaher, B., & Brent, D. A. (2003). Major depressive disorder in adolescents exposed to a friend's suicide. *Journal of the American Academy of Child and Adolescent Psychiatry, 42*(11), 1294.

Brown, B. V., & Bzostek, S. (2003, August 1). *Violence in the lives of children.* Cross Currents: Child Trends Databank, Pub 20031-15. Retrieved May 28, 2008, from www.childtrendsdatabank.org/PDF/Violence.pdf

Brown, G. K., Ten Have, T., Henriques, G. R., Xie, S. X., Hollander, J. E., & Beck, A. T. (2005). Cognitive therapy for the prevention of suicide attempts: A randomized controlled trial. *Journal of the American Medical Association, 294*(5), 563–570.

Bureau of Justice Statistics Crime Data Brief. (2003). *Intimate partner violence, 1993–2001.* Washington, DC: Author.

Cain, A. C. (1972). *Survivors of suicide.* Springfield, IL: Charles C. Thomas.

Centers for Disease Control and Prevention, National Center for Injury Prevention and Control. (2007). *Injury statistics query and reporting system* (WISQARS). Retrieved May 28, 2008, from www.cdc.gov/ncipc/wisqars

Crissman, J. K., & Parkin, J. (2003). *Epidemiology of homicide.* Retrieved May 28, 2008, from http://findarticles.com/p/articles/mi_gx5214/is_2003/ai_n19132168

De Leo, D. (2007). Suicide by the elderly. *Encyclopedia of death and dying.* Retrieved May 28, 2008, from www.deathreference.com/index.html

Doka, K. J. (2007). Grief and suicide. *Encyclopedia of death and dying.* Retrieved May 28, 2008, from www.deathreference.com/Gi-Ho/Grief.html

Donatelle, R. J. (2002). *Access to health.* New York: Benjamin Cummings.

Dunne-Maxim, K., Dunne, E. J., & Hauser, M. J. (1987). When children are suicide survivors. In E. J. Dunne, J. L. McIntosh, & K. Dunne-Maxim (Eds.), *Suicide and its aftermath: Understanding and counseling the survivors.* New York: Norton.

Fox, J. A., Levin, J., & Quinet, K. D. (2004). *The will to kill* (2nd ed.). Boston: Allyn & Bacon.

Galai-Gat, T. (2004, April). *Early interventions with survivors of terrorist attacks in Jerusalem.* Paper presented at the 28th Convening of Crisis Intervention Personnel and 2nd Collaborative Crisis Centers Conference, Chicago.

Garbarino, J. (1999). *Lost boys: Why our sons turn violent and how we can save them.* New York: Ballantine Books.

Gilligan, J. (1997). *Violence: Reflections on a national epidemic.* New York: Vintage Books.

Green, E. (2007, April 19). Shootings show need for preventing, coping with violence in the workplace. *Pittsburgh Post-Gazette.* Retrieved May 28, 2008, from http://www.highbeam.com/doc/1G1-162284674.html

Kahne, M. J. (1968). Suicide among patients in the mental hospital. *Psychiatry, 31*, 32–49.

Kastenbaum, R. J. (2004). *Death, society, and human experience* (8th ed.). New York: Pearson.

Kessler, R. C., Borges, G., & Walters, E. E. (1999). Prevalence of and risk factors for lifetime suicide attempts in the National Comorbidity Survey. *Archives of General Psychiatry, 56*(7), 617–626.

Kleespies, P. M., Penk, W. E., & Forsyth, J. P. (1993). Suicidal behavior during clinical training: Incidence, impact, and recovery. *Professional Psychology: Research and Practice, 24*, 293–303.

Knox, K. L., Yeates, C., & Caine, E. D. (2004). If suicide is a public health problem, what are we doing to prevent it? *American Journal of Public Health, 94*(1), 37–45.

Leek, S. D. (Ed.). (1999). *Hate crimes resource manual* (4th ed.). Retrieved May 28, 2008, from http://www.in.gov/icrc/2346.htm

Leenaars, A. A., & Wenckstern, S. (1991). *Suicide prevention in schools.* New York: Hemisphere.

Lester, D. (1990). Surviving a suicide. In A. H. Kutscher et al. (Eds.), *For the bereaved: The road to recovery.* Philadelphia: The Charles Press.

Linehan, M. M., Comtois, K. A., Murray, A. M., Brown, M. Z., Gallop, R. J. Heard, et al. (2006). Two-year randomized controlled trial and follow-up of dialectical behavior therapy vs. therapy by experts for suicidal behaviors and borderline personality disorder. *Archives of General Psychiatry, 63*(7), 757–766.

Luoma, J. B., Pearson, J. L., & Martin, C. E. (2002). Contact with mental health and primary care prior to suicide: A review of the evidence. *American Journal of Psychiatry, 159*, 909–916.

Madhani, A. (2007, April 20). Students struggle to deal with pain. *Chicago Tribune.* Retrieved May 28, 2008, from http://www.accessmylibrary.com/coms2/summary_0286-30363887_ITM

McIntosh, J. L. (1989). How many survivors of suicide are there? *Surviving Suicide, 1*, 1–4.

Meltzer, H. Y., Alphs, L., Green, A. I., Altamura, A. C., Anand, R., Bertoldi, A., et al. (2003). International Suicide Prevention Trial Study Group. Clozapine treatment for suicidality in schizophrenia: International Suicide Prevention Trial (InterSePT). *Archives of General Psychiatry, 60*(1), 82–91.

Miller, A. (1983). *For your own good: Hidden cruelty in child rearing and the roots of violence.* New York: Farrar, Straus & Giroux.

Miller, M., Azrael, D., Hepburn, L., Hemenway, D., & Lippmann, S. J. (2006). The association between changes in household firearm ownership and rates of suicide in the United States, 1981–2002. *Injury Prevention, 12*(12), 178–182.

Mishara, B. L. (2007a). Suicide by adolescents and youths. *Encyclopedia of death and dying.* Retrieved May 28, 2008, from www.deathreference.com/index.html

Mishara, B. L. (2007b). Suicide by children. *Encyclopedia of death and dying.* Retrieved May 28, 2008, from www.deathreference.com/index.html

Moscicki, E. K. (2001). Epidemiology of completed and attempted suicide: Toward a framework for prevention. *Clinical Neuroscience Research, 1*, 310–323.

National Center for Injury Prevention and Control. (2006). *Intimate partner violence: Fact sheet.* Retrieved May 28, 2008, from http://www.cdc.gov/ncipc/dvp/ipv_factsheet.pdf

National Institute of Mental Health. (2007). *Suicide in the U.S.: Statistics and prevention.* NIH Publication No. 06-4594.

Paulozzi, L., & Sells, M. (2002). Variation in homicide risk during infancy: United States, 1989–1998. *Morbidity and Mortality Weekly, 51*(9), 187–189.

Petronis, K. R., Samuels, J. F., Moscicki, E. K., & Anthony, J. C. (1990). An epidemiologic investigation of potential risk factors for suicide attempts. *Social Psychiatry and Psychiatric Epidemiology, 25*(4), 193–199.

Rynearson, E. K. (2001). *Retelling violent death.* Philadelphia: Brunner-Routledge.

Schwartz, M. (2003). Investigating deaths in the field. *Association for Death Education and Counseling, 29*(3), 1–15.

Scogin, F. (2007). *Introduction: Depression and suicide in older adults resource guide.* American Psychological Association. Retrieved May 28, 2008, from www.apa.org/pi/aging/depression.html

Terror Nine to Five: Guns in the American Workplace, 1994–2003. (2004). Arlington, VA: Handgun-Free America.

U.S. Department of Health and Human Services. (2001). *Appropriateness of minimum nurse staffing ratios in nursing homes.* Report to Congress. Washington, DC: Health Care Financing Administration.

Van Dongen, C. J. (1990). Agonizing questioning: experiences of survivors of suicide victims. *Nursing Research, 39*, 224–229.

Chapter 16

After Life, Then What?

Sleep after toil, port after stormy seas,
Ease after war, death after life does greatly please.
—Edmund Spenser (1552–1599)

Objectives

After reading this chapter, you will be able to answer the following questions:

- What were the ancient Greek philosophers' views toward life after death?
- What are some contemporary religious views on life after death?
- What are some of the characteristics of near-death experiences, and what are some potential causes of the phenomenon?
- How many people have experienced after-death communication?
- How do older Americans view the after-life?

All of us know (although most of us do not want to admit it) that our lives will end in death. Thomas Lynch (1997), the poet and funeral director, said that the death expectancy rate is 100%. But, if we believe that life exists after death, are we denying the finality of death itself? Does belief in an afterlife simply serve to buoy hopes, rather than confront the possibility that, after death, there is nothing? Tony Snow (2007) said that, for him, there is "an intuition that the gift of life, once given, cannot be taken away" (p. 32).

Views on Immortality in Ancient Greece

Even though it is reasonable to believe that humans have always thought about **immortality** (survival of the self after physical death), the first recorded attempts to answer afterlife questions were made by Greek philosophers.

Plato supported the idea of reincarnation (that the soul, in a new body, comes back to earth after death), an idea introduced by Pythagoras, another Greek philosopher, who said that he remembered eight of his past lives. Plato was the first philosopher to point out that considering life after death was a developmental process, meaning that the older people become, the more they think about life after death. About 600 B.C., Hermotimus, an ancient Greek philosopher who was considered a past life of Pythagoras, was known for his claimed

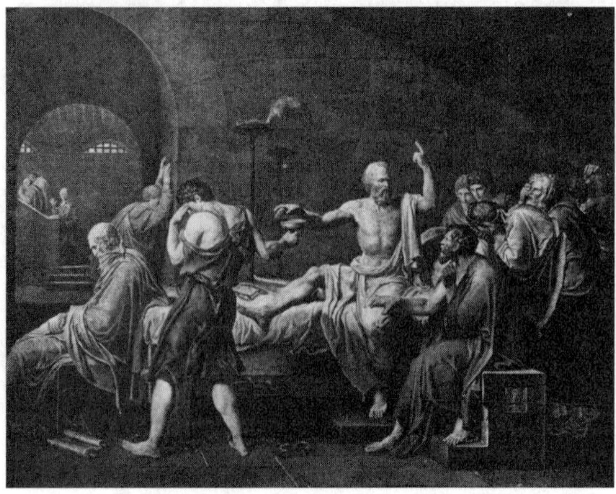

ability to leave his body at will. Supposedly, during these out-of-body experiences, Hermotimus's soul traveled to faraway places in search of knowledge. At that time, Greek philosophers knew that whether life existed after death depended on whether the conscious self could exist independently of the physical body. Whether the [conscious] mind and [physical] body can separate remains one of the primary issues in today's debates about the afterlife.

Contemporary Religious Views on Life After Death

Exploring others' views about the afterlife might help you appreciate multiple views of the afterlife. Also, by developing a supportive philosophy about death and the afterlife, perhaps you can develop a better philosophy about life and living. I enjoy wondering what I would say and how exciting it would be to meet Abraham Lincoln or Babe Ruth or Albert Einstein, as well as my deceased family members. This desire is well expressed by Edgar Allan Poe in *The Raven* (1845/1998):

> Tell this soul with sorrow laden, if, within the distant Aidenn,
> It shall clasp a sainted maiden whom the angels name Lenore—

Hinduism and Buddhism

Most religions, including the most primitive, claim that life continues after death. Descriptions of life after death vary considerably, though. For example, being *born again* after death (i.e., reincarnation) is part of the Buddhist and Hindu traditions. In this view, the soul remains the same but the person's body changes after death. Buddhists and Hindus believe that a person's last thought of his or her previous life determines the makeup of the next incarnation. In Buddhism, a person's actions affect the kind of body he or she will receive in the next life, and animal bodies are among the possibilities. In Hinduism, a person has the power to influence the quality of the next life, with the best possible option being a release from the chore of rebirth (Denosky, 2006).

In Hinduism, the world's oldest religion, death in this life is defined as *mahakala*, or the personification of time, and the process of passing the soul from one body to another is referred to as *samsara*, or journeying. The linkage of these incarnation experiences is *karma*, or the moral law of cause and effect wherein past actions and thoughts determine the present state of being, which in turn present choices for future states. Therefore, no occasion should exist to rejoice over birth or grieve over death (Long, 1977). In the Hindu *Veda* it is written, "From unreality lead me to reality; from darkness lead me to light; from death lead me to immortality" (Yajur Veda, Brhadaranyka Unpanishad 1.3).

Not only does karma in Hinduism refer to the endless cycle of birth and death, it also refers to action-to-action moments in everyday life. For example, if you ask a friend to tell her professor about a person she saw cheating on a test, your friend might answer, "No, that's bad karma," meaning that what you do (good or bad) comes back to you the same way.

Death holds a prominent place in Buddhist teachings, with the ultimate aim of **nirvana**, or extinction. In this view, no self exists to survive after death. Therefore, one cannot be reborn. Everything is in continual transition. In the Buddhist view, karma is the universal principle of moment-to-

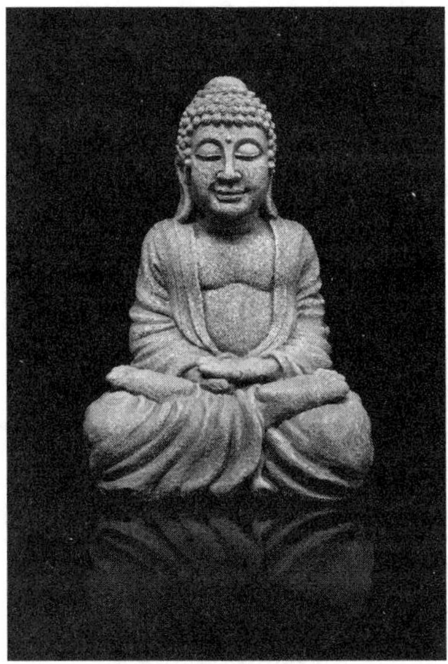

moment causality. This transmigration can be likened to transferring energy in a game of billiards when the cue ball strikes the cluster of balls on the table (DeSpelder & Strickland, 2005).

Abrahamic Religious Traditions

An alternative to the Buddhist and Hindu traditions regarding the number of lives one has is found in Judaism, Christianity, and Islam—the *Abrahamic* religious traditions. These religions are so grouped because they stem from the biblical patriarch Abraham. According to these religions, a human being consists of one mind, one body, and one life. When a person dies, that person's life will continue in some other place.

The idea of a final judgment is found in many religions, with the belief that good people will be rewarded for their moral behavior and bad people will be punished. In Christianity, wrongdoers in this life might end up in hell or, if Catholic, bad people first go to purgatory (the place of temporary punishment for those who have not lived moral lives; Figure 16.1). According to Jews, wrongdoers and sinners will be punished on the Day of Judgment.

How one can reach heaven, or paradise, varies among religions. According to Protestants, after death, the soul goes immediately to heaven. Jesus said to one of the robbers on a cross next to Him as they died, "I tell you the truth, today you shall be with me in paradise" (Luke 23:43). The Catholic idea is that there will be a resurrection of the dead on the Day of Judgment, and only after that will good people be rewarded. According to the Bible, believers in Jesus Christ go to heaven and nonbelievers go to hell. In Matthew 25:34, it is written to believers, "Come . . . take your inheritance, the kingdom prepared for you since the foundation of the world" (Mat. 25:34). For the nonbelievers, it is written, "Depart from me, you who are cursed, into the eternal fire prepared for the devil and his angels" (Mat. 25:41).

Figure 16.1 A Depiction of Hell.

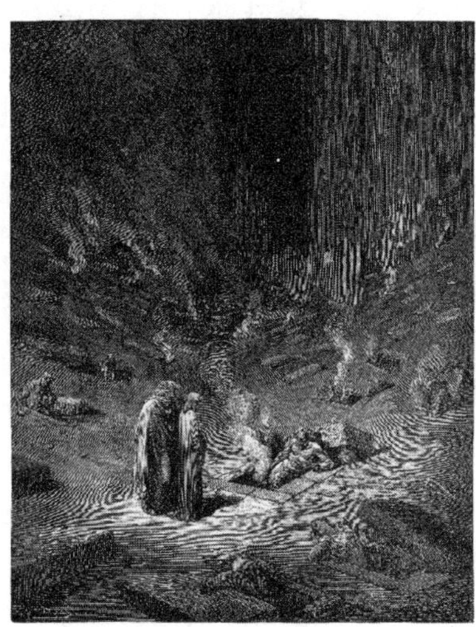

Interestingly, the Bible also gives examples of living on Earth again after death. In the book of Matthew, Jesus restores a girl to life, and in the book of John, Jesus raises Lazarus from the dead. Foremost, though, is that after his burial, Jesus made himself known as he walked the Earth and talked to people (Luke 24). Nevertheless, from biblical accounts, God seems to be concerned mostly with the living—not the dying.

Similar to Judaism and Christianity, Islam refers to one God who makes people accountable on a Day of Judgment. Muslims, so named for the prophet Muhammad, are believers who have accepted Islam as a way of life in this world and in "the other life." According to the holy book of Islam, the **Koran**, or **Qur'an** in Arabic, the basic premise is that God determines the span of a person's life and, at death, "It is Allah that takes the soul of men" (Koran 39:42). When the Book of Deeds, wherein all good and bad actions of people are recorded, is opened on the Last Day, and accompanied by bodily resurrection, people will be consigned either to everlasting happiness or eternal torment.

Near-Death Experiences

A life-after-death experience, or **near-death experience** (**NDE**; see Moody, 2001), has been reported by some people after they have been revived from clinical death. Most people who report having an NDE describe feelings of peace and joy, seeing a bright light, or entering another world. Some, however, report bad NDEs, involving torture by elves, giants, or demons (Figure 16.2).

Although individual experiences differ, reports from those who have had NDEs while ill can be summarized as follows (Greyson, 1993). The person:

- learns that he or she has died;
- leaves or rises from the body;
- meets with dead loved ones or people who were close;
- returns to the body.

Figure 16.2 THE FAR SIDE.

THE FAR SIDE® By GARY LARSON

Before
After
And then suddenly I saw this bright light at the end of a tunnel!
Larson
© 1992 FarWorks, Inc. All Rights Reserved/Dist. by Creators Syndicate

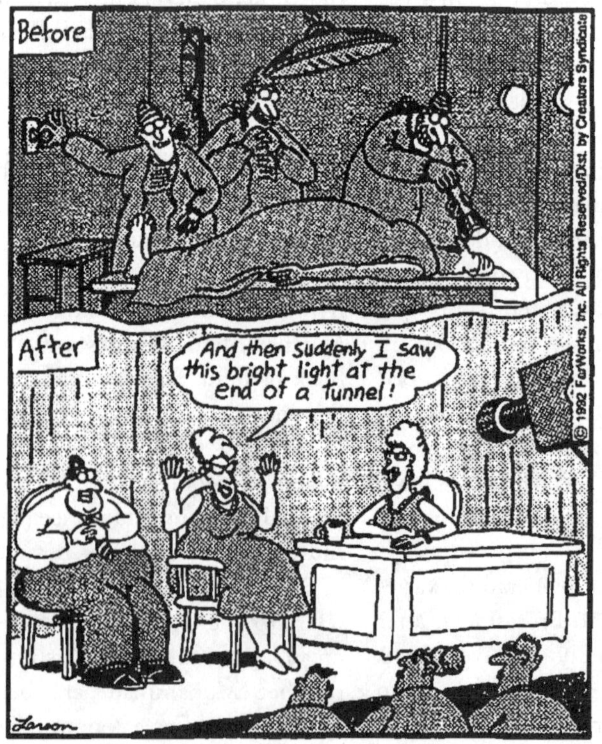

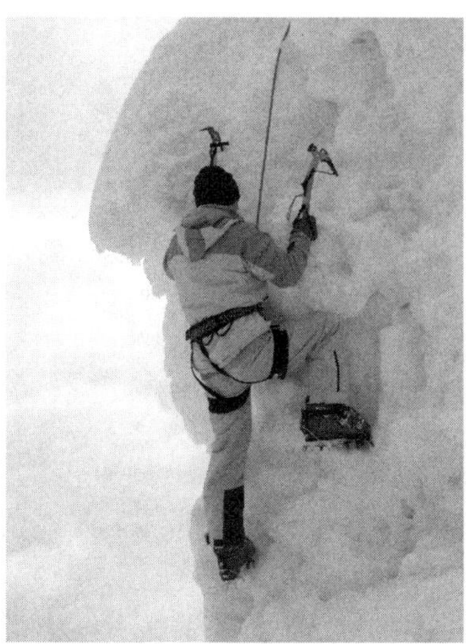

Questions & Answers

Question: Are all NDEs heavenly?

Answer: No. In fact, some NDEs reported by people who experience them are described as hellish and frightening. In the aftermath of these NDEs, people feel emptiness and despair. But most people associate what they saw and felt in their NDE as a life-changing religious experience. Furthermore, their fear of death was lessened after the event.

An NDE resulting from confronting a seemingly fatal danger involves different stages (Noyes, 1981). These stages include:

- *Resistance*: recognizing the danger, struggling against it, and then accepting the likelihood of death.
- *Life review*: as the self leaves the body, a panorama of memories survey the whole of the subject's past life.
- *Transcendence*: an expanding, cosmic awareness replaces the narrower, egoistic sense of self.

The implication of NDEs for many people is that consciousness exists after clinical death, but there is an ongoing debate regarding whether this phenomenon is actually the case. For example, whereas some argue that NDEs prove the existence of life after death, others maintain that these experiences are nothing more than a neurological event.

Some theories used to account for NDEs include the following (DeSpelder & Strickland, 2005):

- Neuropsychological theories:
  1. Temporal lobe paroxysm: seizure-like neural discharges in the temporal lobe.
  2. Cerebral anoxia: shortage of oxygen in the brain.
  3. Endorphin release: release of certain neurotransmitters associated with pain-killing effects and a sense of psychological well-being.
  4. Massive cortical disinhibition: loss of control over the random activity of the central nervous system.
  5. False sight: hallucinatory imagery arising from structures in the brain and nervous system.
  6. Drugs: side effects.
  7. Sensory deprivation.
- Psychological theories:
  1. Depersonalization: psychological detachment from one's body from a defensive reaction to the perceived threat of death.
  2. Motivated fantasy: a type of defensive fantasy wherein the person has an impression of surviving death because they desire to survive death.
  3. Archetypes: images associated with various elements of the near-death experience are wired into the brain as mythological archetypes of common humanity.
- Metaphysical theories:
  1. Soul travel: transitional journey of the soul or spirit to another mode of existence or realm of reality (e.g., heaven).
  2. Psychic vision: glimpses into another mode of reality, though not necessarily providing proof of soul-survival after death.

Researchers in the Netherlands (Van Lommel, Van Wees, Meyers, & Elffench, 2001) interviewed 344 patients who had been resuscitated after suffering clinical death (i.e., the heart stopped beating). They interviewed the patients within 5 days of the NDE experience and checked them at 2 years and 8 years after the event. The study was not conducted as an attempt to prove anything about the reality of NDEs (which some researchers have tried to do); rather, these researchers simply said that the NDEs of the patients they followed did not correlate with any psychological, physiological, or medical measurements, meaning that their NDEs were unrelated to the processes of a dying brain.

Don Piper (2004) said that he used to listen to NDE stories and testimonies with skepticism. Experiencing his own apparent death changed his mind. Piper said that, although he has no intention of trying to end the debate on the actuality of NDEs, he *knows* he went to heaven on January 18, 1989. While seemingly dead for 90 minutes, Piper reported that he did not flow through a long, dark tunnel or have a sense of fading away or of coming back. He did not feel his body being transported into the light. Neither did he hear voices.

What Piper felt at his moment of death was the envelopment of a brilliant light beyond earthly comprehension or description. After being enveloped in the light, he reported standing in heaven. He felt joy as he looked around and became aware of a large crowd of people, whose faces radiated a serenity he had not seen on earth. They were people who had been special to him and died in his lifetime. He saw colors that he never believed existed. He says, "I've never ever felt more alive than I did then" (p. 33) and "I felt as if I had never seen, heard, or felt anything so real before" (p. 25). What he cherishes most was the music he heard. "It was the most beautiful and pleasant sound I've ever heard, and it didn't stop. It was like a song that goes on forever" (p. 29).

Certainty about NDEs is difficult to establish other than by faith. For example, how do we know that a NDE is not just a stopover to a final destination? Possibly, minutes into the NDE, the bright light could dim and the euphoria could fade. NDEs, in this account, are analogous to going through Paris, thinking you will see France.

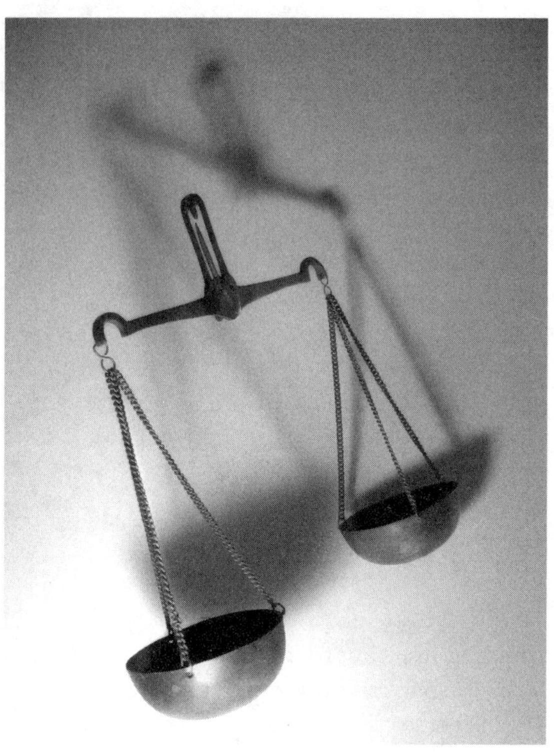

If the soul had weight, the person should weigh less immediately following death. Even if the soul had mass, though, how practical is it to weigh someone immediately before and after death?

After-Death Communication

Numerous faith traditions have taken it for granted that some type of communication can occur between the living and the essence of a dead person. Such assumptions underlie ancestor worship, Buddhist practices, and prayer involving a Roman Catholic saint. Also commonplace for people who have lost loved ones is to sense their presence. In opinion polls, up to 40% of Americans report having felt in touch with someone no longer alive at least once. These sensations do not come often, though, and to some, they do not come at all.

My Story: The Afterlife

I wonder often if there's a heaven. I sure hope so. I don't like the thought of hell or even nothingness. When my best friend, Jenny, was killed in a car wreck, though, I may have gotten a clue. Because I was in the car behind hers, I was the first one on the scene. It's funny, but, there, in this terrible hellish scene, while I was holding Jenny's hand as we waited for the ambulance, there was this beautiful butterfly that wouldn't go away. I kept swatting at it, but it kept coming back. Suddenly, I wondered if the butterfly was Jenny holding on to me as she was leaving earth. Then, I wondered if the thoughts about Jenny and the butterfly—uncommon thoughts—were given to me so that I would *know* that she's okay and that there's a heaven. Now, every time I see a butterfly, I think about Jenny and I think about a future time where we'll be best friends again.

Studies (Guggenheim, 2004) conducted on after-death communication (ADC) have established common modes of ADCs that seem to offer clues to the afterlife. Some researchers have used what they considered scientific methods to test and evaluate evidence of the afterlife. In the 1890s, the British Society for Psychical Research (SPR) conducted a Census of Hallucinations to explore what it called "spontaneous hallucinations of the sane" (Wright, 2002). In its study, 17,000 people were asked if, when awake, they had ever heard a voice or had an impression of seeing or being touched by a living being or inanimate object. Of the reports, almost 300 reported some sort of contact with the dead.

In 1899, Camille Flammarion (1901), a distinguished astronomer, set out to replicate the 1890s SPR work. He arranged for three popular French journals to publish a request for personal accounts of "cases of apparitions (ghosts) and manifestations on the part of the dying and the dead." Unlike the SPR study, he welcomed accounts of phenomena involving dreams and other sources of communication aside from sight, hearing, and touch. He received almost 1900 responses. Over the next two decades, Flammarion received thousands of letters in which people gave first-person reports of psychic experiences, including many hundreds dealing in detail with ADCs. Flammarion (1923) concluded that these occurrences prove that there is no final death.

Although none of Flammarion's research took place in a laboratory, his findings can be compared to contemporary polling techniques. Researchers who collect modern accounts of ADCs are replicating his work. Again and again, their data "reveal" that people are describing something real—to them.

Sylvia Wright (2004) believes that the three most common routes for ADCs are telepathy, dreams, and a sense of presence. The most common explicit communications reported are something like, "Don't worry about me; I'm okay" or "You need to move on with your life." Wright believes that these ranges of phenomenon, including NDEs and ADCs, provide evidence that an afterlife exists.

Older Americans' View of the Afterlife

In a survey, 1011 multicultural Americans aged 50 and over were asked about their beliefs about death and afterlife (Newcott, 2007). Nearly three-fourths (73%) reported that they believe in life after death. More women than men reported believing in an afterlife, 80% to 64%. About two-thirds of the survey respondents explained that their confidence in an afterlife increased as they grew older. One 90-year-old woman summarized the thoughts of most of the survey group by saying, "I'm looking forward to seeing my husband and my family and all those who have gone to their rest before me." (p. 70)

Visions of the Afterlife

Although most of the surveyed elders in Newcott's (2007) report believe that life exists beyond the grave, their visions regarding heaven and hell differ. For one, the survey results indicated that the richer the respondents were, the less likely they were to believe in heaven. In households with an income of $75,000 and more per year, 78% believe in heaven; among elders earning $25,000 or less, 90% believe in heaven. The same was found to be true of those who were better educated. Of college-educated people, 77% reported that they believed in heaven, compared with 89% of those who had a high school diploma or less. In the Bible, it is written, "It is easier for a camel [actually, the Aramaic word for camel also meant rope, the more likely intended meaning] to go through the eye of a needle than for a rich man to enter the kingdom of God." Maybe the same thing could be said for those who are better educated.

Abut 40% of survey respondents (Newcott, 2007) who believe in heaven believe that it is a real place—just as Clarksville, Tennessee, is a place. Another 47% of that group said that heaven is a state of being. Of hell, 42% believe it is a place, and 43% believe it is a state of being. Survey respondents' ideas about what heaven is like seem similar to an ideal retirement home:

- It's better place than this one.
- Everyone gets along with each other.
- Daytime is always beautiful, clear, and sunny.
- Pleasure abounds, and there will be sex.
- Humor will exist.
- Continuing education will be available.

The Price of Admission

Elders in the AARP survey (Newcott, 2007) disagree about what it takes to get into heaven. The largest group (29%) responded that a person has to believe in Jesus Christ; presumably most of the respondents were Christian. Another 25% believe that people have to be "good" to get in. Another 20% were split regarding admittance into heaven: 10% believe it is for those who believe in God and 10% believe that everyone gets into heaven.

Regarding hell, 40% believe it's for "bad" people or people who have sinned. Another 17% believe that hell is for people who do not believe in Jesus Christ. One person suggested that hell is probably a place where people continually engage in activities that they do not like. Obviously, that would differ, depending on what a person disliked. (While dining with my daughter and two small grandchildren at a popular pizza place where lights were flashing, sounds were loud, large stuffed animals sang and played musical instruments, and children were running wildly from one game/toy to the next, I told my daughter that, if I go to hell, I will find myself having all of my meals at a similar place!)

Back to Earth

Twenty-three percent of survey respondents (Newcott, 2007) said that they believe in reincarnation, meaning a return trip to earth. Survey members of the boomer generation, people born from 1946 to 1964, were more likely to believe in reincarnation. One survey respondent revealed, "We're intended to come back until we get it right" (p. 72). Although the idea of reincarnation might be controversial among Americans, it is a mainstay among Eastern religions, such as the Hindu.

More than half of the surveyed elders (Newcott, 2007) believe in ghosts, with women (60%) believing moreso than men (44%). Boomers are more likely to believe in ghosts (64%) compared to elders in their 60s (51%) or 70 and older (38%). As many as 38% of survey respondents reported that they have felt a presence or have seen "something," which they believe may have been a ghost. One respondent revealed that, when secure things unexpectedly fell, he believed that someone on the other side was trying to get his attention.

The English writer C. S. Lewis (1946) wrote about a man on a commuter bus who finds that he is on a tour of heaven and hell. Lewis's message is that, regardless of what view people have regarding

MAKING SURE

As many as 47 researchers have tried to determine if an afterlife exists (Roach, 2006). Some were physicians, physicists, or psychologists. Two of them were Nobel-prize winners. Only one man, Thomas Lynn Bradford, tried to "know for certain." On February 6, 1921, Bradford sealed the doors and windows of his rented room in Detroit, Michigan, blew out the pilot on his heater, and turned on the gas. But before this event, Bradford secured the presence of an accomplice to solve the mystery by having their two minds properly attuned. His plan was to die and she, being "properly attuned," would report back to others about the afterlife. Afterwards, though, the accomplice was silent. Obviously, reporting back was a challenge she couldn't overcome.

the afterlife, the reality of it is heading toward them. Their view is either dead right or dead wrong. But how can it be known before death? Maybe it is much better to fully live life with enjoyment without worrying about the afterlife, knowing that, one day, life will hand you the answer.

SUMMARY

- The first recorded attempts to answer questions about the afterlife were made by Greek philosophers.
- Being "born again" (i.e., reincarnation) is part of the Buddhist and Hindu traditions wherein the soul remains the same but the person's body changes after death. Not only does karma (the law of cause and effect) in Hinduism refer to the endless cycle of births and deaths, it refers to action-to-action moments in everyday life.
- Judaism, Christianity, and Islam are referred to as the Abrahamic religious traditions because they stem from the biblical patriarch, Abraham. How to reach heaven, or paradise, varies among religions. According to Protestants, after death, the soul goes immediately to heaven. Similar to Judaism and Christianity, Islam refers to one God who makes people accountable on a Day of Judgment.
- Near death experiences (NDEs) are sometimes reported by people after they have been revived from clinical death. NDEs have been described by those who have experienced them as either heavenly or hellish. Controversy exists over whether NDEs are real, imagined, or the result of a physiological occurrence. Controversy exists regarding whether after death communication (ADC) is possible.
- From results from one survey, about three-fourths of Americans aged 50 and over reported that they believe in life after death; more women than men reported believing in an afterlife. Also, those richer were less likely to believe in heaven. Controversy exists regarding whether heaven, if it exists, is a real place or a state of being.
- Many people believe in ghosts. Of a group of elders who were surveyed, boomers are more likely to believe in ghosts compared to older elders.

ADDITIONAL RESOURCES

Books

Albom, M. (2006). *For one more day.* New York: Hyperion. Albom tells a ghostly tale about a retired baseball player who gets a chance to spend one more day with his dead mother to glean understanding about his childhood and get his life "right."

Piper, D. (2004). *90 minutes in heaven.* Grand Rapids, MI: Revell. Don Piper recounts the dramatic story of his almost-fatal car crash and subsequent 90 minutes in heaven.

Movies

Ghost. (1990). This movie is a story of a love that transcends life.

Meet Joe Black. (1999). This movie is about the personification of death in people's lives.

Over Her Dead Body. (2008). This movie is about a woman who discovers that her new boyfriend is being haunted by the ghost of his former fiancée.

Sixth Sense. (1999). As a psychological horror film, this movie tells of a troubled, isolated boy, who claims to be able to see and talk to the dead, and an equally troubled child psychologist who tries to help him.

CRITICAL THINKING

1. Explain how you would try to convince someone that life exists after death. Be specific, using evidence, experience, and reasoning in your explanation.
2. Explain how you would convince someone that life does *not* exist after death. Be specific, using evidence, experience, and reasoning in your explanation.
3. What you think about NDEs? Are they evidence of life after death? Of a soul? A neurological event?

CLASS ACTIVITY

Invite leaders of a number of different faiths (e.g., Protestant, Jewish, Muslim, Buddhist, Hindu, and so on) to class to serve on a panel in which class members take turns asking them about their beliefs of an afterlife. Possibly, this activity could involve the attendance of all students across campus.

REFERENCES

Denosky, J. (2006). *A Buddhist practice of purification dealing with reincarnation.* Retrieved June 8, 2008, from http://www.many-lives.com/

DeSpelder, L. A., & Strickland, A. L. (2005). *The last dance: Encountering death and dying* (7th ed.). New York: McGraw-Hill.

Flammarion, C. (1901). *The Unknown.* New York: Harper.

Flammarion, C. (1923). *Death and its mystery: After death.* New York: Century.

Greyson, B. (1993). Varieties of near-death experiences. *Psychiatry, 56*, 390–399.

Guggenheim, B. (2004, June 17). *After-death communication: A new field of research.* Address delivered at the 30th annual conference of the Academy of Religion and Psychical Research.

Lewis, C. S. (1946). *The great divorce.* New York: Macmillan.

Long, J. B. (1977). Death as a necessity and a gift in Hindu mythology. In F. E. Reynolds & E. H. Waugh (Eds.), *Religious encounters with death: Insights from the history and anthropology of religions.* University Park: Penn State University Press.

Lynch, T. (1997). *The undertaking life: Studies from the dismal trade.* New York: Penguin.

Moody, R. (2001). *Life after life* (rev. ed.). San Francisco: HarperCollins.

Newcott, B. (2007, September–October). Life after death. *AARP The Magazine,* 69–73.

Noyes, R. (1981). The encounter with life-threatening danger: its nature and impact. *Essence: Issues in the Study of Ageing, Dying and Death, 5*(1), 21–32.

Piper, D. (2004). *90 minutes in heaven.* Grand Rapids, MI: Revell.

Poe, E. A. (1998). The Raven. In *Collected poems.* Ann Arbor. MI: Lowe & B. Hould Publishers. (Original work published 1845)

Roach, M. (2006). What happens after you die? *New Scientist, 192*(2578), 66–69.

Snow, T. (2007). Cancer's unexpected blessings. *Christianity Today, 51*(7), 30–32.

Van Lommel, P., van Wees, R., Meyers, V., & Elffench, I. (2001). Near-death experiences in survivors of cardiac arrest: A prospective study in the Netherlands. *Lancet, 358*(1998), 2039–2045.

Wright, S. H. (2002). *When spirits come calling: The open-minded skeptic's guide to after-death contacts.* Nevada City, CA: Blue Dolphin.

Wright, S. H. (2004). Clues to the nature of the afterlife from after-death communication. *The Journal of Spiritual and Paranormal Studies, 29*(3), 149–159.

Chapter 17

The Past, Present, and Future of Death Education

The wave of the future is coming
And there is no fighting it.
—ANNE MORROW LINDBERGH

Objectives

After reading this chapter, you will be able to answer the following questions:

- What is the history of death education?
- What is the role of death education in elementary and secondary schools?
- What are university students' views toward death?
- What lessons have university students learned from death education courses?
- What are some ideas about the future of death and dying?

History of Death Education

Death education arose along with an academic interest in death in the mid-1950s, specifically with Herman Feifel's 1959 book, *The Meaning of Death*. V. R. Pine (1977) identified three periods in the history of death education: exploration (1928–1957), development (1958–1967), and popularity (1967–1977). It is probably reasonable to assume that death education is still in the popularity period. Pine said that the three periods can be further divided into pure and applied approaches. *Applied* death education refers to an interest in the management of dying or adjustment following bereavement. The work of Elisabeth Kübler-Ross exemplifies the applied interest approach. By contrast, the *pure* approach involves educating people about attitudes toward death, understanding grief and mourning, euthanasia and suicide, the effect of parental death on children, and the meaning of one's own death.

Thirty-two years ago, in *The Scope of Death Education* (1977), Daniel Leviton identified the goals of death education and defined **death education** as a developmental process in which death-related knowledge and the implications resulting from that knowledge are transmitted. He identified the following goals of death education: *primary prevention* (preparing individuals for eventual death events), *intervention* (helping people face personal aspects of death), and *rehabilitation* (understanding and learning from death-related crises). More specific goals included promoting comfortable interactions with the dying, removing taboos, and reducing anxiety. In his article, "Death Education: An Outline and Some Critical Observations," William Warren (1981) suggested, from having read syllabi and course aids used in death-education courses, that the expressed goals of the courses were incorporated to defuse death of the "socially disruptive consequences that might flow from the acceptance of personal mortality" (p. 38).

Sometimes, though, according to Simone de Beauvoir (1964), the goal of death education is to create anxiety rather than to reduce it. In so doing, a student becomes painfully aware of the need to confront death. As de Beauvoir wrote,

> There is not such thing as a natural death: nothing that happens to a man is ever natural, since his presence calls the world into question. All men must die; but for every man his death is an accident even if he knows and consents to it, an unjustifiable violation (p. 106).

Knight and Elfenbein (1993) conducted a study to determine anxiety and fear of death among 103 college students, some who had and some who had not taken a course in death education. They found that students enrolled in the death education course reported increased anxiety and fear about death relative to those who had not taken the course. Students from the death education course also reported an increase in thinking about their own death. Whether that thinking was good or bad is unknown. Increased anxiety about death and more thoughts about death might be positive in that it might cause students to appreciate their lives more. Did this course in death education increase or decrease your anxiety about death and dying?

Death Education in Elementary and Secondary Schools

A growing movement exists among educators to implement death education programs in elemen-

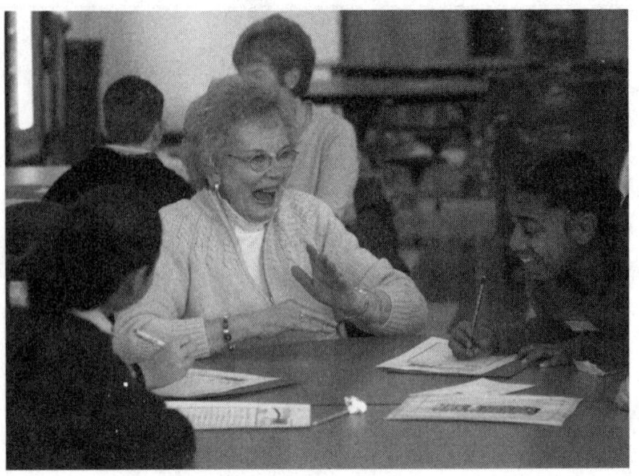

tary and secondary public and private schools. One driving force is the incidence of suicide among children and adolescents; one of every three adolescents reports to have contemplated suicide and one in six reports having attempted suicide (Thompson, 1993). According to a government survey (U.S. Department of Health and Human Services [USDHHS], 2000), 2.6% of adolescents in grades 9 through 12 attempted suicide in 1999. Because the finality of death in seeking a solution to a problem is not always clear to adolescents, death education can be seen as a preventive measure because, according to Eddy and Alles (1983), death education causes adolescents to think about death in more realistic ways.

Another important factor driving the death education movement in schools is that the death of a classmate is becoming common among school-aged children. The leading causes of death among children and adolescents are accidents, homicide, and suicide—in that order (USDHHS, 2000). Many students' peers are dying premature and violent deaths. Along with confronting these deaths, children and adolescents often do not have adequate opportunities to grieve.

Many theorists believe that death education has replaced sex as the "last taboo" (Chadwick, 1994; Wagner, 1995; Warren, 1981). Herman Feifel (1972) pointed out that death education is as necessary as sex education, and perhaps more so because death is universal and sex is not. Even though children understand death to varying degrees, many adults do not believe, as some do

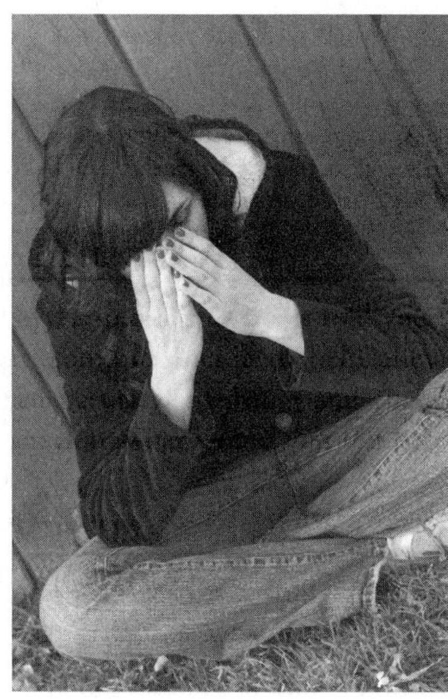

regarding sex education, that death education is an appropriate subject for discussion at either home or school.

Getting parents to agree to allow death education in schools is important. In a survey of parents of 375 youth, Jones, Hodges, and Slate (1995) found that parents were generally supportive of death education programs in schools. Furthermore, 77% of these parents reported that they did not perceive death education programs as interfering with their parental responsibilities.

To determine whether death education is appropriate for students in the primary grades, Lynn Bowie (2000) conducted a study among students and teachers in an elementary school setting. Results supported the inclusion of death education in the primary curriculum because it is a natural part of life, with one-third of students agreeing. The main ingredient for successful teaching of death education to young children, however, has to do with teachers' comfort with it. Therefore, it seems important for college students, especially those who plan to be schoolteachers, to familiarize themselves with the issues of death, dying, and grieving and to be able to talk about them.

Corr, Morgan, and Wass (1994) reported that death, dying, and bereavement are fundamental aspects of the human experience. By appreciating the reality of death, dying, and bereavement, they argue that individuals can more fully live; without this understanding, unnecessary suffering and a diminished quality of life are likely. Therefore, these authors believe that education about death, dying, and bereavement is an essential component of the educational process at all levels.

University Students' Views of Death

Have you ever wondered how your thoughts about death compared to your peers? Results from a study conducted by Dennis, Muller, Miller, and Banerjee (2004) revealed that college-age males and females (from a mostly Caucasian population) accepted death as another life experience. Differences existed, however, between male and female responses to the following statements:

- I am less concerned about death than others.
- I am not concerned about the inevitability of death.
- I neither fear death nor welcome it.
- I am not frightened of death like others.

For each statement, males' scores were significantly higher than females' scores, meaning that males were less concerned about death and its inevitability; feared death less, but did not welcome it; and were less frightened of death than they believed others are.

When interpreting these results from Dennis et al. (2004), it is important to know that males also reported more often engaging in risky behaviors (e.g., less likely to use seat belts and more likely to drive a vehicle after drinking, more likely to engage in a physical fight, and more likely to smoke cigarettes). Although males might not welcome death, given their risky behavior, premature death for them appears more probable.

In a similar study, Dennis, Hicks, and Banerjee (2005) asked the same questions of a predominately African American group of college students. Overall, death acceptance scores were similar to those cited previously, although no significant differences existed between African

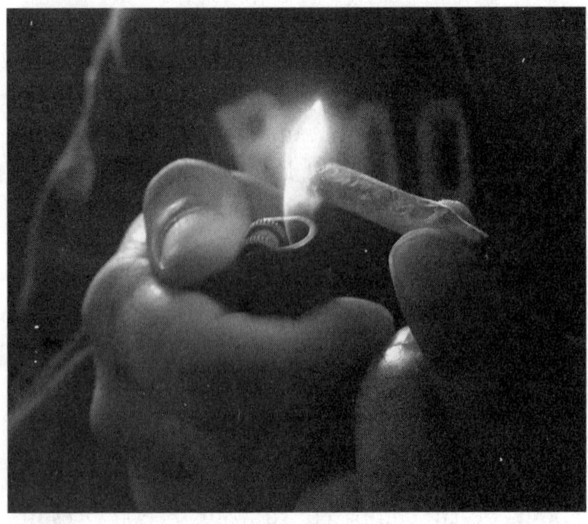

American males and females on the inevitability of death. African American males' scores were significantly higher than females' scores on being concerned about death or frightened of death.

Generally, research results from studies about death anxiety reveal that females score higher than males, but because African American males have a very high rate of death by homicide (USDHHS, 2000), it is possible that they know that premature death is more probable for them.

Lessons Learned from Death Education Course Assignments

In an evaluation survey of a death education course taught by Edwin Stefan (1978), students said that the course was valuable because they were allowed to talk with one another about their fears of and curiosities about death. Of the 36 students in the course, 18 said they had a greater acceptance of their own death, and 14 reported that they were more accepting of the death of others. Also, one-half of the students reported that the value of the course was the awareness that life needs to be lived daily.

Asking for Forgiveness

Forgiveness is not easy, whether one is trying to forgive others or oneself. A student in one of my death education courses, a nurse, had the assignment to interview someone who works with death and dying on a daily basis. She chose a minister. The minister told her that there is one question he always asks someone who is dying, "Is there anyone you need to forgive?" Forgiveness appears to be needed for peace in life and peace at death's door.

The minister's question implies that many people hold on to emotional pain too long. If you have anyone to forgive, do it now. Possibly, that someone is yourself, as was the case with Tonya, another student in a death education class, who, when asked to write to someone dead for the purpose of resolving an issue, wrote a letter to her lost baby of 25 years before. I spoke with her after she submitted the assignment, and she told me that, for the first time in her life, she had begun to forgive herself and have peace about what happened. There is power in the intent of forgiving, oneself—or others—for mistakes and hurts. If you have something you want to write or say to one of your loved ones, do it now.

Coming to Terms with Living and Dying

Another student in one of my death education courses wrote about her learning experience from volunteering at a local hospital. She wrote:

> One of the patients in the hospital was close to death, and we [the student and her supervisor] did not want her to be alone. So, I decided to go to provide support. It was so peaceful. She exhaled gently and then, in less than a minute, she gently exhaled again. And she was gone. . . . I had another patient who was swinging her

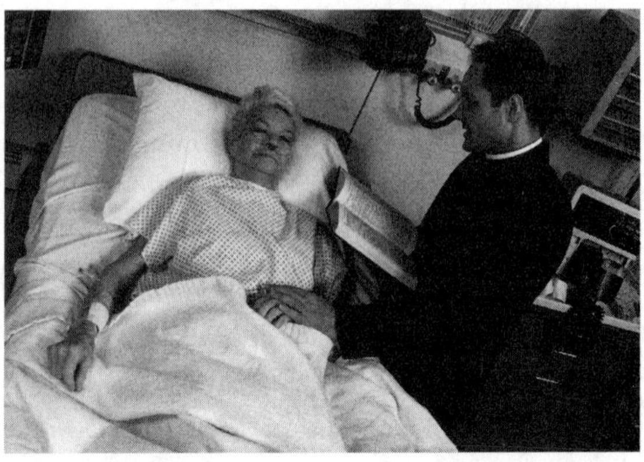

My Story: What I Learned from Death Education

When I, as a doctoral student, took a course in death education with components similar to the ones in this text, my world was opened—to forgive, to say goodbye, and to embrace the inevitability of my own impending death. At the forefront of my experiences in death education, however, was the sense that I needed to fully live my life. Since I began developing and teaching courses in death education, I have been privileged to witness others doing likewise. As others' learning experiences (e.g., forgiving someone, saying I'm sorry or I love you to someone who is dead or dying, or learning to appreciate life) are presented in this chapter, see if, after coming to end of your course in death education, you have similar experiences.

> arms in the air and screaming, "Leave me alone; I do not want to go!" It just so happened (divine intervention) that her pastor stopped by, and he prayed with her. She calmed down, and then she died. . . . Each day when I leave the hospital, I reflect on life itself. We know we are not here to stay, but facing death can be so devastating. It is one thing not knowing about it, but it is another thing to have to come to terms with it. I hope my hospital experiences will allow me to be able to come to terms with it for myself.

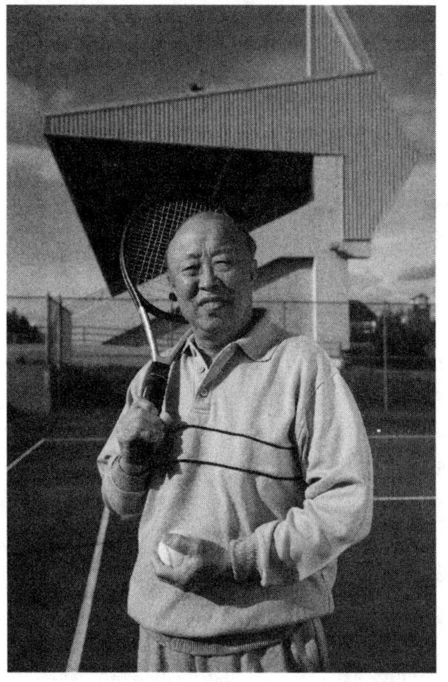

Hector, another student, wrote about what he learned from interviewing an elderly gentleman who spoke about the lessons he had learned through his life. Hector wrote:

> After my interview, I looked at many things in life differently. The man I interviewed was four times my age, and he still walks, talks, and lives like he is living life to the fullest. He certainly was a role model. This interview was something that profoundly changed my life forever.

Overcoming Feelings that Death Is Creepy

In addition to lessons in forgiveness, resolving old emotional pains, or choosing to live a better life, an assignment in a death education course can help alleviate fears of death's strangeness. In her assignment to go to a cemetery and write about the experience, Sarah wrote:

> For as long as I can remember, I have thought cemeteries are spooky places, and you definitely don't want to go by yourself at night. I guess I still had those feelings about cemeteries, because I REALLY did not want to do this assignment. Just the thought of being in a place where hundreds of dead bodies below me really gives me the creeps. My aunt loves to go to the cemetery and put flowers on her husband's grave. Often, she has asked me to go with her, and I go just to pacify her. But I don't like it. I have to admit, though, that the longer I walked around looking at the tombstones, the more comfortable I got with being there. I couldn't help but continue to look around and see what the earliest date I could find. The oldest one I found was from a person who was born in 1710 and died in 1742.

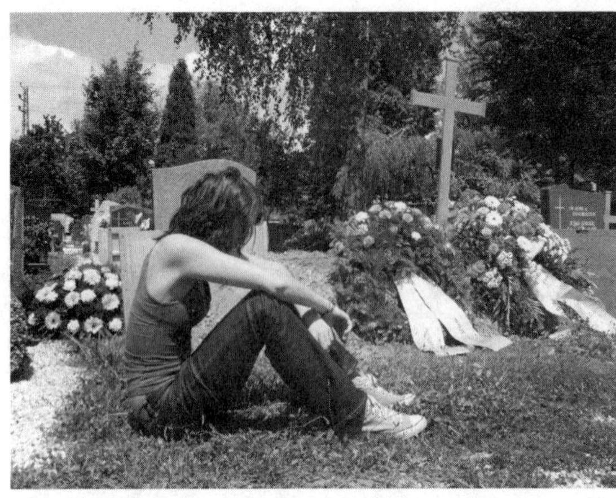

It's just hard to imagine that something from so long ago is still around—the tombstone, I mean. I guess this assignment wasn't so bad after all. I have no plans to hang out in a cemetery any time soon, but I don't think it will make me nearly as uncomfortable the next time I go.

Thank You for Living

Another assignment, again to write a letter to someone dead or alive, was for the purpose of saying thank you to someone. Sonya, Angie's aunt, wrote her such a letter:

> Dear Angie,
>
> Your unexpected illness and death was devastating for your mommy and daddy and all of us who loved you so much. We anxiously anticipated your arrival and just could not wait for you to come into this world. You were so beautiful and looked so healthy. I saw you when you were only two days old. By that time, you had tubes and machines on your little body to help you feel better. You did not get better, though. You died five days after you were born. But, Angie, you brought so much joy to us. I watched as your grandmother, Dolly, rocked you the night before you went to Heaven. She had such a big smile on her face—so tender.
>
> You have a new brother now—Justin Tyler. He's really cute, nothing like you, though (just between the two of us!). He keeps your mommy hoppin' every day, and she isn't as sad anymore. She talks about you often. You'll always be Mommy's and Daddy's little angel, and I know you are one of God's favorites! I love you, Angie. Thank you for coming to see us.

Although it is true that baby Angie may never have known how much Sonya thanked her for being born, it is also true that many people need to hear a thank you now—from you.

Meaning in Life

In summing up what she learned in her online death education course, one student wrote:

> I believe that the movie [she was required to view], along with the book [she was assigned to read] went hand in hand with this Death Education Course. . . . Throughout the course, I have been molded into a better person who is more aware of the difficulties of life, how to encourage myself and others to succeed in hard times instead of being defeated by insecurities. Every paper I have written, every discussion question that I have answered has brought back memories (some good, some bad) that have shown me where I have strayed from my original life goals. Morrie [in the book, *Tuesdays with Morrie*] gave me the courage and strength to withstand the most devastating news, while Sam [in the movie *My Life*] gave me the belief that unconditional love exists and is worth protecting. Without this course, I would never have realized any of this. But, because I was extremely lucky to run across it, I have enabled myself to stand strong and take a long look at my life and continue on the right path. Who knows, maybe one day I will be able to have a conversation with Morrie and meet a real-life Sam. With the renewal of my beliefs in myself and others, I do not only think that this could happen—I KNOW it will.

While this student wrote how her life was enriched by taking a death and dying course, another student wrote how the assignment to read the book, *Tuesdays with Morrie*, came at a perfect time for her. The student wrote:

> At first glance of this book, *Tuesdays with Morrie*, I thought to myself, "At least it is a short book." Little did I realize that what this book would come to mean to me. At first, I

thought the book was going to be slow and boring—not that a story about an old man dying wasn't necessarily interesting, but old people do die eventually. So what really could be that interesting? I soon came to find out that this book would mean more to me than I ever thought possible.

I was at my parents' home recovering from a hysterectomy when I noticed this small book on my Mother's desk. As I examined it, I realized it's the book that I was required to read in my "death" class. Hum . . . I was surprised that my mother had that book. I asked her why she had the book and if I could read it. Of course, she told me to read the book. She explained that one of her friends from church brought it to her and suggested that she and my sister read it. You see, my older sister was fighting a cancer battle.

While reading this book, I came to love this old man. His words of wisdom actually touched my heart as I thought about his feelings, knowing that he would soon die. Some of his moving remarks were: "Accept what you are able to do and what you are not able to do"; "Accept the past as past without denying it or discarding it"; "Learn to forgive yourself and to forgive others"; and, "Don't assume that it's too late to get involved."

While reading the book, I watched my sister gradually deteriorate. My sister had always been so healthy, participating in many athletic endeavors. Also, she had her dignity, you know. Please, don't get me wrong. The dignity is still there even in the darkest days of her cancer, but the sight of seeing this sickening disease consume her life was very difficult to watch. I soon knew, after reading this book, that there were things that must be said.

I cannot tell you how many people I have recommended to read this book. I realize now that a day, just one day, can make a difference. My sister's physician explained to my mother how my sister likely had only two weeks left but that, as many physicians say, "You never know, though, because I'm not God." Because of reading *Tuesdays with Morrie*, I began telling my sister some of the things I needed to say, things as simple as, for example, "I love you"; "Thanks for helping pay for my college"; "Thanks for going to see me cheerlead." Next, I prepared something for my sister's funeral. I would tell people that Ann Lee loved horses and the Kentucky

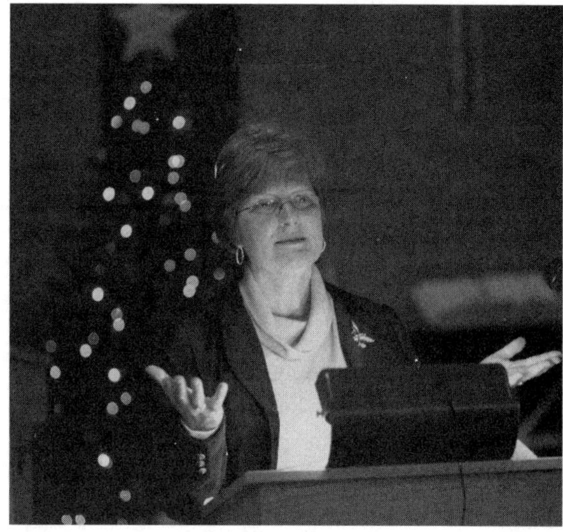

Derby, she loved to ride a motorcycle, and she had a hang-up for my Grandmother Carver's brownies. I would tell them how she played continuously with her grandchildren. I want people to know my sister—not her cancer.

The day came. On one the darkest days of my life, *Tuesdays with Morrie* helped me tell a group of people the little things I cherish most about my sister. That small, non-attractive book has been such a blessing to me over the last year. I have heard that when the student is ready, the teacher will come. I was ready; Morrie was there.

Those who have read *Tuesdays with Morrie* will know that Morrie would be happy to know that he made a positive impact on this person's life. Specific to what one should focus on in life, though, is what Jon wrote on the meaning of life and death:

> Nobody is certain about how much life is left to live, and life is too short to be focused on our death. Young people of all ages die every day. The point is that we should live life to the fullest no matter how much is left. I have been hit by death so much in my life. I need to focus on living, enjoying, and doing my best with what I have and whenever it is my time to go, so be it. Negative thoughts almost killed me when I lost my dad, and it made me make bad choices when I lost my first partner at age 27. Death is just a

transition. It is scary because we do not know what is afterwards with certainty, but if we were supposed to focus on death, why live then? I treasure my life and because of the inevitability of death, I choose to live!

The Future of Death, with Some Very Odd Ideas

Chronic conditions, such as those related to heart, cancer, stroke, and Alzheimer's, are the primary causes of death for elders. By 2025, the number of people age 65 and over in the United States is expected to grow to 62 million (Hoyert, Kung, & Smith, 2003) even as 77 million baby boomers begin hitting 65 in 2011 (Samuelson, 2007). Therefore, the number of deaths related to chronic diseases among elders is expected to rise. Care of the dying is likely to become a big health business for Americans, and the future of death and dying, as well as staying alive, might be very different from what it has been.

William Bainbridge (2006) proposes a foreseeable future in which all of a person's memories can be preserved. Using the technique he describes, it would be possible to record and classify all of a person's episodic memories and thereby build, in digital format, a network of mental associations connecting all of a person's life events with his or her related physical and emotional significance, which, in essence, is a process to duplicate a person's personality and preserve it in digital form. Even after physical death, a person would, in effect, be alive.

Lane Jennings (2005) offers a similar idea. Jennings proposes that the elderly, or those with life-threatening illnesses, could use hallucinogenic drugs and electrical stimulation of the brain to prepare for death. He calls this process *statutory death* or *reversible suicide*. The person would, while alive, write and sign a legal will to renounce all worldly rights and responsibilities. The person would act as though he or she was legally dead while physically being alive. At a medically supervised "pleasure hospice," the person would be maintained in a "twilife" condition. Through drugs/brain stimulation, the person would mimic real-life situations of his or her own choosing. In other words, the person would continue in a physically passive but mentally enhanced state. The procedure would be reversible in that the patient could go back to regular life in intervals at choice. Jennings believes that one advantage of statutory death is that a person could attend his or her own funeral. When the time for actual death arrived, the person would smoothly and painlessly exit with goodbyes and grieving already done.

Christopher Buckley (2007) has another idea about future death issues that is especially relevant to the increased financial burden of having aging Baby Boomers on Social Security. In his novel, Buckley tells about a plan wherein financial incentives are advertised for elders who agree to kill themselves at the age of 70. Even greater incentives would be offered to elders who agreed to kill themselves at age 65. He calls this suicide plan "voluntary transitioning." Although this plan exists only in Buckley's fictional, outrageous, and hilarious novel, *Boomsday*, the potential issues involving finances are real for Americans. Younger Americans will be faced with paying the bills for increased numbers of elders. Could life, eventually, possibly imitate fiction? If so, death (and health) education will definitely be different than it is today.

SUMMARY

- Death education arose from Herman Feifel's 1959 book, *The Meaning of Death.*
- Death education is a process in which death-related knowledge and the implications resulting from that knowledge are transmitted.
- Death education sometimes creates anxiety about death rather than reducing it.
- Death education causes adolescents to think about death in more realistic ways.
- Parents are generally supportive of death education programs in schools.
- Many college-aged males and females accept death as another life experience.

- Students previously enrolled in college death education courses report learning about important life necessities, such as forgiving, asking for forgiveness, saying "I love you," coming to terms with one's own death, accepting the death of a loved one, saying "Thank you," accepting a regrettable past, and becoming determined to fully live the one and only life each person is given.

Additional Resources

Books

Buckley, C. (2007). *Boomsday*. New York: Hachette Book Group USA. This hilarious, cynical, and entertaining book, which is sure to please Baby Boomers, is about corruption in Washington, DC.

Pausch, R., & Zaslow, J. (2008). *The last lecture.* New York: Hyperion. As a college professor who had pancreatic cancer, Randy Pausch wrote his "last lecture."

Movie

Dead Poet's Society. (1989). A film about how a teacher inspired his students to live extraordinary lives.

Critical Thinking

If your 90-year-old grandparent told you that she wanted to commit suicide to help alleviate the U.S. Social Security dilemma, and thereby help your generation, what would you tell her?

Class Activity

Form groups of five to six students. Each group should make a list of what activities, readings, movies, and/or material in this course about living, dying, and grieving has been the most helpful. Share lists/discussion with all groups.

References

Bainbridge, W. S. (2006). Cyberimmortality: Science, religion, and the battle to save our souls. *The Futurist, 40*(2), 25–29.

Bowie, L. (2000). Is there a place for death education in the primary curriculum? *Pastoral Care in Education, 18*(1), 22–26.

Buckley, C. T. (2007). *Boomsday.* New York: Hachette Book Group USA.

Chadwick, A. (1994). *Living with grief in school: Guidance for primary school teachers.* Biggin Hill, Kent, UK: Family Reading Centre.

Corr, C. A., Morgan, J. D., & Wass, H. (1994). *Statements on death, dying, and bereavement.* London, Ontario, Canada: International Work Group on Death, Dying, and Bereavement.

de Beauvoir, S. (1964). *A very easy death.* London: Deutsch, Weidenfeld, & Nicolson.

Dennis, D. L., Hicks, T., & Banerjee, P. (2005). Spirituality among a predominately African American college student population. *American Journal of Health Studies, 20*(3–4), 135–142.

Dennis, D. L., Muller, S. M., Miller, K., & Banerjee, P. (2004). Spirituality among a college student cohort: A quantitative assessment. *American Journal of Health Education, 35*(4), 220–227.

Eddy, J. M., & Alles, W. F. (1983). *Death education.* St. Louis, MO: Mosby.

Feifel, H. (1959). *The meaning of death.* New York: McGraw-Hill.

Feifel, H. (1972). The meaning of death in American Society, Tape 5. *Cassette Tape Program in Death, Grief, and Bereavement.* Minneapolis: University of Minnesota.

Hoyert, D., Kung, H. C., & Smith, B. L. (2003). *National vital statistics report. Deaths: Preliminary data for 2003.*Retrieved June 9, 2008, from www.cdc.gov/nchs/data/nvsr/nvsr53/nvsr53_15.pdf

Jennings, L. (2005). Finding better ways to die. *The Futurist, 39*(2), 43–47.

Jones, C. H., Hodges, M., & Slate, J. R. (1995). Parental support for death education programs in the schools. *School Counselor, 42,* 370–376.

Knight, K. H., & Elfenbein, M. H. (1993). Relationship of death education to the anxiety, fear, and meaning associated with death. *Death Studies, 17,* 411–425.

Leviton, D. (1977). The scope of death education. *Death Education, 1*(1), 41–56.

Pine, V. R. (1977). A sociohistorical portrait of death education. *Death Education, 1*(1), 57–84.

Samuelson, R. J. (2007, April 16). 'Boomsday' is approaching. *Newsweek,* 44.

Stefan, E. (1978), Perspectives on death: An experimental course on death education. *Teaching of Psychology, 5,* 142–144.

Thompson, R. A. (1993). Posttraumatic stress and posttraumatic loss debriefing: Brief strategic intervention for survivors of sudden loss. *The School Counselor, 41,* 16–21.

U.S. Department of Health and Human Services. (2000). *Healthy people: 2010.* Washington, DC: Author.

Wagner, P. (1995). *Schools and pupils: Developing their responses to bereavement.* In R. Best, P. Lang, C. Lodge, & C. Watkins (Eds.), *Pastoral care and personal–social education entitlement and provision.* London: Cassell.

Warren, W. (1981). Death education: An outline and some critical observations. *British Journal of Educational Studies, 29*(1), 29–41.

Glossary

Abortion. Termination of a pregnancy after, accompanied by, resulting in, or closely followed by the death of the embryo or fetus.

Active euthanasia. Acting to end the life of a terminally ill person.

Advance care directive (living will). Written document that reveals what a person wants or does not want if, in the future, he or she cannot make known his or her wishes about medical treatment.

Algor mortis. Fall in body temperature immediately after death.

Alzheimer's disease. Mental dysfunction in an elderly person that is characterized by irreversible memory loss, reduced ability to use language, loss of problem-solving skills, and reduced mobility.

Anticipatory grief. Distress at losses to come; a pulling away from the expectations of a future with, and for, a dying person.

Apnea. Inability to breathe spontaneously.

Artificial hydration and nutrition. A medical treatment that allows a person to receive nutrition (food) and hydration (fluid) when he or she is no longer able to take them by mouth.

Assisted suicide. Knowingly providing someone the means, such as with a supply of drugs or a weapon, to commit suicide.

Asthma. Chronic lung disorder marked by recurring episodes of airway obstruction.

Atherosclerosis. Fibrosis of the inner layer of the arteries.

Autopsy. Examination of the body after death to determine the cause of death.

Bereavement. Period after a loss during which grief is experienced.

Bibliotherapy. Reading self-help literature.

Bioethicist. Person trained to judge the ethical implications of biological research and applications, especially in medicine.

Biological death. The third and final stage of death, immediately following brain death, in which body cells begin to die (also called *cellular death*).

Blood alcohol concentration (BAC). Percentage of alcohol per volume of blood.

Brain death. The second of three stages of death in which no brain activity is detected for at least 12 hours.

Calacas. Mexican skull mask symbol used to represent the dead.

Cancer. A group of diseases that has one thing in common—cells in the body that grow abnormally and out of control.

Cardiopulmonary resuscitation (CPR). Treatments used to keep alive a person whose heart, and/or breathing, has stopped.

Caregivers. People who provide care for people who cannot care for themselves.

Caregiving. Providing care (e.g., physical, emotional, and/or financial) for people who cannot care for themselves.

Casket. A more or less ornate rectangular box in which a dead body is buried.

Cellular death. The third and final stage of death, immediately following brain death, in which body cells begin to die (also called *biological death*).

Cerebral blood flow (CBF). Radioactive isotope injected into the blood stream and used to determine, with a radioactivity counter, blood flow. No blood flow means the brain is dead.

Clinical death. First of three stages of death; it occurs when the heartbeat stops.

Codicil. A legal document used to modify a will.

Coffin. Box, wider at the shoulder than at head or foot, usually made of plain wood, for burying a dead body.

Cognitive therapy. Treatment which emphasizes substitution of desirable patterns of thinking for maladaptive or faulty ones.

Columbarium. A wall, usually in a church or as part of a mausoleum, with niches (small spaces) for placing cremated remains in urns.

Conditional will. Type of will in which what must occur after the testator's death, before the will is valid, is specified.

Congestive heart failure. When the heart is unable to maintain adequate blood circulation.

Conservator. Person or institution designated, usually by a court, to take over and protect the interests of someone who is incompetent.

Coroner. Elected official, not usually a physician, who conducts inquests into the causes of unnatural deaths. Also conducts or supervises autopsies in such cases.

Corpse. Dead body.

Cortical death. Result of severe brain damage, leading to a state of wakefulness without awareness. Also called *persistent vegetative state* (PVS). Not the same as brain death.

Cremains. The remains ("ashes") from the cremation of a corpse.

Cremation. Process of burning a dead body and its container and processing the resulting bone fragments to a uniform size and consistency.

Crematory. Place where cremations take place.

Dances of Death (*dances macabre*). Artistic expressions of the fear of sudden death brought on by the Bubonic plague in medieval Europe.

Day of the Dead. A Mexican and Latin American festival held on November 1 (All Saints Day) and November 2 (Souls Day) with emphasis on honoring the lives of the dead and celebrating death as the beginning of a new stage in life.

Dead-donor rule. Widely accepted ethical norms that govern organ procurement for transplant: (1) vital organs should be taken only from dead patients and (2) living patients should not be killed for or by organ procurement.

Death. Loss of all brain function (as defined by the 1981 Uniform Determination Death Act, used by all states).

Death education. Developmental process in which death-related knowledge and the implications resulting from that knowledge are transmitted (*see also* Thanatology).

Death investigator. Police officer who specializes in determining the cause and manner of a death.

Dementia. Severe memory loss and confusion, usually in older people.

Depression. Mental disorder characterized by sadness; inactivity; difficulty in thinking and concentration; a significant increase or decrease in appetite and time spent sleeping; feelings of dejection, inadequacy and hopelessness; low self-esteem; and sometimes a tendency to contemplate suicide.

Diabetes. Chronic disease that is characterized by either the body's failure to properly use or make the hormone insulin, which is needed to store or use glucose.

Dialectical behavior therapy. Treatment that is focused on helping a patient develop skills for coping with everyday life crises.

Disenfranchised grief. Grief that cannot be openly displayed or formally expressed because society does not acknowledge it.

Do Not Resuscitate (DNR). A physician's written order instructing healthcare providers not to attempt cardiopulmonary resuscitation (CPR) in case of cardiac or respiratory arrest.

Doll's eye (oculocephalic) reflex. The manner in which a live person's eyes move opposite the way the head is turned. A dead person's eyes do not move in this way.

Double effect. When a physician provides medication to relieve pain, knowing that it could hasten death.

Durable power of attorney (healthcare proxy). A type of advance directive that is used to designate an individual to make decisions for a person no longer competent to do so.

Electroencephalogram (EEG). Measurement of brain voltage. No voltage denotes brain death.

Embalming. Process of replacing the blood in a dead person's blood vessels with a preservative so that the body can be viewed during the funeral service.

Epitaph. Words written on, or engraved in, a grave marker (tombstone or monument).

Escheat. Taking of property by the state when there are no legal heirs.

Estate. All of a person's assets and possessions.

Estate tax. After-death tax imposed by the federal government and some states on the value of the dead person's property and assets; subject to various deductions and exemptions.

Euthanasia. Hastening the death of a person suffering a fatal, incurable illness. (*See also* Voluntary euthanasia; Nonvoluntary euthanasia; Passive euthanasia; Physician-assisted suicide.) Withholding or withdrawing life-sustaining treatment is an accepted practice if specified in advance care directives.

Executor. Person appointed by a testator to manage the process of seeing that the terms of a will are met.

Fair market value. A price at which buyers and sellers with reasonable knowledge, and who are not compelled, are willing to buy and sell.

Funeral director. Person who carries out the activities of a funeral home, including receiving the body, embalming the body, preparing the body for viewing, conducting the viewing, providing a casket, and performing a burial.

Funeral home. Place where the funeral director prepares the dead body for viewing and burial.

Funeral service (funeral). A service commemorating the dead person, with the body present.

Funeral visitation. An event usually a day or two before the funeral service when friends and loved ones of the dead person visit with each other (usually at the funeral home) and view the dead person. Funeral visitation is sometimes referred to as a *wake.*

Good death. Dying whereby the patient is able to make choices during the last days and months.

Grave. A six-foot deep rectangular hole in the ground, usually in a cemetery, for burying a dead body.

Grave liner. A concrete cover over the top and sides of a casket in a grave; minimizes ground settling.

Grave vault. Concrete or water-resistant metal container that completely encloses a casket in a grave.

Graveside service. A service to commemorate the dead person, which is typically held at the cemetery before burial.

Grief. How one reacts to a loss, usually deep distress. Might be experienced in response to physical losses, such as the death of someone close, or social losses, such as divorce or loss of a job.

Guardian. Someone responsible for taking care of the person or property of another.

Hate crime. Crime committed on another person for reason of race, national origin, religion, sexual orientation, or disability.

Holographic will. A will that is written in the testator's own handwriting.

Homicide. Act of one person killing another.

Hospice. A program for delivering supportive and pain-relieving care to individuals diagnosed with life-limiting illnesses or who are near the end of life. Includes support for the person's family. The hospice location can be at home or in a hospital.

Hypertension. Abnormally high blood pressure, especially arterial; the systemic condition accompanying high blood pressure.

Immortality. The state of being exempt from death; living forever.

Inheritance tax. An estate tax or gift tax.

Interment. Burial in the ground.

Intestate. Term given to describe a person who dies without a will.

Intubation. Insertion of a tube through the mouth or nose into the trachea (windpipe) to create and maintain an open airway to assist breathing.

Joint will. A will that two people make together, each leaving all their property and assets to the other; also is used to stipulate what happens when the second person dies.

Koran/Qur'an. Book of sacred writings accepted by Muslims as revelations made to Muhammad by Allah through the angel Gabriel.

Life expectancy. The number of life years projected for people born in a given year.

Lifetime taxable gifts. Cumulative total of money and property given to someone else over the donor's lifetime that exceed the applicable estate-tax exclusion amount.

Living will. Advance directive specifying medical treatment for a person who is at the end of life and unable to communicate.

Livor mortis. A bluish tint to the face and purple-red to other body parts after death that occurs because blood no longer circulates throughout the body.

Mausoleum. An above-ground building in which remains are buried or entombed.

Medicaid. Government program that provides medical and residential care for U.S. citizens whose financial resources and other assets are below a certain level of value.

Medical power of attorney (healthcare proxy). A document that allows an individual to appoint someone else to make decisions about his or her medical care if he or she is unable to communicate.

Medicare. Government program that provides medical benefits to all U.S. citizens over the age of 65.

Memorial service ceremony. Commemorating the dead without the body present.

Memorial society. An organization that provides information about funerals and disposition but that is not part of the state-regulated funeral industry.

Monument. Engraved stone (with name, birth date, death date, and epitaph) placed at the head of a grave for the purpose of memorializing the dead.

Morgue. Place where bodies of persons found dead are kept until identification is made or an autopsy completed.

Mortuary. Place dead bodies are readied for viewing and burial.

Mourning. Culturally defined ways of expressing grief.

Mutual will. The type of will in which each person who signs the will leaves everything to the other person.

Myocardial infarction. Medical term for *heart attack*; an acute episode of heart disease usually as a result of a coronary thrombosis or occlusion.

Near death experience (NDE). Experiences of various kinds, usually involving body–spirit separation, reported by people who were clinically dead and then revived.

Niche. A space in a columbarium, mausoleum, or wall to hold an urn.

Nirvana. Generally, a state of mind in which one is unaware of worry, pain, or external reality; specifically, the final beatitude that transcends suffering, *karma*, and *samsara* and is sought especially in Buddhism through the extinction of desire and individual consciousness.

Nonvoluntary euthanasia. Termination without the consent or against the will of the recipient. Might be done when believed consistent with the person's prior wishes.

Novena. Catholic tradition wherein a rosary is said for a dead family member for 9 consecutive days.

Nuncupative will. A person orally tells another person how his or her estate is to be distributed.

Obituary. Newspaper notice of a person's death.

Oculocephalic reflex. *See* Doll's eye reflex.

Oculovestibular reflex. Violent eye twitching.

Osteoporosis. Condition characterized by a decrease in bone mass, which produces frailty, particularly among women.

Pallbearers. People (usually six) who carry the casket from the funeral service to the vehicle that takes the body to the burial site.

Palliative care. Compassionate care (pain management as well as emotional and spiritual support) for a terminally ill patient.

Passive euthanasia. Withholding or withdrawing life-sustaining treatment to allow death to occur naturally.

Persistent vegetative state (PVS). Result of severe brain damage leading to a state of wakefulness without awareness; also known as cortical death, although it is not the same as brain death.

Physician-assisted suicide (PAS). A physician assists a mentally competent but terminally ill person to end his or her life.

Probate. The process of proving in court that a will is the valid last will and testament of a dead person.

Processes of death. What happens to bodies after death: immobility, uncertainty, isolation, and decomposition.

Processes of dying. Activities, thoughts, and feelings with which a person must deal when anticipating his or her own death while he or she is alive.

Reincarnation. A Hindu-Buddhist philosophy of an eternal birth–death–birth cycle, during which a soul moves from body to body.

Remains. Dead body or corpse.

Respiratory arrest. When an individual stops breathing. If breathing is not restored, the individual's heart will eventually stop beating, which is called cardiac arrest.

Rigor mortis. Stiffening of muscles, usually occurring within a few hours after death.

Risk behaviors. Daily habits that positively or negatively affect a person's health.

Rituals. Repeated practices that have become customary or traditional.

Senile dementia. Loss of mental function in the elderly.

Shiva. Seven days of mourning for Orthodox Jews.

Social death. When a person is treated as an outcast; considered no longer a member of the group to which he or she belongs.

Stroke. When blood clots, or traveling cholesterol clumps, become lodged in blood vessels, cutting off blood supply to the brain.

Sudden infant death syndrome (SIDS). When a baby suddenly dies from no apparent cause.

Suicide. Intentional taking of one's own life.

Superstitions. Practices or beliefs, which are due to ignorance or fear of the unknown.

Survivor. People who are left behind after a loved one's death.

Suttee. The live cremation of a Hindu widow on the funeral pyre of her husband.

Technological imperative. Because a particular technology makes something possible, it ought to be done, or must be done because it is needed, or inevitably will be done in time.

Terminal disease. Progressive disease that ends in death.

Terrorism. Violent or destructive acts, such as suicide or other bombing, committed by groups in order to intimidate a population or government into granting their demands.

Testator. The maker of a will; the person who, before death, owned the property that is distributed according to specifications outlined in his will.

Thanatology. The study of psychological and social behavior related to death, dying, and bereavement.

Tombstone. Grave marker.

Transient Ischemic Attack (TIA). Mini-stroke.

Type I diabetes. Also referred to as *juvenile* or *insulin-dependent* diabetes, characterized by the body's inability to produce insulin. Type I diabetes mainly occurs in children and adolescents 18 years and younger.

Type II diabetes. A disease characterized by the body's inability to use the limited amount of insulin that it has. Type II diabetes usually occurs in adults over 30 years of age and also is referred to as *adult-onset* or *non-insulin-dependent* diabetes.

Unified credit. A deduction that can be taken from the combined federal gift and estate taxes.

Urn. A container to hold cremated remains.

Viewing. A time, usually a day or two before a funeral service, when family and friends gather at the funeral home to be together and view the dead person.

Violence. Behaviors that bring on injury or death.

Voluntary euthanasia. When a competent dying individual has given voluntary, informed consent to actions that will result in death.

Wake. Funeral home visitation or gathering at the home of the dead person to celebrate the life.

Widow. Woman whose spouse has died.

Widower. Man whose spouse has died.

Will. A document made out before a person dies wherein exactly how his/her assets and possessions are to be distributed is outlined.

Appendix

Help in Funeral Planning

Planning for a Funeral: Summary

1. *Plan ahead.* It allows you to compare without time constraints, creates an opportunity for family discussion, and lifts some of the burden from your family. Bear in mind that you can honor a loved one without buying the fanciest casket or the most elaborate funeral.
2. *Shop around in advance.* Apply the same smart shopping techniques you use for other major purchases. Resist pressure to buy goods and services you don't really want or need. Laws regarding funerals and burials vary from state to state, so it's important to know which goods or services the law requires you to purchase and which are optional.
3. *Compare prices from at least two funeral homes.* Ask for a price list: the law requires funeral homes to give you written price lists for products and services. You can cut costs by limiting the viewing to one day or one hour before the funeral and by dressing your loved one in a favorite outfit instead of costly burial clothing. Remember also that you can supply your own casket or urn.

Source: Federal Trade Commission. *Funerals: A Consumer Guide, 2007*. Available online at http://www.ftc.gov/bcp/conline/pubs/services/funeral.shtm.

Helpful Funeral Organizations

Most states have a licensing board that regulates the funeral industry. You may contact the board in your state for information or help. You also can contact other groups.

AARP Fulfillment

601 E Street, NW
Washington, DC 20049
1-800-424-3410
www.aarp.org

AARP is a nonprofit organization whose publications, *Funeral Goods and Services* and *Pre-Paying for Your Funeral,* are available free by writing to the above address. This and other funeral-related information are posted on the AARP Web site.

Council of Better Business Bureaus, Inc.

4200 Wilson Blvd., Suite 800
Arlington, VA 22203-1838
www.bbb.org

Better Business Bureaus are private, nonprofit organizations that promote ethical business standards and voluntary self-regulation of business practices.

Funeral Consumers Alliance

33 Patchen Road
South Burlington, VT 05403
1-800-765-0107
www.funerals.org

The Funeral Consumers Alliance (FCA) is a nonprofit, educational organization that supports increased funeral consumer protection. It is affiliated with the Funeral and Memorial Society of America (FAMSA).

Cremation Association of North America

401 North Michigan Avenue
Chicago, IL 60611
(312) 644-6610
www.cremationassociation.org

The Cremation Association of North America (CANA) is an association of crematories, cemeteries, and funeral homes that offer cremation.

International Order of the Golden Rule

13523 Lakefront Drive
St. Louis, MO 63045
1-800-637-8030
www.ogr.org

OGR is an international association of about 1,300 independent funeral homes.

Jewish Funeral Directors of America

Seaport Landing
150 Lynnway, Suite 506
Lynn, MA 01902
(781) 477-9300
www.jfda.org

The Jewish Funeral Directors of America (JFDA) is an international association of funeral homes serving the Jewish community.

National Funeral Directors Association

13625 Bishop's Drive
Brookfield, WI 53005
1-800-228-6332
www.nfda.org/resources

The National Funeral Directors Association (NFDA) is the largest educational and professional association of funeral directors.

National Funeral Directors and Morticians Association

3951 Snapfinger Parkway, Suite 570
Decatur, GA 30035
1-800-434-0958
www.nfdma.com

The National Funeral Directors and Morticians Association (NFDMA) is a national association, primarily of African American funeral providers.

Selected Independent Funeral Homes

500 Lake Cook Road, Suite 205
Deerfield, IL 60015
1-800-323-4219
www.selectedfuneralhomes.org

Selected Independent Funeral Homes is an international association of funeral firms that have agreed to comply with its Code of Good Funeral Practice. Consumers may request a variety of publications through the association's affiliate, Selected Resources, Inc.

Funeral Service Consumer Assistance Program

PO Box 486
Elm Grove, WI 53122-0486
1-800-662-7666
www.funeralservicefoundation.org

The Funeral Service Consumer Assistance Program (FSCAP) is a nonprofit consumer service designed to help people understand funeral service and related topics and to help them resolve funeral service concerns. FSCAP service representatives and an intervener assist consumers in identifying needs, addressing complaints, and resolving problems. Free brochures on funeral related topics are available.

Funeral Service Educational Foundation

13625 Bishop's Drive
Brookfield, WI 53005
1-877-402-5900
www.funeralservicefoundation.org

The FSEF (Funeral Service Educational Foundation) is a nonprofit foundation dedicated to advancing professionalism in funeral service and to enhancing public knowledge and understanding through education and research.

Source: Federal Trade Commission. *Funerals: A Consumer Guide, 2007*. Available online at http://www.ftc.gov/bcp/conline/pubs/services/funeral.shtm.

Index

D

Photo Credits

Page 1 © Rob Marmion/ShutterStock, Inc.; **page** 2 © PureStock/age fotostock; **page** 11 (left) © Daniela Schraml/ShutterStock, Inc.; **page** 11 (right) © Photos.com; **page** 16 © Claudio Rossol/ShutterStock, Inc.; **page** 20 © Jose Gil/ShutterStock, Inc.; **page** 21 © Chin Kit Sen/ShutterStock, Inc.; **page** 24 © Bobby Deal/RealDealPhoto/ShutterStock, Inc.; **page** 30 (left) © LiquidLibrary; **page** 30 (right) © Photos.com; **page** 31 © Corbis Collection/Alamy Images; **page** 34 © Elena Ray/ShutterStock, Inc.; **page** 52 © Galyna Andrushko/ShutterStock, Inc.; **page** 53 © www imagesource.com/Jupiterimages; **page** 54 © Jack Dagley Photography/ShutterStock, Inc.; **page** 55 © BananaStock/age fotostock; **page** 58 © Anita/ShutterStock, Inc.; **page** 69 © Dina Rudick, Boston Globe/Landov; **page** 87 © LiquidLibrary; **page** 89 © Ron Nickel/age fotostock; **page** 91 © Photodisc; **page** 92 Courtesy of Bill Branson/National Cancer Institute; **page** 93 © Jamie Wilson/ShutterStock, Inc.; **page** 94 © Marcin Balcerzak/ShutterStock, Inc.; **page** 96 © LiquidLibrary; **page** 97 © plastique/ShutterStock, Inc.; **page** 101 © Joshua Roberts, Reuters/Landov; **page** 105 Library of Congress, Prints & Photographs Division, [reproduction number LC-USZ62-1234]; **page** 108 © AbleStock; **page** 110 © Art-Line Productions/Brand X Picture/Alamy Images; **page** 120 © Ron Hilton/ShutterStock, Inc.; **page** 132 © AP Photos; **page** 133 (left and right) © Photos.com; **page** 134 (top) © PA Photos/Landov; **page** 134 (bottom) © Aron Hsiao/ShutterStock, Inc.; **page** 136 (top left) © Nicola Gavin/ShutterStock, Inc.; **page** 136 (top right) © Pat Canova/Alamy Images; **page** 136 (bottom right) © Geir Olav Lyngfjell/ShutterStock, Inc.; **page** 137 (top) © Natalia V. Guseva/ShutterStock, Inc.; **page** 137 (bottom) © vario images GmbH & Co.KG/Alamy Images; **page** 141 (top left) © mauritius images/age fotostock; **page** 141 (bottom left) © Eric Etman/ShutterStock, Inc.; **page** 141 (right) © Chris Carlson/AP Photos; **page** 146 © Evrensel Baris Berkant/ShutterStock, Inc.; **page** 147 © signorina/ShutterStock, Inc.; **page** 152 © Christopher Michot/ShutterStock, Inc.; **page** 153 © Simone van den Berg/ShutterStock, Inc.; **page** 158 © Tim Shaffer, Reuters/Landov; **page** 162 © Photos.com; **page** 177 © Kevin Dietsch, UPI Photo/Landov; **page** 179 © AP Photos; **page** 180 © Taolmor/ShutterStock, Inc.; **page** 181 Courtesy of Andrea Booher/FEMA News Photo; **page** 188 © SuperStock/age fotostock; **page** 189 (left) © Stephen Coburn/ShutterStock, Inc.; **page** 189 (right) © Photos.com; **page** 191 © prism_68/ShutterStock, Inc.; **page** 192 © Falko Matte/ShutterStock, Inc.; **page** 198 © Enigma/Alamy Images; **page** 199 © Jason Stitt/ShutterStock, Inc.; **page** 200 (top) © Tiburon Studios/ShutterStock, Inc.; **page** 200 (bottom) © Corbis/age fotostock; **page** 201 © Supri Suharjoto/ShutterStock, Inc.; **page** 202 © Bilderbox/age fotostock; **page** 203 © Steve Skjold/Alamy Images.

Unless otherwise indicated all photographs are under copyright of Jones and Bartlett Publishers, courtesy of Maryland Institute for Emergency Medical Services Systems or have been provided by the author.